Anti-racist Health Care Practice

Anti-racist Health Care Practice

Elizabeth A. McGibbon
and
Josephine B. Etowa

Canadian Scholars' Press Inc.
Toronto

Anti-racist Health Care Practice
by Elizabeth A. McGibbon and Josephine B. Etowa

First published in 2009 by
Canadian Scholars' Press Inc.
180 Bloor Street West, Suite 801
Toronto, Ontario
M5S 2V6

www.cspi.org

Copyright © 2009 Elizabeth A. McGibbon, Josephine B. Etowa, and Canadian Scholars' Press Inc. All rights reserved. No part of this publication may be photocopied, reproduced, stored in a retrieval system, or transmitted, in any form or by any means, electronic, mechanical, or otherwise, without the written permission of Canadian Scholars' Press Inc., except for brief passages quoted for review purposes. In the case of photocopying, a licence may be obtained from Access Copyright: One Yonge Street, Suite 1900, Toronto, Ontario, M5E 1E5, (416) 868-1620, fax (416) 868-1621, toll-free 1-800-893-5777, www.accesscopyright.ca.

Every reasonable effort has been made to identify copyright holders. CSPI would be pleased to have any errors or omissions brought to its attention.

Canadian Scholars' Press Inc. gratefully acknowledges financial support for our publishing activities from the Government of Canada through the Book Publishing Industry Development Program (BPIDP) and the Government of Ontario through the Ontario Book Publishing Tax Credit Program.

Library and Archives Canada Cataloguing in Publication

McGibbon, Elizabeth Anne, 1955–
    Anti-racist health care practice / Elizabeth A. McGibbon and Josephine B. Etowa.

Includes index.
ISBN 978-1-55130-355-0

    1. Discrimination in medical care—Canada. 2. Minorities—Medical care—Canada. I. Etowa, Josephine B., 1965– II. Title.

RA563.M56M35 2009   362.1'08900971   C2009-900245-0

Interior design and layout: Brad Horning and Stewart Moracen

09 10 11 12 13   5 4 3 2 1

Printed and bound in Canada by Marquis Book Printing Inc.

Canadä

For our children,

Emily and Sophie Gardner (Elizabeth)
and
Ntami and Deval Enang (Josephine)

whose patience and loving support continue to ground us.

Table of Contents

Preface 1

Chapter 1
Introduction to Anti-racist Health Care Practice 3

Chapter 2
Racism as a Determinant of Health: Evidence for Change 31

Chapter 3
Beyond Cultural Competence: A Critique of Diversity and
Multicultural Health Care Models 63

Chapter 4
Theoretical Foundations for an Anti-racist Framework 81

Chapter 5
An Anti-racist Framework to Guide Practice 111

Chapter 6
Engaging in Everyday Anti-racist Health Care Practice 139

Chapter 7
Racism, Public Policy, and Social Change 165

Further Reading 193

Related Websites 201

Glossary 209

References 217

Copyright Acknowledgements 237

Index 239

Preface

When we met during graduate school almost 15 years ago, we became increasingly dismayed that the health fields were lagging so far behind the social sciences and humanities regarding knowledge about racism, sexism, and classism, to name a few of the -*isms*. This pushed us to the edge, to some extent. We were used to being on the edge in clinical practice, where the overarching focus was (and still is) biomedical—identify the problem, find the solution, apply the solution, evaluate its effectiveness, and go from there. Who wanted to complicate already very complex clinical situations with yet another layer of thinking and acting? Why were we being so negative? Couldn't we try to be more positive?

Although the racism we were trying to fight remained a serious and thorny business, we had great laughs about some of these experiences because they were so similar across our differences in race and ethnicity and geographies of origin. We found in each other someone who could take the "straight goods" without the sugar-coating; someone who didn't need the half-dozen careful caveats before saying what she actually meant. The same holds true today.

Somewhere along the way, as we began our applied health research programs in critical health studies, we realized that there was no cohesive collection of work, however small, that could bring together critical social science ideas with knowledge in the health fields to fight oppression, and racism in particular. This realization was the genesis of *Anti-racist Health Care Practice*. While completing doctoral studies at the University of Calgary and the University of Toronto, along with raising our children, the book took shape more and more, at least in our minds. Ultimately we pulled together the threads of our many conversations to produce this book. It is tethered in the many long days and nights we have spent in our clinical work with people in crisis, with people mending themselves and their families, and, of course, with people shepherding a brand new life into the world—in the birthing room. Our starting point for this book was, and continues to be, one of hope for transformation.

Acknowledgements

This book would not have been possible without the inspiration, contributions, enthusiasm, and support of many people during the various stages of its preparation. We are indebted to those whose intellectual work has inspired and influenced us as cited throughout the book. We owe a debt of gratitude to the many students with whom we have worked with over the past ten years. We developed many of the book's application exercises in the classroom setting, and students' intellectual curiosity and their passion for social change continues to keep us moving along this path. Their work emphasizes the need not only to promote cultural competence, but to transcend to a level of health care that embraces anti-oppressive health practice. In particular we want to thank our colleagues, Sharon Davis-Murdoch, Charmaine McPherson, and Adele Vukic, who have so generously provided us with their work to use as examples in the book. We thank our mentors, Nancy Edwards, Barbara Keddy, Dennis Raphael, and Sarla Sethi, to name but a few, who have challenged us to develop our understanding of the forces of societal oppression, including racism.

We would like to thank the many people who provided us with invaluable suggestions and ongoing support throughout the writing of the book, including Kate Edu, Emily Gardner, Chris Pauley, Patty Smith, and Joannne Tompkins for their careful reading of drafts. We offer a special thank you to Charmaine McPherson, who painstakingly considered each chapter in such fine detail, and whose intellectual and moral support grounds much of the book, and to Patrick Gardner, who has shepherded many a project with his careful support and encouragement.

We thank the people at Canadian Scholars' Press Inc., especially Megan Mueller for her enthusiasm and support of the project, and we gratefully acknowledge supportive funding from the Centre for Regional Studies (SSHRC) at St. Francis Xavier University.

CHAPTER 1

Introduction to Anti-racist Health Care Practice

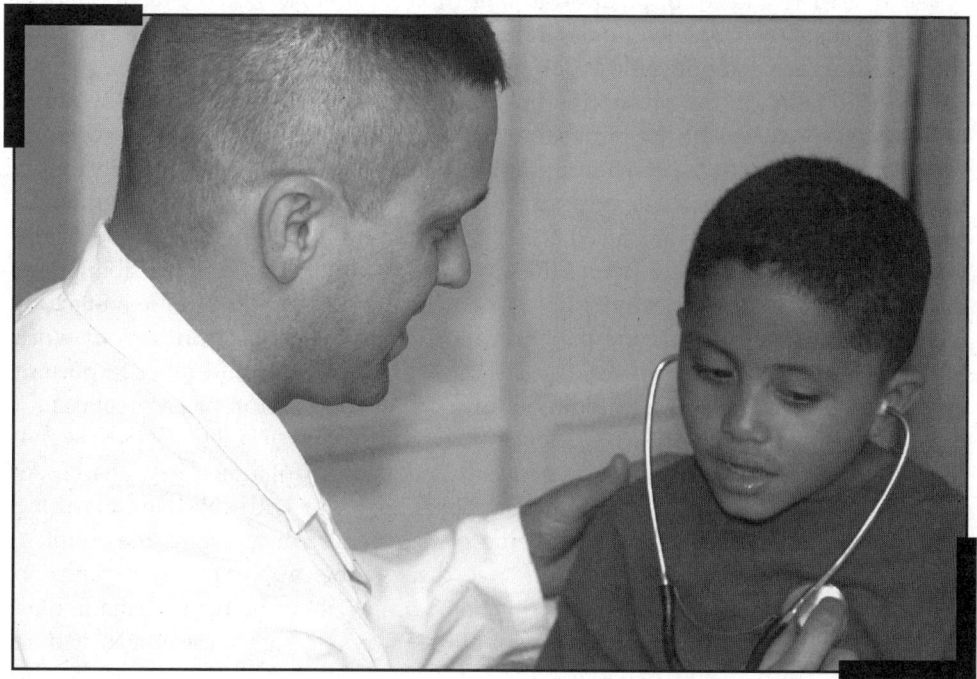

To the memory of my ancestors, who managed to ensure the survival of the Mi'Kmaq People by their awe-inspiring tenacity and valour in the face of virtually insurmountable odds! For more than four centuries these courageous, dignified, and heroic people displayed a determination to survive the various hells on earth created for them by Europeans with a tenacity that equals any displayed in the history of mankind. May their brave accomplishment inspire the Mi'Kmaq and other oppressed peoples to meet the challenges of today and tomorrow. (Daniel Paul, 2007, p. vii)

This introductory chapter describes the foundations for the book. Learning how to engage in anti-racist practice is a worthy journey for practitioners in a field that espouses compassion for fellow human beings, regardless of their life situation, colour, or beliefs. The chapter provides the foundations to begin this journey. If you are already on this journey, this chapter will affirm some of your struggles. Our framework for anti-racist practice is presented, along with descriptions of key terms such as race, culture, religion, and White privilege. We describe our social locations as a Black woman and a White woman in order to provide the reader with some of the contexts that shaped the book. The chapter concludes with an overview of the organization of the book.

Why is there a need for an anti-racist health care practice book? Practitioners in most fields usually have the understanding that everyone should be treated equally, regardless of race, religion, culture, ethnicity, and age. The health fields in particular have a foundation in the promotion of so-called scientific objectivity, and learning to leave personal bias at the door when working with patients or, more recently, "clients," which includes the family and community. The same generally holds true for students, researchers, educators, and policy-makers. After all, who would support biased research or biased teaching or biased policy-making? One of the main goals of this book is to upend this mythical thinking about the possibility and desirability of scientific objectivity in everyday health care practice — of leaving your identity in a basket outside the patient's door, or on the porch during your work in the community. *Anti-racist Health Care Practice* brings these and other important contexts into plain view as a foundation for social change to stop racist practices.

There is a pressing need to develop a critical, action-oriented perspective regarding the relationship between racism and health outcomes in Canada. As we illustrate throughout the book, racism bears itself out with solid and alarming evidence about the health and well-being of people of colour across the country. White is, of course, a colour too, and we discuss this apparent discrepancy in later chapters. During the writing of this book, a new set of Statistics Canada data became available, so we updated many of our statistics. In some cases the 2006 data was even worse than the 2001 data. These numbers tell a chilling story across the country. Individuals and families of colour have the most overall poverty and the worst overall health outcomes in the country. In some provinces, almost 30 percent of children of colour live in poverty (Ministerial Advisory Council on Rural Health, 2002). Why are we letting this injustice happen in a country that traditionally sees itself as taking pride in collective responsibility and in creating the conditions for a fair and decent life for its citizens? This book is a challenge to meet this evidence head-on, and to take action for change.

Although there are a growing number of academic works that address racism and health, there is not yet any comprehensive analysis of the links among theoretical ideas, systemic racism, and how racism unfolds in everyday clinical practice in the health fields. Although Canada lags behind other countries in its attention to compiling an evidence base that relates race and ethnicity to racism in provision of care and in policy, however there is little reason to think that the same troubles are not present in Canada.

Our aim is to raise ongoing questions about the inseparable and dynamic flow between racism, as an individual act, and systemic racism. For example, while there is clear evidence of the individual racist attitudes of health care professionals when doing postnatal work with Black moms and babies (Enang, 1999), acts such as not offering routine sickle cell anemia screening to these babies are rooted in systemic racism. In the case of prenatal and postnatal care of young Black women, Enang found evidence that the maternity care system actively excluded these young women from care. The women told stories about standing at the nurses' station, waiting to be heard, while the concerns of White mothers, who had arrived after them, were addressed. The truth is that it is difficult for health clinicians to believe this research finding. In fact, when Enang attempted to publish her results in a world-renowned health journal, a reviewer suggested that the nurses were perhaps just busy, and that it was not likely that they were actually ignoring the young Black women. Disturbingly, Enang's research also contained uncannily similar stories from elder women in the same Black community, and many of the elders' struggles were the same regarding the births of their own babies many decades ago. It was as if time had stood still.

This book provides a hands-on guide for students, practitioners, educators, researchers, and policy-makers in the health field who wish to understand and engage in anti-racist practice. Although the book is directed chiefly at practitioners, it provides a solid theoretical foundation for anyone interested in the context of racism and health and avenues for anti-racism work, including anti-racist policy-making and anti-racist research. After all, how can policy-makers engage in anti-racist policy-making without knowing the cycle of oppression? How will applied health researchers understand and incorporate anti-racist research strategies without knowing about the interlocking nature of inequities in the social determinants of health? Specifically, the book provides a much-needed practical and theoretically grounded perspective for anti-racist practice in the area of human health in Canada.

Although we emphasize application in the health fields, the ideas are very much applicable to any field where practitioners are engaged in human services. There is no existing book, to our knowledge, that addresses racism and health from an everyday clinical practice perspective in the health fields. In particular, this book provides the reader with clear and detailed definitions of concepts and terms related to racism and health, as well as descriptions of their application to everyday practice in the health professions. Another unique feature of this book is that it is action-focused, with numerous examples of what racism looks like in the health care system, along with clearly articulated strategies to interrogate and address racism. Although theoretical in nature, the book can be used for undergraduate and graduate courses with students in the health professions, many of whom have had limited exposure to critical social science. Throughout the book, the reader will notice that both the terms Aboriginal and Indigenous are used. We use the term Aboriginal when we are describing, quoting, or referring to literature that uses the term, in order to correctly reflect the various authors' terminology. However, in our discussions we use the term Indigenous to reflect our own understanding of the context of first peoples in the geography of colonialism.

Overview of the Foundations of the Book

Our presentation of anti-racist health care practice is based on a broad definition of health that incorporates biologic and genetic endowment, as well as the social determinants of health. We view health as inseparable from the social and political context that encompasses the everyday lives of individuals, families, communities, and nations. Health is also intimately connected to our spiritual and psychological selves, however we define them. Overall, the book is designed to be an introduction to thinking critically about the many forms of oppression, with key terms and concepts clearly presented. We focus on racism, and discuss the interlocking nature of oppressions, including those related to race, social class, and gender. Although we stress that racism operates as a well-developed societal system, we include first-person examples of how racism operates for people of colour in their day-to-day lives. These stories form a foundation for raising consciousness about the everyday nature of racism and other oppressions. For White people, this means understanding White privilege, something that few White people have thought about. It is difficult for White people to see how racism unfolds. This is because whiteness brings with it the privilege of not noticing. Box 1.1 offers a description of how White people might begin to notice.

Box 1.1: The Many Sides of Poverty: Some Reflections on Racism and Health

The issue of where racism fits into health and health care has received little attention in the health care system or among health care providers. We have a tough time getting our heads around why this should even be a concern. I guess this isn't surprising since "we" are predominately white-skinned. A few years ago, I presented at large three-day workshop for students of the health professions in Halifax, Nova Scotia. The topics were pretty standard fare, with various invited speakers from the community. One of the presenters was a man who described his experiences growing up as a Black Nova Scotian. "John" talked about many things, including some of his experiences with the health system. I was struck by the fact that this was the first time I heard anyone speak about this issue from their own experience for more than a few minutes.

After the presentation, the entire group of over four hundred students and facilitators met in smaller groups of about a dozen students. I facilitated one of these groups. The students soon began to discuss John's presentation and "what the heck did that have to do with anything?" I later learned from the other facilitators that most of the students did not like John's presentation and that they wanted to have "more relevant" speakers.

There are many possible reasons for why this happened. It is unlikely that there was any anti-racism content in the course work of any of these students; they were hearing about it for the first time from John. It is likely that health issues related to racism, if discussed at all, were placed under the heading of multiculturalism and health. Notions of privilege and power were probably never addressed. It has been my experience as a white person that, since we live in a profoundly racist society, I could not begin to understand racism, or even to accept that racism exists until people began to help me *see* racism.

> This continues to be a challenge for me because my whiteness allows me to look the other way; I can choose to not notice that Band-Aids are the colour of my skin, that when I buy pantyhose with "skin colour" written on the label, it is my skin colour, that when I buy shampoo, it is shampoo that is specially formulated for my hair. When I buy these items at the drug store, I can be pretty sure that the faces of the cashiers and the pharmacists, the people stocking the shelves, and the pictures of the people looking back at me from almost all the products will have my skin colour. I have the privilege of not having to think about these things. This, unlike my friend Althea, who has very dark brown skin and was recently told at a local drug store that the hair products for "her type of hair" were locked up and she would have to get the key from the manager if she wished to buy these products.
>
> I give these examples because I believe they are at the core of how racism operates in a health care system that has been designed by white people, and some would argue, *for* white people. Perhaps we could shift our attention and look at the ways we educate health professionals—from anatomy books that have exclusively white bodies depicted in their pages to the disturbing lack of Black and Native students and practitioners. How about a health professional's version of the Indigenous Black and Mi'kmaq program that increases diversity in the graduates at the Dalhousie University's Law School? Most importantly of all, let's examine the link between racism and health. What are the specific health effects for families trying to access the health system? What is the result of producing a fairly long hospital patient booklet that depicts only white faces? What are the specific health effects for those who experience racism first hand on a daily basis? These effects include, and go beyond, the results of lack of access to good hair care products. I think that the bottom line is that we need to start somewhere. From my experience as a white health professional, one of the best ways to get focused is to challenge ourselves to continually *notice* and *see* racism. Then, I think that we are ethically and professionally bound to act based on what we see.
>
> *Source:* McGibbon, E. (1998). The many sides of poverty: Health issues (The Nurse is in) Racism and health: Some reflections. *Street Feat—"The Voice of the Poor"* (June/July 1998), p. 7.

These kinds of examples show how we can bring White privilege forward for analysis as a key foundation for anti-racist practice. White privilege is the other side of the coin, the most often-hidden side of the racism equation. Without White privilege, racism cannot sustain itself. In other words, White privilege is the core pillar of racism. It can manifest in individual acts of racism, such as treating people unfairly in the emergency department, or it can manifest in systemic racism, such as Canadian government policies that set in motion Indian residential schools for the annihilation of Indigenous culture and language. It is important to note that when the government of South Africa began to build a system of apartheid, they visited their counterparts in the Canadian government to obtain a successful template for the exploitation and subjugation of Indigenous peoples.

Understanding White privilege is a tricky business because it involves "nice" people's complicity in racism, even if they are not aware of their role. This is why White privilege is so often referred to as invisible. We take up these discussions further throughout the book. Christopher Spence's (2000) work regarding racism and sports is an excellent example of the relationships among racism, White privilege, and the fact that the experience of racism runs all along the life course. Spence's story in Box 1.2 offers a bird's-eye view of everyday racism in the life of a Canadian boy.

> **Box 1.2: The Skin I'm in: Christopher M. Spence and Racism, Sports, and Education**
>
> Kids can be the most innocent but also the meanest creatures on the face of the earth. Let me tell you a personal story. If you looked at me now, you would never know it, but I used to compete in gymnastics. I still remember my last competition as a gymnast representing my hometown of Windsor, Ontario, at the provincial championships. At the time, two gymnastic teams were operating in the city. I will refer to one team as the A team and the other as the B team. Now, the A team was much more established than the B team and had all the frills of a successful program—the finest coaches the city had to offer, uniforms, and a generous sponsor. The B team, my team, on the other hand, was a new team that had not yet created an identity for itself. As a result, our practice times, facilities, and the like were all second-rate compared to those of the A team, but that did not deter us from competing and training just as hard. In fact, most of us hoped to someday be a part of the A team. However, for me that thought quickly disappeared one day.
>
> It was perhaps my rudest awakening as a Black athlete. Although it came at the innocent age of twelve, the experience still makes me shake my head in disbelief. It all began with a phone call from my coach, telling me I had qualified for the provincial championships. That was the good news. The bad news was I was the only one from the B team who had done so. After thinking about it and discussing it with my parents, we all felt that it was too good of an opportunity to pass up. Although my parents couldn't make it to the championships, which were being held in Ottawa, about a six-hour drive away, they gave me a send-off that left me as high as a kite. My coach could not make it to the competition either and had arranged a ride for me with the A team. I was instructed to meet them at Central Park at 6:30 a.m., which I did, and that is when the problems began.
>
> Clearly I was an outsider. No one volunteered to take me in their car. This after the other fellows had been wooed to cars of parents driving. I had never in my young life felt so uncomfortable. I honestly did not know what to do, so I just stood there hoping someone would notice. Luckily, someone did notice and asked if I would like to ride with them. I will call her Mrs. Green. Her decision to ask me to ride in their car was not a popular one. In fact, her son became so agitated that she had to pull him over to the side and talk to him privately. But it was too little, too late; the damage was done. I still recall him telling his friends he didn't "want no coon" in his car and pleading with his mother, "Why, oh why, do we have to take him?" In fact, some of the other boys who were to ride in the same car threatened to ride with someone else if I came along. As it turned out, the only room left in their station wagon was at the back of the luggage. At the time, as far as I was concerned, the roof of the car would have been ok. But being at the back wasn't so bad; it allowed me to put on my headphones and shed a few tears without drawing attention myself. The six-hour car ride seemed like twelve hours, especially when the other boys didn't even attempt to include me in their conversation. And if it wasn't for Mrs. Green shouting the occasional, "How you doing back there?", I probably wouldn't have said a word. Even when we stopped for food and fuel, I was on my own. The A team members were a tight-knit group who didn't give me the time of day.

> When we finally reached our destination and were given our room assignments, I was on my own again. Now part of that must have come from the fact that I was the only one from the B team, and the A team had had room assignments before I arrived. But part of me thinks the skin I'm in didn't help either. That night all the members of the team gathered for dinner. I overheard their coach saying he would call the rooms and tell everyone what time they would be meeting in the morning. I never did get that call, which led me to believe they might forget me. After spending the night in a room by myself, tossing and turning and contemplating whether to call home (which I decided not to do out of fear that my parents would be on the next plane and make a scene any twelve-year-old would be embarrassed about), I got dressed and went down to the lobby at about 5:30 a.m. and waited. The coaches, parents, and gymnasts arrived in the lobby at about 7:30 a.m. and coyly asked where I had been. Like they really cared.
>
> It didn't take long for me to notice that I was the only Black gymnast competing in the championships. I'm not sure if it made a difference, but it was by far my worst performance. It was ironic that while competing I was positioned right after a member of the A team, which meant the opportunity to give me a little applause and wave the hometown banner was there if they wanted to. They certainly made some noise for Bobby, but my routine ended in utter silence. Not even a clap? Even today, as I reflect back on my days as an athlete and all the lessons I have learned through sports, I cannot help wondering if the skin I'm in has been a major factor.
>
> *Source:* Spence, C.M. (2000). *The skin I'm in: Racism, sports, and education* (pp. 7–8). Halifax, NS: Fernwood Publishing.

This book differs from most other efforts to address notions of difference in health practice as we consciously locate racism and health within an anti-racism framework. In this framework, White privilege, power, and oppression are central. This contrasts markedly with frameworks now in common usage, where concepts of cultural competence, multicultural care, celebration of diversity, and working with the "other" are dominant. Although we have learned a great deal from some of these frameworks, with a few notable exceptions, the fact that they gloss over racism is a major flaw. White privilege is barely mentioned at all, yet White privilege continues to be the largely unacknowledged mechanism for perpetuating racism, the glue that continues to hold colonization and oppression together. We emphasize the continued centrality of colonialism in the health of Canadians of colour. Power/power over and oppression/domination are ever-present systemic aspects of every health care situation. Notions of power and power over carry additional and important meanings in clinical practice, where physical and psychological vulnerabilities are already central to health care encounters. Here we have the compounding of the power and privilege of everyday racism, with the power and privilege of the therapeutic relationship. This mixture is potent and can have dangerous consequences for the health of people of colour.

This book uses a teaching to transgress (hooks, 1994) approach to learning, based on author and Black teacher and scholar bell hooks's works, *Teaching to Transgress: Education as the Practice of Freedom* (1994) and *Teaching Community: A Pedagogy of Hope*

(2003). When teachers and students transgress, they actively challenge commonly held ideas and meanings. The overall goal is social change through self-examination and questioning the taken-for-granted everyday world of racism around us. Our work has also been greatly informed by the works of Carl James, most notably his *Perspectives on Racism in the Human Services Sector: A Case for Change* (1996), and *Seeing Ourselves: Exploring Race, Ethnicity, and Culture* (2003). James provided the first detailed application of anti-racist principles to the context of human services, including front-line care and in policy. Agnes Calliste and George Sefa Dei's (2000) *Anti-racist Feminism* provided a clear compass for situating sexism and racism as central aspects of the lives of women of colour.

We have also drawn upon Grace-Edward Galabuzi's (2006, 2008) theoretical and statistical work throughout the book, particularly *Canada's Economic Apartheid: The Social Exclusion of Racialized Groups in the New Century*. Frances Henry, Carol Tator, Winston Mattis, and Tim Rees's germinal book, *The Colour of Democracy: Racism in Canadian Society*, informs much of this book. George Dei's *Anti-racism Education: Theory and Practice* (2000) also grounds our work, particularly in the area of translating anti-racism theory into anti-racism practice. Dei's *Spiritual Knowing and Transformative Learning* (2002) helped to provide foundations in teaching to transgress as a political stance. Transgression encourages actively challenging taken-for-granted social and political structures. The moment we step out of commonly held meanings, we engage in a lively questioning of the attitudes and knowledge we already have. We know when this happens because we will feel resistance, sometimes within ourselves, and very often from the people around us.

For example, one of our most common experiences with resistance is in the context of large gatherings of academics, practitioners, and policy-makers in the health fields. Over the course of the day at these conferences or forums, it is relatively unusual to hear words of transgression such as racism, oppression, social injustice, policy-created poverty, power and privilege, and White privilege. We have always felt compelled to bring these ideas out into the open, so by the time there is a morning break, we have usually found a place to bring the discussion into the reality of oppressive forces in the health care system. At the first mention of these words, the reaction is usually a patient silence, perhaps an *Isn't that interesting for her to be thinking about it?* stance. At the second mention, some of the body language in the room relays an open discomfort. This usually takes the form of shuffling papers, poring over the conference agenda, and crossing and uncrossing legs.

It is important to note that these behaviours are also common when people are bored or need a break. However, it does not matter what time of the day, what topic, or what type of conference we attend. The persistent mention of the words of anti-racism makes people uncomfortable. If we bring up the issue a third time in the context of the discussion at hand, we might see people rolling their eyes or leaving the room. At the lunch break, people might have difficulty making eye contact, or will not speak to us, as was the case at a recent national health policy gathering.

This open hostility is a sign of resistance to the ideas and the political implications of anti-racist talk. These experiences are still encouraging for us because almost every time they happen, one or more people make it a point to tell us privately at the break that they were "relieved" or "delighted" that we brought the discussion into a socio-political or anti-racist realm. The reactions to these transgressions feel similar for both of us, but the different colours of our skin situate us very differently. Although White people who engage in anti-racist acts are often the target of subtle and not-so-subtle hostility, the moment they walk out of the conference hall, they enter a world where their *whiteness alone* will never invoke hostility from other White people.

The following list provides some of the ways that White privilege operates in the health fields. We have adapted Peggy MacIntosh's *White Privilege: Unpacking the Invisible Knapsack* (1990) for practitioners in the health fields:

- When I seek health care, I can be pretty sure that I will encounter a practitioner of my own race.
- When I ask to speak to the "person in charge" when I am in the hospital, I can be pretty sure that I will be facing a person of my own race.
- When I read health promotion literature in the waiting rooms of hospitals, clinics, or pharmacies, I can be pretty sure that many, if not most, of the faces in the pamphlets will reflect my skin colour.
- If I need special bandages, splints, or prosthesis, I can be pretty sure that the colour of the materials used will reflect my skin colour.
- When I attend professional association meetings, I can be pretty sure that most of the people in positions of importance and decision making in my association are people of my race.
- Whether I work in a hospital or in the community, I can be pretty sure that the board of directors who govern my workplace will be mostly people of my race.
- If I decide to lobby my local or national political representatives about a health-related issue, it is more than likely that that I will be talking to a person of my race.
- If I decide to further my education in the health fields at the baccalaureate, master's, or doctoral level, I can be pretty sure that most of my professors will be people of my race.
- When I study for my exams, my textbooks will depict mostly people of my race.
- In my class about the historical influences on health, when I speak up about the discrimination and near-starvation of Irish people at the hands of the British in the Potato Famine, I can be pretty sure that I will not be accused of making an issue of something that is long past and no longer worth dwelling on, or of "taking things too seriously."
- As a student, when I go to the clinical skills lab, I can be pretty certain that the demonstration models will reflect my skin colour.
- When I apply for research funding, I can be pretty sure that most of the decision makers will be people of my race.

- When I read professional magazines, I can be pretty sure that most of the faces depicted in its patient advertisements will be people of my race.

Examples such as these bring whiteness in the health fields forward for discussion and integration into working for change.

Introduction to the Book's Anti-racist Framework to Guide Practice

Anti-racism work has many possible avenues of reflection and action. The framework that lays the foundation for this book is based in the linkages among *seeing* the paths from biased thinking to oppression, *understanding and connecting* these paths of oppression to the policies that create and sustain them, and, finally, *acting* for change. We describe the framework in detail in Chapter 5, and the following discussion provides a brief overview of its main ideas.

Seeing the Paths from Stereotype to Oppression

Oppression is rooted in biased thinking and stereotypes that persist across time. In terms of seeing the paths from biased thinking to oppression, consider the example of social (income) assistance recipients. Starting with *biased information* about the nature of social assistance recipients, we may develop a stereotype such as the commonly held belief that people receiving assistance are lazy. These stereotypes can lead us to think in a particular way that demonstrates *prejudice* (McGibbon, Etowa & McPherson, 2008).

For example, we may hold the prejudicial view that people receiving assistance don't want to work because they are lazy. Then, when we *act* in a particular way based on our prejudice, we are participating in *discrimination*. When we treat people on welfare disrespectfully during a clinical assessment, we are discriminating. In this way, we are contributing to lack of full access to competent and compassionate health care. When our discriminatory actions are supported by the health care system, this is an example of *oppression*—our discriminatory acts are condoned by our facility, and the systemic power within the facility. For example, if substandard intake assessments of people who are receiving social assistance are not challenged, discrimination is being supported by institutional power. In fact, the reasons for unemployment among social assistance recipients are multiple and complex (McGibbon, Etowa & McPherson, 2008).

Connecting Paths of Oppression to Policy

Once we see some of the particular paths from biased information to oppression, we must move toward understanding and connecting these paths of oppression to their origins in policy at many levels, including governmental; in individual health care and educational institutions; and in professional association policies. The policy cycle shows us that anti-racism issues must be on the policy agenda at each of these levels and many others. They must also stay on the policy agenda and be translated into policies that address systemic racism. Policy implementation, and indeed all phases of the policy cycle, must involve individuals and communities who will benefit from, or be harmed by, policies. Evaluation of policy should provide evidence to move forward, including statistical evidence as well as rich qualitative data regarding the lived experience of racism.

Acting for Social Change

Action is a central feature of each of the three areas described in the Anti-racist Framework to Guide Practice—seeing, understanding and connecting, and acting for change. Action involves educating ourselves, educating others, supporting and encouraging others who speak up, initiating change, and preventing racism. We consider the three areas to be fluid, overlapping, and interconnected. Action for change is necessarily linked to *seeing* racist oppression and its genesis at various points in policy-making. Similarly, understanding forms of racism such as environmental racism will, at the same time, bring our attention to racist municipal government policies. We emphasize the notion of intersectionality, where, for example, being a woman and being an Indigenous woman creates a compounding of injustices—a "double jeopardy" based in racism and sexism. Being a Black adolescent boy and being a Black adolescent boy from a working-class or poorer family similarly creates an intersection of racism and classism that create powerful barriers to educational and employment related achievement. Figure 1.1 illustrates the components of the Anti-racist Framework to Guide Practice.

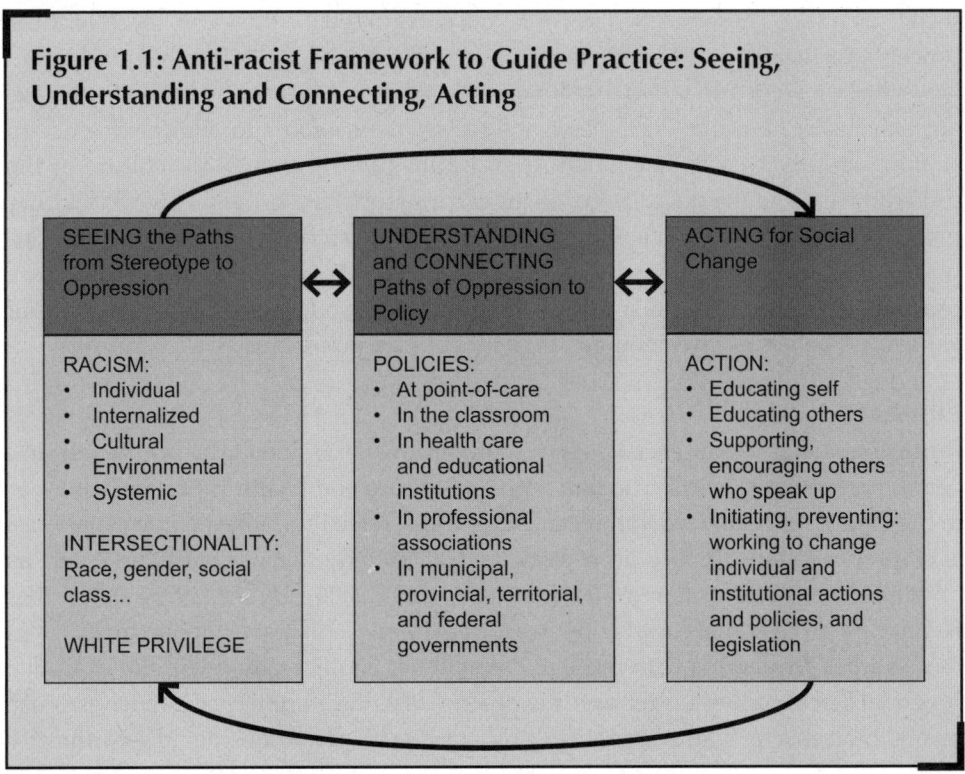

Figure 1.1: Anti-racist Framework to Guide Practice: Seeing, Understanding and Connecting, Acting

Ethnicity, Culture, Race, Religion: Concepts Informing Racism Discourse

As health care professionals learn more about the meaning and effect of racism on the health and health care of racialized peoples, we have an ethical imperative to enrich our knowledge. This process involves negotiating boundaries across differences. One of the most fundamental features of cross-cultural interaction is a basic appreciation of the cultural norms, values, and beliefs that health care professionals carry as part of the human race. An examination of concepts such as ethnicity, culture, race, and religion is central to discussions of racism and its health impact. Notably, these concepts have been used in the health literature for decades. They provide an evolutionary and cultural context within which the health care experiences of racialized peoples may be better understood in the Western world. This understanding is key to developing policies and health services that are more responsive to the cultural and social contexts of racialized peoples. Although defining these concepts can be a subject of much debate due to lack of consensus on their meanings, we provide some definitions to facilitate progression through the chapters of the book from a common reference point. There are many other important terms and concepts that are central to anti-racist practice, and these too are introduced and debated.

Ethnic, cultural, racial and religious influences are not easily demarcated by social scientists. Therefore, while we take a broad view of the importance of these concepts for health and health care access, we also recognize that they overlap in ways that are often difficult to disentangle. This discussion is meant to be illustrative, not exhaustive. We use examples from our own research and clinical practice to explore various aspects of the culture of health care recipients, the culture of the professionals, and the organizational culture in which care providers work. Culture provides us with a way of viewing our world and how it represents the assumptions we make about our everyday life. Rodriguez-Wargo (1993) noted that as health care providers, practitioners must acknowledge, understand, and incorporate cultural values and beliefs as an ongoing component of care provision.

Culture

Culture is a significant social aspect that can overarch and influence health and health care in many ways. The link between culture and health is particularly clear in the case of marginalized and racialized groups. Racially visible people experience a disproportionate impact of negative social and economic conditions such as unemployment and underemployment (Galabuzi, 2006). Miller (1995) stated that health care professionals need to be aware of their own cultural values because, when these values are at odds with those of their clients, conflict may occur. For example, pregnant Black women who engage in a practice of using home remedies such as goose fat and molasses for cold symptoms, or other substances not considered scientifically beneficial, may not share common beliefs with the health care professional. This is because health care professionals' beliefs originate from a Eurocentric health care culture in which biomedical science is the main way of knowing, and beliefs that differ are often viewed as superstition. Eurocentric means being centred on belief systems, languages, cultures, and ways of thinking that have their historical origins in Europe. People's confidence in health care often depends to a large extent on whether care fits in with what they have come to expect. They tend to have faith in the system they have grown up with (Schott & Henley, 1996). Differences in cultural values also bring with them power differentials. In the aforementioned case of the pregnant Black women, professionals' superstitious attitudes can convey a clear message that the women's ways are inferior to conventional health care practices: " ... culture cannot be conceptualized in terms of unified systems of meanings, but rather as conflicting, contradictory, ambiguous, dynamic, and full of contending discourses, all of which are mediated by power" (James, 2003, p. 28).

Ethnicity and Religion

"Ethnicity" and "culture" are often used interchangeably. Ethnicity refers to belonging to a group that shares the same characteristics, such as country of origin, language, ancestry, and culture. Ethnicity is drawn from the recognition that an individual's thoughts, perceptions, feelings, and behaviours on a given situation are often congruent with those of other members of the same ethnic group. It is one of the basic aspects of our being and is fundamental to our identity (McAdoo, 1993). Ethnicity is primarily about symbolism, group cohesion, and personal identity. It involves being aware of some particular difference between oneself and others, being able to identify the significance and relevance of the difference, and being able to organize and mobilize around that difference. The concept of culture is used to illustrate issues that cross both ethnic and cultural boundaries because, fundamentally, ethnicity refers to membership in a culturally defined group. Nationality is based on the country where people are citizens, so nations such as Canada have a multitude of ethnicities and cultures, and all of these people have the same nationality—Canadian.

Religion is a system of faith and worship, such as Islam, Catholicism, Hinduism, and Protestantism. It is the formalization of a collection of faith-based principles. Religion is sometimes confused with ethnicity, and both have been used as a reason to brutalize individuals, families, and whole peoples. Powerful modern examples include the Holocaust perpetrated against Jewish people, and the recent conflation of Islam with terrorist political parties. The Holocaust remains one of the most egregious acts against a people in modern times. It resulted in the murder of 6 million Jews, 1.5 million of whom were children, and the destruction of 5,000 Jewish communities. These deaths represented two-thirds of European Jewry and one-third of the world's Jewish people. Jewish people were gradually denied any legal rights as citizens, and eventually they were subject to attempted annihilation. Hitler and his supporters put forward racial theories claiming that Germans with fair skin, blond hair, and blue eyes were the supreme form of human, or master race. The Jews, according to Hitler, were the racial opposite. This arbitrary and socially constructed discrimination was to have a deadly impact on Jewish people. By the end of World War II, 4 million Jewish people had been gassed in the death camps while another 2 million had been shot dead or died in the ghettos (Bauer, 2001). Immigration policies in Canada meant that many Jews were denied access to Canada, and racial discrimination against Jewish people carries an enduring legacy:

> *In 1938, thirty-two nations, including Canada, attended the Evian Conference to discuss the problem of Jewish refugees fleeing Nazi Germany, but refused further Jewish immigration. In 1939, a shipload of German Jewish refugees aboard the S.S. St. Louis, were refused sanctuary in Canada and forced to return to Europe. During the Holocaust, Canada admitted only about 5,000 Jews – one of the worst records of any of the refugee receiving countries. (Virtual Museum Canada, 2008)*

The relationships among religion, ethnicity, and racism is also illustrated by more recent events. For example, Islamic people in Canada experienced much increased racism after the 9/11 terrorist attacks on the World Trade and Convention Center in New York. Islam is the religion and faith of approximately one-fifth of the world's population—more than 1.2 billion people. Its adherents are called Muslims. Islam, which means "to submit to the will of God Almighty," is the last in an ancient continuum of God's messages revealed to humanity through chosen messengers, from Adam to Muhammad (Canadian Islamic Congress, CIC, 2008). There are about 650,000 Muslims in Canada, and half are Canadian-born. About one-third trace their origins to the Indian subcontinent, one-third from Arab and Middle Eastern countries, and the remaining third are from more than 30 other nations. The CIC's third annual study of anti-Islam in the Canadian media had the goal of evaluating anti-Islam media coverage, an issue that the Muslim community and the CIC consider a serious problem affecting virtually every household of Muslim Canadians (CIC, 2008).

The study found that words associated with the adjective Islamist were dictatorship, extremist, extremist group, extremism, fighters, fundamentalist, fundamentalism, hard-liner, insurgency, insurgent, Jihad, guerrillas, militia, hijacker, militant, militant group, radical, separatists, suicide bomber, terrorist, terrorism, and violence. These words infer that Islam is an intolerant and extreme religion that teaches, endorses, or condones acts of violence (CIC, 2008). These discriminatory practices in the media reflect powerful modern-day racism in Canada. The examples show us so clearly how racism is deeply embedded in modern Canada, rather than something that we have somehow gotten over as we move to a more pluralist, multicultural society. The bombing of the World Trade and Convention Center was a catalyst that sparked a wave of hatred toward Islamic people that continues today. Box 1.3 provides definitions of some key terms in anti-racist practice.

Box 1.3: Definitions of Some Key Terms in Anti-racist Practice

Culture	Refers to a group's shared set of beliefs, norms, and values. It is the totality of what people develop to enable them adapt to their world, which includes language, gestures, tools, customs, and traditions that define their values and organize social interactions.
Ethnicity	Refers to belonging to a group that shares the same characteristics, such as country of origin, language, ancestry, and culture. Ethnicity is drawn from the recognition that an individual's thoughts, perceptions, feelings and behaviours on a given situation are often congruent with those of other members of the same ethnic group. People of the same race can be of different ethnicities. For example, Asians can be Japanese, Korean, Thai, or many other ethnicities.
Religion	Refers to a system of faith and worship, such as Islam, Catholicism, Hinduism, and Protestantism. It is the formalization of a collection of faith-based principles. Religion is sometimes confused with ethnicity, and both have been used as a reason to brutalize individuals, families, and entire peoples. Powerful modern examples include the Holocaust perpetrated against Jewish people, and the recent conflation of Islam with terrorist political groups.
Race	Refers to a group of people who share the same physical characteristics such as skin tone, hair texture, and facial features. The transmission of human genes from one generation to another is a complex process that is examined in the field of genetics. Since people can be grouped by any number of physical differences (height, foot size, resistance to certain diseases), race is an artificial way to categorize people. The salience of the term race lies in its use to signify and symbolize socio-political conflicts and interests in reference to different types of human bodies. Race is an important concept because people use racial differences as the basis for discrimination.
Nationality	Refers to country of citizenship. The concept of nationality is sometimes used to mean ethnicity, even though the two are technically different. People of one ethnic group do not necessarily live in one geographic location (such as a Chinese person residing in China and a Chinese Canadian living in Canada). Because of this, ethnicity and nationality are not always the same.
White privilege	Refers to a set of unearned advantages, opportunities and authorities that are based solely on having White skin and which confer life long increased access to the goods and services of society. White privilege is a key to the perpetuation of injustice based on race. An understanding of the ways that White privilege operates in an everyday way is central to undertaking anti-racist practice.

Stereotype	Refers to an exaggerated belief, image, or distorted truth about a person or group, a generalization that allows for little or no individual differences or social variation; a fixed image.
Bias	Refers to a way of thinking based on a stereotype or fixed image of a group of people. A common stereotype is that people who receive social assistance are lazy. When we begin to think that people on social assistance should be denied coverage for medications because they are lazy and don't deserve assistance, we are demonstrating biased thinking.
Prejudice	Refers to a negative way of thinking and attitude toward a socially defined group and toward any person perceived to be a member of the group. Like biases, prejudice is a belief and it is based on a stereotype.
Discrimination	Discrimination is an action that typically results from prejudice. Inaction in the face of need is also considered discrimination. Discrimination can occur at the individual, organizational, or societal level.
Oppression	Refers to discrimination backed by systemic power. Discrimination occurs and is supported through the power of public systems or services such as health care systems, educational systems, legal systems, and/or other public systems or services. Denying people access to culturally competent care is a form of oppression. See also "-isms."
-isms (e.g., racism, classism, sexism)	Refers to the use of social power to systematically deny people access to resources, rights, respect, and representation on the basis of gender, race, age, income, or membership in any other group; "-isms" are based on the false belief that one group is superior to another group.

Race

Houston and Wood (1996) described race as a social construction involving the classification of individuals into arbitrary groups, and assigning disparate meaning and value to the created groups. Such classifications affect the personal, social, political, and material circumstances of people's lives, and consequently shape how they view themselves, others, and their relationships (Houston & Wood, 1996). According to Witzig (1996), race is a social construction that is created from prevailing social perceptions without scientific evidence. Begley (1996) stated that the term race "can have a biological significance only when a race represents a uniform, closely inbred group, in which all family lines are alike—as in pure breeds of domesticated animals. These conditions are never realized in human types and impossible in large populations" (p. 68). A medical dictionary by Anderson, Anderson and Glanxe (1994) defined race as "a vague unscientific term for a group of genetically related people who share some physical traits" (p. 657). According to Witzig (1996), only 0.012 percent of the variation between humans in total genetic material can be attributed to differences in race.

Logan (1990) described race as an emotionally laden word that evokes deep feelings and triggers stereotypical images about certain groups of people. For example, the physical identity and social categorization, which is the essence of race, determines the predominant perceptions of Blacks in the Western world. Thus, when people think of Black families, they immediately think of a racial group (Logan, 1990). Although scientific evidence rejects the use of the social construct of race, it is still used in the health literature. Authors in some of the medical literature have even employed race "to attribute not only physical characteristics, but also psychological and moral ones to members of given categories, thus justifying or naturalizing a discriminatory system" (Begley, 1996 p. 68). Institutional racism is common in society and arbitrary race groupings are part of this kind of racism (Witzig, 1996). Our moral responsibility as health professionals is to invest in an approach that enables clients to define themselves rather than labelling them according to a social construction that "masquerades as a scientific fact" (Witzig, 1996, p. 678).

Freeman (1990) noted that care providers should endeavour to identify and understand the world view of Black people as being distinct from that of the larger society. This process is important because care providers often have a distorted view of Black people's behavioural patterns and many label the behaviours as deviant, rather than viewing them as natural responses to institutional racism. This notion is supported by Welshing (1991), who argued that when Black children are not supported in their basic development through Erikson's (1959) eight stages of development into adulthood, including basic trust, autonomy, initiative, industry, identity, intimacy, generativity, and integrity, their basic development occurs in the form of the counterparts. The counterparts to these eight stages are mistrust, shame and doubt, guilt, inferiority, role confusion, isolation, stagnation, and despair. Welshing (1991) further noted that denying Black children equal opportunity to develop psychosocially creates "dependency, negative self-image, negative self-concept and vulnerability" (p. 256). These stages pose disturbing questions about the relationships among race, racism, and health. In addition to the above possible psychosocial effects, Black children may experience a sense of powerlessness, rejection, self-hatred, fear, and general inadequacy, all of which are manifestations of failed psychosocial development (Benton, 1997).

Because race has such real consequences in people's lives, it is necessary for caregivers to explore the reasons behind some of these differences so that they can better understand how race influences people's perceptions. At the very least, health professionals' misunderstanding can result in ineffective care, which is a manifestation of racism. For example, "the traditions, values, and belief systems of First Nations and other Aboriginal people are poorly understood by many providers and often are not respected or considered. Aboriginal knowledge tends to be devalued or marginalized" (Smye & Mussell, 2001, p. 3). Areas of particular concern for Aboriginal mental health in Canada include the lack of a core Aboriginal health program federally or provincially and the lack of coordinated services related to the well-being of children (Smye & Mussell, 2001). There are insufficient resources to meet mental health concerns related to residential schools. These schools, and the Indian Act that created them in 1920, remain a powerful example of the outcomes of categorization based on race.

Racism, which is a set of attitudes and behaviours toward people of another race, is often based on the belief that races can be superior or inferior (Benton, 1997). Racism is a form of discrimination and prejudice, which is enhanced by institutional power and can be used to the advantage of one ethnic group and to the disadvantage of another ethnic group (Boyd, 1998). Racism is very complex because, although all races may discriminate to some extent, only those races who possess the power to oppress a subordinate group can practise racism (BLAC Report, 1994a). The subordinate group must then withstand the unequal treatment given them by the dominant group. This subordination includes the underrepresentation of people of colour in many workplaces and in the professions. Although there are no Canadian studies identifying health professionals by racial backgrounds, anecdotal evidence suggests significant underrepresentation of Indigenous peoples and people of African descent in the health professions, especially in leadership positions.

The lack of Indigenous peoples and people of African descent in the health professions has been associated with the often diminished accomplishments of young Indigenous and Black people. Their vision of being successful citizens is greatly limited by lack of inspiration from role models. Box 1.4 describes first-hand stories about race, racism, culture, and ethnicity. These stories are taken from Enang's (1999) research on African Nova Scotian women's pregnancy and childbirth experiences. The study was the first of its kind in Canada, and it documented historical and present-day racism specifically associated with health care during the childbirth experience.

White Privilege

White privilege is the other side of the coin when we examine the disadvantages experienced by people of colour. Discussions about White privilege are integrated throughout the book since it is a key aspect of working for social change to stop racism. Box 1.3 provided a brief definition of White privilege.

The Writers' Social Location

We discuss social location at several points in this book. It is from our social location(s) that all of us can situate ourselves to work for change. The ideas in this book are rooted in our social locations and our clinical practice, among other aspects of our identities. We describe some of these roots briefly. Our narratives were written independently of each other, and they are in no way intended to be parallel, or to be a sort of comparison between the two of us. They simply are what they are. We encourage the reader to approach them as stories, rather than an attempt to root ourselves in the theoretical foundations of the book. It turns out that they do describe some of these connections, but this is not our aim here.

Box 1.4: Voices from the Margins on Culture and Racism in Health Care

Culture

"I know I was sick. I had high blood pressure, but they used to come in and just kick my family and friends out. I never had a lot of friends down there. They used to just come in and kick anybody out. Those are my friends. I mean, they are not more important than me having a stroke or something like that. But they came down to see me. They took their time and now you're...."

"If our family comes in, they shouldn't get frustrated because we have extra one or two family members around. That is just the way we are. And if they are finding that they are having problems understanding our culture or understanding our needs, then they need to first of all attack their administration to get some workshops or sessions. There are people that can come in and to do sessions with them—both patients and other professionals. And then they can also attack the training institutions that they came from ... and say, 'Well, you didn't tell me this. What are you doing for people that are coming through now?' Because you've got to stop the cycle somehow."

"To make sure they are sensitive to the people's needs, they should know a bit about our culture, a bit about us. And if they don't know ... there are ways to find out. There [are] probably ... some of the nursing staff or other staff that could answer our questions."

Ethnicity and Religion

"You know, some people have different religions. I think there should be more awareness in the hospital to be nice to people of African, Chinese, or Indian descent. A lot of people that live here now do things differently in their country ... so there should be people of their culture in the hospital that they could talk to, can relate to and share religious beliefs."

Race and Culture

"It would be beneficial for women from different races to be able to have the information they need. If one nurse doesn't have the information, it would be nice to say, 'Well, we have someone else on staff from your culture that could help answer your questions better than I can.' We need more cultural diversity awareness. I think it will be helpful for everyone to see the different cultures because not everybody is Black and White."

Racism

"They were taking my blood. She got the student nurse to take my blood. But she couldn't find my vein. And she kept plucking around on me, and it was hurting me. So I told her, 'No, you can't keep doing this.' And the nurse said, 'No, just try it one more time.' I said 'No, you're not trying it no more. Why can't you do it?' She said, 'Well, it's known that Black people have tougher skin than White people.'"

"I felt that they wanted me to do what they made me do because I was a 'strong Black woman.' And I thought 'You've got to live to that image.' Looking back, I feel like they were thinking, 'You're a Black woman. You're tough. You need a drink of water? You walk up the hall for it. You need a painkiller, you come to the nurse's station and ask for your pain killers.' It was really tough."

"I think everybody is different in their own way.... I find that everybody have [sic] a different background, culture, or race. But it seems like when you go into the hospitals, everything you see is just White ... White babies' pictures, cards, magazines."

> "It seemed like every time the nurses would come in, it was like, 'Oh, do you want me to bring a social worker for you or anything like that?' I was like, 'No.' I didn't need no social worker. But they just kept coming in: 'Oh, do you need the social worker?' I was like, 'No, I don't need a social worker. Why would I need the social worker?' (Implicit assumption: Black women are dependent on welfare, unemployed, and unmarried.)
>
> "If a White person says something, it is automatically accepted. What they have to say is always important, and so it's spoken about and dealt with. But if it's a young Black person, they are like, 'Oh, they are trouble makers anyway. They're always in trouble.' It makes it harder for young Blacks who want to speak up on how they feel because they don't want to be looked down upon."
>
> "We need more of our people in the health care professions. And if it means we're going to have to start fighting to allow our young people into medical school, then we'll have to start doing that. I think that we need to attack some of the training institutions for change in their curriculum and in their approach. Then we need to attack our school, especially high schools and elementary schools, to get some mentors into the schools to encourage children to go into health care professions."
>
> Source: Enang, J. (1999). *Childbirth experiences of African Nova Scotian women.* Master of Nursing thesis, Dalhousie University, Halifax, NS.

Josephine: As a first-generation African-Canadian woman and a health care professional who has witnessed how Black people's lives are shaped by multiple interlocking systems of oppression, understanding the issues affecting the health of visible minority people in Canada has been my long-standing interest. Critically speaking, my personal and professional journey as a middle-aged Black woman places me on a path of constant negotiation within the spaces of difference at the intersection of race, gender, and class. Engaging in racism discourse has enhanced my understanding of the complex ways in which institutionalized systems of oppression such as racism and other forms of discrimination interact to create inequities in health and health care. In its most subtle, everyday form, racism is a razor within the psyche, slicing into self-confidence and self-love, an inner wound that is constantly being reopened by covert and sometimes overt messages that Black people are inferior to the dominant White race.

As one of my study participants noted several years ago, "Racism in Canada is like slow poison.... I see it as poison that invades the Black psyche, the Black experience ... and unless we can get rid of that poison, we're not going to be totally healthy.... It's insidious. It's slow. It's sly.... It doesn't get you right away." Having lived and worked as a health care professional in two very different societies, Nigeria and Canada, it appears that health care can be very much what the society makes of it. It can be an ordeal, a procedure, an event, or a spectacle. It can also be medical, empowering, belittling, spiritual, humiliating, joyous, painful, terrifying, and/or routine. It is widely acknowledged that while overt racism has become less socially acceptable across the Western world, racist values have not really changed. Rather, racism has largely become "quiet," "closeted," "subtle," "disguised," "hidden," and "covert." Visible minority people shoulder a heavy burden as targets of racism in Canada and North America generally. The racism that lingers in the Canadian society is still powerful enough to place people of colour under the pressure of always being on the watch for the sharp edge of discrimination.

My own experiences of living in Canada for the past 17 years have created in me a realism that I often find disturbing and confusing. My reaction to this new reality varies; sometimes it gives me a feeling of fear, anger, and helplessness for my inability to make a difference in the face of racism (especially that affecting my children), and at other times I feel a burning desire to continue the struggle to dismantle prejudice and discrimination. Most mainstream people are divorced from the real-life experiences of people on the margins of Canadian society, and they find it easier to recognize racism as an issue experienced by poor Black people. It is much more difficult for them to acknowledge that Black people of their own social class experience racism. Perhaps it is easier to think that problems experienced as a result of poverty and class can be eliminated by the victim's individual effort to change his or her own situation. Of particular concern are the ways in which the victims of oppression are silenced from making efforts to combat the harsh reality of these forms of social injustice that are fundamentally structured in power relations.

Without doubt, the history of Africans in the diaspora has been one of dealing with challenging circumstances and struggles for survival. Undertaking graduate studies in Canada gave me the impetus to examine the complex health needs of visible minority people. Some of the findings revealed in my graduate studies were the limited Canadian research available regarding the health of Black people, and the prevalence of racism in health care. An additional finding was that the under-representation of minority groups, such as Black people in the health professions, creates a barrier to effective health care for minority groups. This motivated me to explore possible connections among Black health status, access to health care, service utilization, and, perhaps most importantly, the underrepresentation of Black nurses in Nova Scotia's health care system. Over the years, I have talked with other Black health care professionals. They, too, find themselves in a health care system where they are marginally represented. Through these conversations, it became obvious that being a Black health care professional in a predominantly White health care system has its difficulties, including rejection by the very patients we desire to serve. The writing of this book is grounded in my lived experiences of racism and a desire to overcome it in health and health care.

At the time of writing this book, I had practised midwifery and nursing for nearly 23 years, 10 of which have been in the academy. I am the only Black faculty member in my department, so I do have an understanding of what it feels like to experience exaggerated visibility and invisibility simultaneously; feeling very conspicuous and yet super-isolated at the same time. Being a Black woman in health care and in academe (especially in the Western world) has its challenges, including the negotiation of everyday problems associated with marginality. In this arena, I am constantly confronted with issues of pedagogy, power, knowledge production, and a myriad of demands (both externally and self-imposed) regarding life on the margins. My often hectic, stressful, frustrating, sometimes painful but stimulating experiences have compelled me to reflect upon issues of pedagogy, the challenge of developing an inclusive and empowering learning environment, and the hardship and contradictions embedded in establishing credibility from the spaces of marginality.

These reflections raise questions that have lingered on unresolved and have provided me the critical and creative moments needed to engage in the writing of this book. This, I believe, is one of the many actions needed to combat inequities in health and health care. I believe that "knowledge is power." As Patricia Hill Collins asserted, Black women have continued to use the knowledge gained at the intersection of race, gender, and class oppression to provide a distinctive angle of vision on current understanding of the reality of being a Black woman. This book makes a contribution in this area. There are challenges and uncertainties along life's journey, but for me these have been overshadowed by the stimulus and intense desire to bring what I have learned over the years to birth in the form of a book on anti-racism practice. It is my hope that our (Elizabeth's and my) numerous dialogues about racism in health and health care, nurtured along the way by the work and experiences of others in the field, will bring new understandings to the Canadian health community.

Elizabeth: Although colonialism is largely viewed as a problem of Canada's past, the dialogue and the evidence in this book show that the master's tools continue to sharpen. Slavery and residential schools no longer exist, but Canada's apartheid against people of colour is inscribed on the bodies and psyche of families and communities around the country. The numbers and the stories are an undeniable testament to the urgent need for books such as this one. White people cannot continue their silence, their complicity, for silence is most certainly assent — inaction in the face of need. We convince ourselves that we are compassionate, non-judgmental, even spiritual in our attitudes and assumptions about these "others," these other than Whites. We are comfortable in this kind of passive benevolence, all the while reveling in the non-biased nature of our silence.

Avenues into social justice work have their own complex paths, and ultimately, many of us, including me, move forward fueled by outrage. Outrage is a beginning point for transgression to move the anti-oppressive project forward. My whiteness has carried me forward in academia in a way that privileges me a great deal. My gender and my working class social origins are my personal avenues into comprehending unfairness, meanness, and misogyny. My heritage is working class Irish on both sides of my family. From my own experience over the years, the social locations that are rooted most deeply in memory are my gender, and my Irish working class heritage. My real name is FitzGibbon. My great great grandmother and grandfather immigrated to New York after the Potato Famine in Ireland — the English attempted to annihilate the Irish by starving them to death. Soon after immigrating, John

FitzGibbon changed his name to John McGibbon to hide his Irish heritage, due to discrimination against the Irish when he immigrated to New York. The Irish were viewed as an inferior species by the British. In the new country, the Irish were still considered to be impure and not fully deserving of being called white.

Eventually, the Irish were "whitened" to the point, where today, we are considered fully white. This process is, of course, entirely a social construction, as are the arbitrary distinctions that White people continue to make about which races are fully worthy, and which ones are not. Even now in Canada, the surname "Mc" denotes Irish heritage, and "Mac" denotes English heritage. All are ancestors of the Celts, so the distinction is arbitrary. I recently watched the film *The Wind That Shakes the Barley*, a film about the brutal genesis of some of the troubles in Ireland today. Intergenerational transmission of trauma is a profound truth that demands reconciliation. How can generations-old brutalization of a people not continue to live on in the collective psyche? I can only guess at the enormity of Indigenous trauma transmission, or the traumatic legacy of slavery, both of which are centrally relevant to an anti-racist discourse in Canada.

I grew up knowing some of the Gaelic language because many grandparents in my area knew the old languages, including Mi'kmaq. I also grew up knowing some Mandarin because Jane, my best friend during grade school and high school, was an immigrant from Hong Kong. I was a devout Roman Catholic until the age of 14. I left the church at that time because I learned that according to the rules of my church, Jane and her family could not go to heaven when they died because they were Buddhist. Such is the clear and passionate logic of adolescence. My childhood social class was mostly an extension of my parents' Irish working class roots from the old country. As far as anybody knows, both sides of my family were from County Cork in Ireland. As the two eldest girls in a large, rural Catholic family, my sister Patty and I grew up cooking and cleaning for the 11 people in our household. So I learned early on how my gender located me in terms of family workload.

My experience throughout my life has been that my social class trumps my gender most of the time when it comes to oppression. The markers of social class are embedded and powerful. Like privilege of any kind, class privilege is taken for granted, and an expose of the nuances of what it is like to grow up "on the wrong side of the tracks" may seem almost petty to persons whose childhoods were not rooted in the everyday experience of classism. Some of my most clear and exact memories include the times I realized all the socially important things I did not know or have, and the enduring barriers that I would continue to experience, by virtue of my social class.

My first recollection of knowledge about the brutality that people experience by virtue of not being White, and the parallel safety of being White, happened when I was 11 years old. Along with the memory of social class described above, it remains with me just as if it happened yesterday. I was walking along the street near the running track in our town. I was a budding track and field star, or so I imagined, and I had just finished an exhilarating two-hour workout involving running up and down the bleachers with two-pound weights strapped to my ankles, along with various carefully counted sets of push-ups, sit-ups and generally gut wrenching activities. In the words of George Bernard Shaw: "Youth is wasted on the young." In the course of strolling up to the main street, my girlfriends and I heard men yelling in a tone that made us instantly afraid. A police a car was parked at the edge of the running field. We ran over, I guess because we thought that we could intervene in some way. Three police officers were attempting to put an Indian man into the back of their police car.

The police kicked this man's head, his arms, his legs. All three of them hit him repeatedly with large sticks, the tools of the trade. He resisted with all his might. I can still hear the thumps as he tried to wedge his legs along the edges of the door frame to avoid being thrown into the car. And they yelled obscenities at him. Even in the chaos of this violence I could clearly hear the man's reasoned pleas for some sort of discussion, some sort of negotiation. I saw, through my 11-year-old eyes, the complete, swift, and brutal price this man paid for being an Indian. Even then I knew that the brutality had everything to do with his Indian-ness. I felt sick. I knew nothing about colonialism or racism or White privilege, mine or others'. But I recognized the self-satisfied enjoyment of inflicting grievous bodily harm that these White police officers were experiencing. Such disgusting bullies I thought. Years later, when I worked at a center for homeless young people, I witnessed similar police treatment of a Métis adolescent. I pleaded the young man's case. The police relented but I later learned that things had not gone well for the young man while in custody. My drive for anti-racism work as a White person is based in these everyday spiritually and physically painful injustices. It simply is wrong. Josephine and I have been on this path together for over 10 years. Our connection is grounded in the injustice of racism. Our identities as mothers and women provide the glue.

Ultimately White people create and perpetuate racism everyday, as individuals and as a collective. We have such a difficult time acknowledging this fact because keeping it hidden is necessary to maintain our privilege. Racism happens to other people. It is out of our lens of experience. Only by crossing the boundaries of our persistent claims that we are not racist can we move the anti-racist project forward. In the health fields we might be particularly resistant to change because the health professions, and I include medical doctors in this group, are rooted in centuries of helping. Racism is entirely inconsistent with how we view ourselves as caring and compassionate. In order to move forward we must stop our magical thinking that being caring, compassionate and non-biased will somehow translate into ethical care of people of colour.

Organization and Outline of the Book

The organization of the book brings the reader from discussion of central concepts in the field of anti-racism to concrete ways in which anti-racist principles may be applied in everyday practice. This chapter, "Introduction to Anti-racist Health Care Practice," discussed the purpose and rationale of the book and provided an overview of some important ideas associated with anti-racism work. We also provided a brief overview of the foundations of this work, including an introduction to the book's Anti-racist Framework to guide practice. A description of our social locations as authors helps to contextualize our passion for social change.

Chapter 2, Racism as a Determinant of Health: Evidence for Change, provides a foundation for critical analysis of the relationships between racism and health. The chapter begins with an overview of some of the historical contexts of racism in Canada. Since little of this information is taught from a critical perspective (if at all) in the elementary and secondary public education system in Canada, it is important to ground this book in a generational context that acknowledges the brutality of colonialism and the historical context of racism in Canada's immigration system. We describe the broad concept of health that underpins anti-racist health care practice using the World Health Organization's (2003) determinants of health, and the Toronto Charter's social determinants of health (2004). We expand on these definitions to include a broader version of identity: race, culture, ethnicity, social class, gender, sexual orientation (lesbian, gay, bisexual, transgendered), (dis)ability, and age, to name a few. Racism is presented as a determinant of mental and physical health through the use of national and international qualitative and quantitative evidence.

The chapter focuses on racism in the health fields, where everything from the chances of being an organ-transplant recipient to the chances of receiving adequate pain medication after surgery are directly related to one's race or, more correctly, racism in the health care system. The links among health inequities, racism, and power relations are described from an individual, everyday perspective and from a systemic perspective. Although health clinicians may engage in racist practices at the bedside, it is systemic racism that creates and sustains these practices.

The systemic nature of racism is further examined in terms of racism toward health care workers, as well as the startling lack of people of colour in the ranks of health care professionals and the teachers of these professionals. Health care access as a social determinant of health is emphasized. This chapter continues to bridge the gap between theory and practice by providing concrete examples of how racism manifests itself in the health and well-being of people of colour, and in their access to the goods and services of society.

Chapter 3, A Critique of Diversity and Multicultural Health Care Models, lays the groundwork for choosing anti-racism as a foundation for change. The chapter provides a history of the development of multiculturalism in Canada, including a description of how people with different cultural views became known as "foreigners." An overview of cultural competence is provided in terms of its contribution to working with diverse populations. The chapter concludes with a critique of the notion of cultural competence and its failure to address racism and White privilege as key processes that sustain racism in health care.

Chapter 4, Theoretical Foundations for an Anti-racist Practice, describes important perspectives on health and health care, and discusses them in terms of their relevance for health care, and for anti-racist practice. These perspectives include: epidemiological, sociological, feminist, anti-racist and anti-colonial, political economy, and human rights. We emphasize the importance of critical perspectives in health practice and in working for change, and we use a case study to explore the practical application of critical perspectives on health and health care. The case study provides a foundation to think about the interconnected layers of intervention that are possible through a critical perspective. Biomedical dominance is discussed to situate anti-racist practice within the dominant mode of thinking in Canadian health and health care. We then provide a comparison of biomedical and critical perspectives on health and health care. Our aim in this discussion is to illuminate paths to move forward.

Chapter 5, An Anti-racist Framework to Guide Practice, presents the underpinnings of our anti-racism framework. This chapter builds on the theoretical perspectives discussed in previous chapters, describing the many forms of racism, with practical examples and first-person narratives. We revisit our intersectionality lens to incorporate the notion of intersecting oppressions and their impact on health outcomes. When oppressions such as racism and classism intersect, they are magnified well beyond a mere additive effect produced by the two oppressions. An intersectionality lens is applied to selected professional practice codes of ethics in Canada. We challenge the notion that ethical care can be provided without a working knowledge of intersectionality as it relates to physical and mental health. We propose the development of social justice-based professional codes of ethics for health care. The chapter concludes with a discussion of important aspects of positioning whiteness in anti-racist practice.

Chapter 6, Engaging in Everyday Anti-racist Health Care Practice, describes central anti-racist principles that are pivotal in working for change: (1) Understanding and addressing the centrality of power; (2) understanding and addressing the facts of oppression; (3) confronting whiteness; (4) engaging in situated practice; (5) confronting the myth of neutrality; and (6) creating a new meaning for critical thinking. Each of these areas is discussed in detail, with numerous practice-based examples. We then discuss working with resistance to anti-racism practice, and strategies to overcome resistance. We emphasize this area because resistance to anti-racism work is relentless and can also be cumulatively exhausting. The chapter concludes with application of an action continuum for social change, based on the work of Wijeyesinghe, Griffin, and Love (1997).

Chapter 7, Racism, Public Policy, and Social Change, provides a concise overview of the policy cycle and its application to anti-racist practice. Some of the ways in which policy-making promotes inequity are described in detail, including policy-created poverty, gender inequity and federal budgets, and democratic racism. We take up health as a human right and build on the human rights perspective described in Chapter 4. A detailed description of how health is a human right is provided by tracing Canadian and global human rights legislation. This information is an important foundation for identifying the ways that racism in the health care system defies Canadian law, and for making anti-racist policy agendas an imperative. The importance of a critical social science view is again stressed, with an emphasis on how this view can inform policy change. We conclude with a discussion of the structural determinants of health, including political ideologies, political parties, and their relationship with public policy.

Conclusions

Each of us has our own starting point along the continuum of working for social change. The urgency of working toward anti-racist health care practice is all around us—in the voices from the margins, and in our own participation in the cycle of oppression. Each of us is positioned differently in this process, and although this position can change over time, it is always our starting point for anti-racist practice. Social change must be a foundation for our everyday practice.

CHAPTER 2

Racism as a Determinant of Health
Evidence for Change

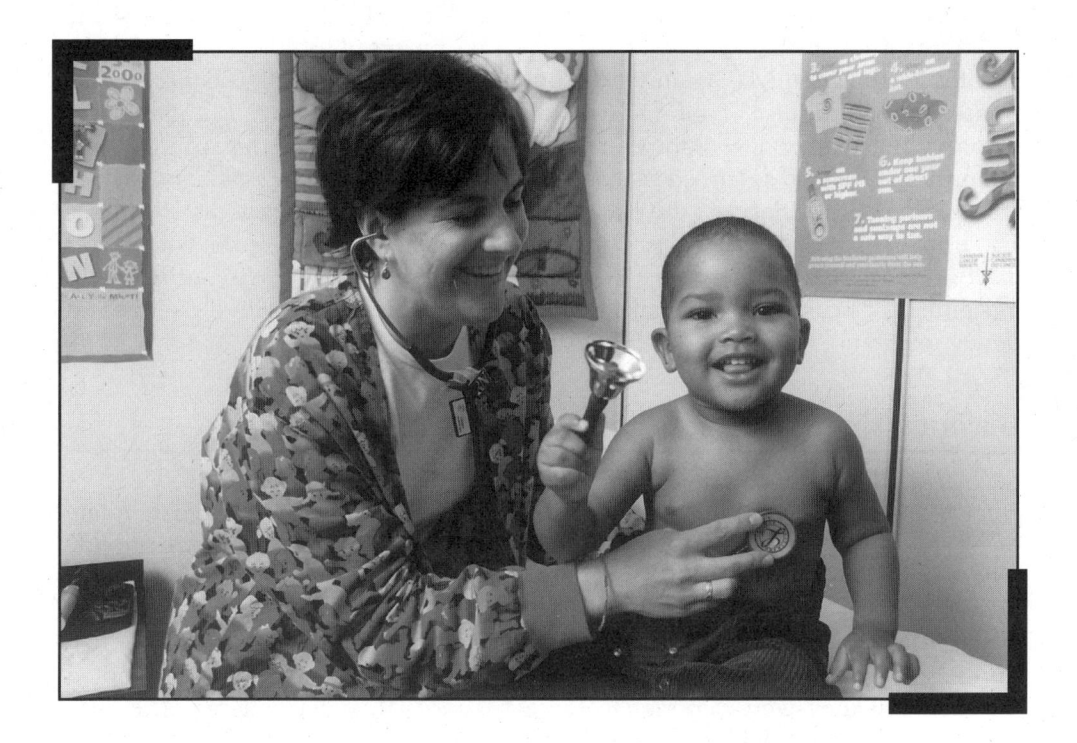

Economic and racial inequality are not abstract concepts, [they] hospitalize and kill even more people than cigarettes. The wages and benefits we're paid, the neighborhoods we live in, the schools we attend, our access to resources and even our tax policies are health issues every bit as critical as diet, smoking and exercise. The unequal distribution of these social conditions — and their health consequences — are not natural or inevitable. They are the result of choices that we as a community, as states, and as a nation have made, and can make differently. Other nations already have, and they live longer, healthier lives as a result. (Larry Adelman, executive producer, Unnatural Causes, March 2008)

Introduction

Differences in the health outcomes of racialized peoples have their roots in the history of racism. The Canadian education system, particularly in the elementary and secondary areas, has largely neglected its responsibility to teach the facts and the sequelae of colonialism, including its impact on immigration. This deficit in education means that health professionals may lack a sound knowledge base to grasp the breadth and depth of racism in Canada. In this chapter we describe brief histories of Indigenous and African Canadians, and immigrant Canadians to provide the context of colonialism that underpins racism. Health is discussed in terms of the determinants of health, including the social determinants of health, using the World Health Organization (2003) and the Toronto Charter (Raphael, 2004) definitions as a base. The significance of anti-racist health care practice in Canada is underscored by providing an overview of the Canada Health Act, and statistics regarding visible minorities. Racism is described as a determinant of health, and intersections such as race, gender, and social class are emphasized as strong multipliers of disadvantage. The impact of racism on physical and mental health outcomes is discussed, and health care access is emphasized as a social determinant of health. We conclude with a beginning discussion of the links among health outcome inequities, racism, and power relations.

Historical Context

History tells us much about ourselves. One of the most successful ways to perpetuate racism is to ensure the erasure of historical facts and stories. In this section we provide a very brief introduction to the historical context of racism in Canada. We return to many of these ideas throughout the book. Much of our current understanding of racism can be traced to the era of colonialism, which began in the 1400s. When Europeans began colonizing Africa and the Americas, the White settlers adopted the idea that they were superior to the other races they encountered. The false notion that Africans and Indigenous peoples were inferior (in addition to the desire for economic power) justified the Europeans' taking land and enslaving people. In this way, naturally occurring racial differences became the basis for systems of exploitation and discrimination. Historically, racial categorization has its roots in racism, and the construct of racism provides avenues to understand racial differences in health. Williams (1999) defined racism as "an ideology of inferiority that is used to justify unequal treatment (discrimination) of members of groups defined as inferior, by both individuals and societal institutions" (p. 176).

It is important to remember that racism is neither natural nor inevitable. Throughout history, people of different racial groups have interacted and coexisted peacefully. In the Middle Ages, for example, Europeans looked up to the people of Africa and China, whose civilizations and cultures were considered to be more advanced. However, these ideas changed significantly during the colonial era. Racism is the systematic practice of denying people access to rights, representation, or resources based on racial differences. As you will learn in this book, racism involves more than personal actions of individuals. It is a comprehensive system of discrimination that involves social institutions and affects virtually every aspect of society. It is important to recognize that racism is a systematic process created by people, and this process can be dismantled by people as well.

Indigenous Peoples

Indigenous peoples are the very first inhabitants of a geographic area. In Canada, White peoples' relations with Indigenous communities created a view of Indigenous peoples as another ethnic minority population that needed to be assimilated into the national whole. Assimilation refers to the process of denying, and erasing where possible, the language, culture, ethnicity, beliefs, customs, and material possessions of a group of people, and forcing them to adopt the systems of the dominant group. Since assimilation involves erasing culture, it is sometimes referred to as acculturation. For example, it is widely thought that the two founding nations of Canada were England and France rather than Indigenous peoples (First Nations, Métis, Inuit). We see ourselves as a bi-cultural nation—English and French. Views of Indigenous peoples are often based in the reasoning that Indigenous peoples are but one of the many ethnic groups that together constitute the cultural backdrop of Canada, and that they should acculturate to facilitate integration into the Canadian norm. One of the most powerful mechanisms for colonial control of Indigenous peoples in Canada was the creation of residential schools. Box 2.1 provides a timeline of the origins of Indian residential schools in Canada.

Box 2.1: A History of Indian Residential Schools in Canada

- **1857:** Gradual Civilization Act passed to assimilate Indians.
- **1870–1910:** Period of assimilation where the clear objective of both missionaries and government was to assimilate Aboriginal children into the lower fringes of mainstream society.
- **1920:** Compulsory attendance for all children ages seven to 15. Children were forcibly taken from their families by priests, Indian agents, and police officers.
- **1931:** There were 80 residential schools operating in Canada.
- **1948:** There were 72 residential schools with 9,368 students.
- **1979:** There were 12 residential schools with 1,899 students.
- **1980s:** Residential school students began disclosing sexual and other forms of abuse at residential schools.
- **1996:** The last federally run residential school, the Gordon Residential School, closes in Saskatchewan.
- **1998:** The Assembly of First Nations establishes the Indian Residential Schools Resolution Unit.
- **2008:** The federal government of Canada issues a formal apology for the atrocities committed in Indian residential schools in Canada.

Source: Assembly of First Nations. (2008). *History of Indian residential schools.* Indian Residential Schools Unit, Assembly of First Nations.

The design and implementation of Canadian residential schools was initiated by a government act that made assimilation of Indigenous peoples a goal of national public policy. These policies were developed to deal with what became known as "the Indian problem." One of the main mechanisms of assimilation was the attempted erasure of Indigenous spirituality and culture through the introduction of residential schools and Christian missionaries. There was compulsory attendance for all Indigenous children ages seven to 15 years, and children were forcibly removed from their homes (abducted) by priests, police officers, and Indian agents. An Indian agent was the chief administrator for Indian affairs, according to the Indian Act enacted in 1876, and Indian agents were assigned districts across the country. The powers of the Indian agents were all-encompassing, and they enforced colonial rule over the lives of all Aboriginal peoples in their jurisdictions. On June 11, 2008, Prime Minister Stephen Harper officially apologized to all Canadian Aboriginal peoples for the government creation and sanction of the residential schools. However, there were mixed responses to the apology:

While many survivors had mixed emotions, many agreed that the apology was long overdue. "I can forgive but I will never forget," says Rose Marie Francis, Yarmouth, Nova Scotia. At the age of six years old the Indian Agent threatened her father that if he didn't let the children go to the Residential School that all of his World War II medals and pension would be taken away. (Bernard, 2008, p. 7)

Colonialism happens in many different ways. Colonizers are groups of people or countries that come to a new place and steal the land from the inhabitants, steal natural resources such as copper, fish, and fur, force the inhabitants to help them develop industries such as mining and farming for cash crops (usually with brutal and inhumane methods), and develop a set of laws and public processes that are designed to violate the human rights of the Indigenous inhabitants and, in some cases, to completely annihilate these inhabitants. Colonizers not only colonized many countries and attempted to destroy Indigenous peoples, but they also implemented a slave trade with its origins in Africa. Slavery was a means for colonizers to make vast fortunes without paying thousands of workers. So, while these same colonizers were colonizing Africa, they integrated their African colonization with North American colonization through the use of slavery. The core of colonization remained the same: "Athough the encounter between colonizer and colonized changes in historically specific ways, and it is always highly gendered, it remains a moment when powerful narratives turn oppressed peoples into objects, to be held in contempt, or to be saved from their fates by more civilized beings" (Razack, 1998, p. 3).

Examples of Indigenous peoples around the globe are the Maori in New Zealand, the Zulus in South Africa, the Mi'kmaq in eastern Canada, the Cree in western Canada, and the Inuit in the north. All of these peoples have a long and disturbing history at the hands of White colonial oppressors. British and other colonizers came to countries such as Barbados, Canada, South Africa, and the United States. The colonial experiences of Indigenous peoples around the globe have rendered them strangers in their own country. The harshness and repression of the colonizers' conquest has been hidden from popular accounts of mainstream history in Canada. This is why many Canadians still hold views such as "We [White people] gave the Natives everything—free houses and free university tuition—and they still can't organize themselves." The brutal attempt at colonial annihilation of Indigenous peoples in Canada is largely kept hidden from view in education, in popular culture, and in the vast literature that we call Canadian. As stated in Chapter 1, most Canadians do not know that when colonial powers in South Africa sought a template about how to subjugate, brutalize, and destroy the many peoples in its nation, they came to Canada and consulted the Canadian government. This was because the White European colonizers were recognized as experts in this horrific process.

> *The relationship between Canada and the First Nations peoples has been marked by social, economic, political, and cultural oppression. Some specific examples of racist policies towards First Nations Peoples are denial of the right to vote, prohibition from purchasing land, outlawing spiritual ceremonies, forced relocation and segregation on reserves, restrictions on civil and political rights, and expropriation of land. (Roy, 2008, p. 1)*

African Canadians

People of African descent have made Canada their home for over 400 years. The legacy of colonialism, although different than that of Indigenous Canadians, bears similarities. The largest migration of Black people were the Black Loyalists, who came to Canada in the late 1700s following the end of the American Revolution, and the independence of the United States of America in 1783 (Carter & Carter, 1993). Like many Canadians, they came in search of freedom and better lives for themselves and their families. Their journeys were full of trials and tribulations, and upon arrival in Canada, they faced many hardships, from failed promises of land to unstable farming and living conditions (Collins, 1993), and later the relocation of whole communities.

One such example is the Black settlement of Africville. Africville was a vibrant African-Canadian community in Halifax, Nova Scotia. The history of Africville has been traced back to 1838 when descendants of American slaves settled in northern Halifax on the shore of Halifax Harbour. The area was originally known as Campbell Road, but it became known as Africville because of its Black population. Under pressure from the White majority in Halifax, municipal officials relocated closed sewage disposal pits to the edge of Africville in 1858. In the 1950s, city officials moved a large open dump to a site just 100 metres from the edge of the area where the houses of Africville were located. Racism intensified in the 1960s when Africville land, increasingly valued for its location on a Halifax waterfront, was expropriated by the city of Halifax and the entire community was "relocated." Many residents were moved in garbage trucks. All their land was taken and their homes were destroyed. Africville remains one of the clearest examples of racism in Nova Scotia

(Boyd, 1998). In spite of all these obstacles, whenever possible, given the institutional barriers, people of African descent moved ahead to obtain work as nurses, teachers, social workers, and other professionals (Carter & Carter, 1993). Box 2.2 provides an exercise for reflecting on some of the ideas presented thus far, and in particular for dismantling some of our beliefs about race and racism.

Box 2.2: Exercise for Dismantling Our Beliefs (and Their Sources) about Race and Racism

Goals

1. To enable participants to reflect on their feelings, beliefs, and understanding of racial discrimination
2. To help participants place their individual behaviours in the context of larger social systems
3. To help participants understand that discrimination is not only the result of individual actions, and that solutions to discrimination need to go beyond individual acts to address systemic issues

Instructions
Reflect on the following questions regarding messages or images you have received about race throughout your life. Record the values or judgments that come to mind, and the sources of your beliefs.

Exercise Questions

Name a group	1. What images come to mind when you think of this group?	2. What values or judgments do you associate with these images?	3. What is the source for these images, values, or judgments?	4. What impact do these images and judgments have on your behaviour?
People of my racial background				
People of racial backgrounds that are not the same as mine				

Immigration

Racism in Canadian immigration policies and processes has been well documented, and many peoples have experienced racism through the immigration process in Canada. Roy (2008) emphasized three groups, in addition to Aboriginal and Black

Canadians, whose history is marked by racism: Chinese, Japanese, and South Asian Canadians. In the 1880s, Chinese labourers were permitted to come to Canada to work in the construction of the railway only when there was a labour shortage. They were subjected to horrific working conditions and were paid only one-quarter of the wages of White workers (Roy, 2008). Living conditions were appalling. After the Canadian Pacific Railway was built, Chinese men continued to be recruited to fill labour shortages caused by new industrial growth. All the while, Chinese people were prohibited from owning property, or voting in municipal or federal elections, even though many had been in Canada for over a decade. During the first two years of World War I, Chinese Canadians, along with all racial minorities and Aboriginal peoples, were refused entry into service for their country. Only when shortages of soldiers began to hamper Canada's war effort were these people permitted entry into the armed forces (Henry, Tator, Mattis, & Rees, 2000).

The Japanese-Canadian experience also reflects racism from the time they first settled in British Columbia in the 1870s. The most blatant act of racism against Japanese Canadians was the internment camps in World War II. Twenty-three thousand people of Japanese ancestry, 13,300 of them Canadian-born, were sent to detention camps and not released until two years after the war was over. Land was confiscated; schools were closed; houses, automobiles, and businesses were sold; and the profits were impounded. There was a mass denial of civil rights, justified through reasons of wartime security because Japan was at war against Canada (Henry et al., 2000; Roy, 2008). In 1988, after years of lobbying, 12,000 Japanese Canadians received $21,000 CAD each as compensation for their internment in the camps.

The consistent mechanisms of legalized racism were also demonstrated in the treatment of South Asian Canadians. South Asians are people who were born (or whose ancestors were born) in India, Pakistan, Sri Lanka, Bhutan, and Bangladesh. They also include people who have immigrated to the Indian subcontinent from Kenya, Tanzania, Uganda, and the Caribbean (Henry et al., 2000). Legalized racism refers to racist practices that are enshrined in the laws and policies of a country. As such, racist acts are made legally defensible and enforceable by the police and other authorities across the region. South Asian Canadians were excluded from the right to vote, denied entry into professional occupations, and subject to restricted property rights and discriminatory housing practices. These exclusions resulted in great difficulty in earning a living and in overt racist acts based on racist stereotypes.

The generational impact of these exclusions, and the others listed above, must be fully acknowledged. We are consistently taught the centrality of history in the shaping of modern-day issues and struggles, in primary, secondary and post-secondary education, and in countless non-academic venues. Yet Canadians, in general, persistently overlook this relatively recent history of overt racism against Indigenous, African, Chinese, Japanese, and South Asian Canadians. If my grandmother and grandfather had all of their hard-earned property and material goods confiscated (stolen) by the government of Canada, would my mother and father not be seriously affected by family financial ruin and the accompanying psychological and spiritual losses? And would my opportunities not be similarly hampered? The painful answer is *yes*. Anti-racist health care practice originates in these concrete comparisons to White people's own humanity, and the acceptance of the longitudinal historical power of racist acts.

These accounts demonstrate a clear and consistent history of racism in Canada. Our inclination as a country is to move on and go about the business of continuing to create a multicultural society where all citizens are welcome. After all, the peoples described above have the right to vote in today's society. The professions such as dentistry, law, medicine, and nursing have no restrictions now, and all professions are open to all Canadians who wish to pursue them. The Canada Health Act guarantees access to health care for all Canadians. When houses go on the market, anyone with sufficient money can buy them. When apartments are for rent, anyone with good references, a solid rental history, and the money to pay rent can get an apartment. However, the evidence we present throughout this book tells a different and disturbing story. This is why historical underpinnings of racism need to be held closely and respectfully in any efforts to ameliorate present day racism. History, rather than being mostly about the past, permeates modern Canadian racism.

Significance of Anti-racist Health Care Practice in Canada

The combined total of numbers of people of colour in Canada is in the millions. However, the significance of anti-racist health care practice in Canada lies not only in the weight of numbers. As the evidence presented in this chapter shows, the unequal distribution of morbidity and mortality in people of colour is cause for great concern. Racism in the health care system has been cited as a significant barrier to receiving needed care and services. For example, in 2000–2001, 20 percent of off-reserve Aboriginal peoples reported an unmet health care need, which is significantly higher than 13 percent for the non-Aboriginal population (Statistics Canada, 2002).

The significance of anti-racist health care practice is underscored by the five principles of the Canada Health Act (CHA): (1) public administration, (2) comprehensiveness, (3) universality, (4) portability, and (5) accessibility. Although readers may be familiar with the Canada Health Act, we encourage a close examination of each of the principles in light of the information presented thus far in the book. The Act sets out the primary objective of Canadian health care policy, which is to protect, promote, and restore the physical and mental well-being of residents of Canada and to facilitate reasonable access to health services without financial or other barriers (Health Canada, 2008). The aim of the CHA is to ensure that all eligible residents of Canada have reasonable access to insured health services on a prepaid basis without direct charges at the point of service for such services. The following list provides a definition of the five criteria set out under the Canada Health Act (Health Canada, 2008).

1. *Public administration:* Provincial and territorial health care insurance plans are administered and operated on a non-profit basis by a public authority, which is accountable to the provincial or territorial government for decision making on benefit levels and services, and whose records and accounts are publicly audited.
2. *Comprehensiveness:* The health care insurance plan of a province or territory must cover all insured health services provided by hospitals, physicians, or dentists (i.e., surgical-dental services that require a hospital setting) and, where the law of the province so permits, similar or additional services rendered by other health care practitioners.
3. *Universality:* All insured residents of a province or territory must be entitled to the insured health services provided by the provincial or territorial health care insurance plan on uniform terms and conditions. Newcomers to Canada, such as landed immigrants or Canadians returning from other countries to live in Canada, may be subject to a waiting period by a province or territory, not to exceed three months, before they are entitled to receive insured health services.
4. *Portability:* Residents moving from one province or territory to another must continue to be covered for insured health services by the "home" jurisdiction during any waiting period imposed by the new province or territory of residence.
5. *Accessibility:* Insured persons in a province or territory have reasonable access to insured hospital, medical, and surgical-dental services on uniform terms and conditions, unprecluded or unimpeded, either directly or indirectly, by charges (user charges or extra-billing) or other means (e.g., discrimination on the basis of age, health status or financial circumstances).

The Act underscores the need to increase knowledge and action regarding anti-racist practice in Canada. According to the definitions above, Canadian law is already losing its ability to enforce the principles of the Canada Health Act. Racism in the health care system and in Canadian society in general is increasingly jeopardizing our country's adherence to the Canada Health Act. Accessibility has already been demonstrated to be a problem for people of colour (Enang, 1999, 2002, 2006; McGibbon, Etowa & McPherson, 2008). Since women, elders, and rural and northern individuals and families also have decreased access, the enormity of the problem becomes apparent. Table 2.1 provides the distribution of visible minorities in Canada. All the terms used in the table are the terms used by Statistics Canada in their 2006 census. As these numbers and the growing loss of adherence to the Canada Health Act demonstrate, anti-racist health care practice is a priority in Canada. Figure 2.1 provides a provincial and territorial depiction of the distribution of combined totals of Aboriginal and visible minority people in Canada in 2006. Figure 2.2 provides a depiction of visible minorities in Canada by origin in 2006. Descriptors are from Statistics Canada.

Table 2.1: Visible Minorities in Canada, 2006

	North American Indian	Métis	Inuit	African Origin	Chinese	South Asian	Arabic
NS	10,485	1,005	180	4,230	3,655	3,215	5,625
PEI	595	45	20	165	200	125	435
NL	6,685	2,280	3,430	475	1,165	1,430	615
NB	9,315	1,005	95	1,295	2,155	1,530	1,225
ON	87,900	9,825	1,055	144,635	543,320	679,875	123,790
MB	80,865	15,625	305	7,250	12,480	14,465	2,265
SK	77,335	10,465	135	3,055	8,410	3,990	1,715
AB	72,075	16,515	750	25,530	110,900	89,805	26,865
BC	80,975	9,655	345	12,300	377,550	231,915	8,995
YT	3,560	140	135	50	245	125	15
NT	10,740	1,105	3,175	290	280	145	80
NU	65	25	22,095	25	55	50	15
QB	3,195	440	55	2,785	1,650	430	3,380

Source: Adapted from Statistics Canada (2008). Ethnic origin, visible minorities, place of work, and mode of transportation. *The Daily*, Wednesday, April 2, 2008.

Figure 2.1: Distribution of Visible Minorities by Province in Canada, 2006

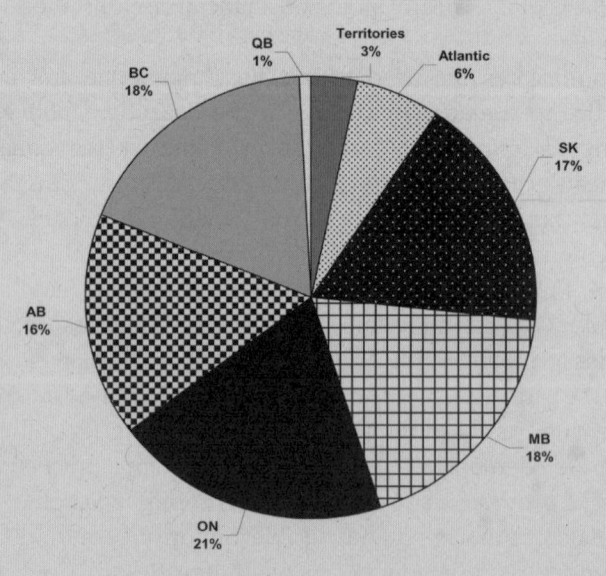

- QB: 1%
- Territories: 3%
- Atlantic: 6%
- BC: 18%
- SK: 17%
- AB: 16%
- MB: 18%
- ON: 21%

Source: Adapted from Statistics Canada (2008). Ethnic origin, visible minorities, place of work, and mode of transportation. *The Daily*, Wednesday, April 2, 2008.

Figure 2.2: Distribution of Visible Minorities in Canada by Origin, 2006

- Arabic 20%
- North Am. Indian 36%
- South Asian 11%
- Métis 4%
- Chinese 13%
- Inuit 1%
- African 15%

Source: Statistics Canada (2008). Ethnic origin, visible minorities, place of work, and mode of transportation. *The Daily*, Wednesday, April 2, 2008.

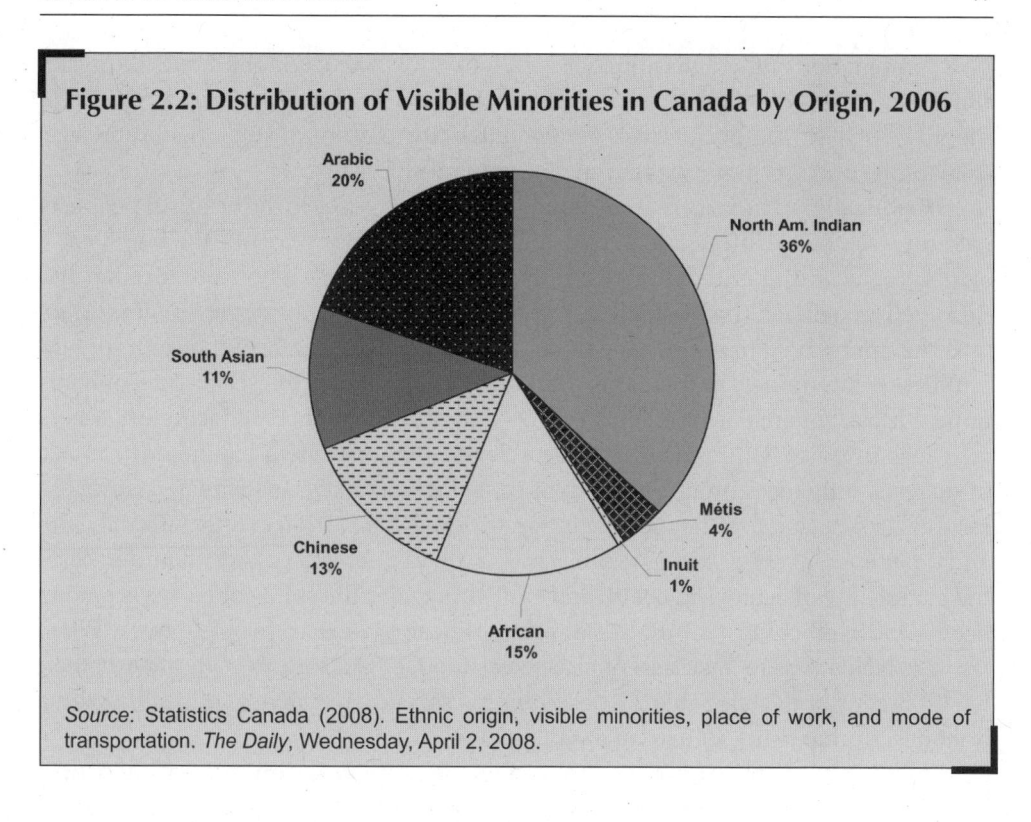

Racism as a Social Determinant of Health

The social determinants of health (SDOH) are well-recognized antecedents to health and well-being, and there is ample evidence that racism is a social determinant of health. Race alone could not account for the substantially worse health outcomes of people of colour. Intersections of the SDOH, and identities such as race, age, and gender, create powerful amplifications of disadvantage. These disadvantages are painfully apparent in the poorer physical and mental health outcomes of racialized and marginalized peoples. The following sections bear testimony to these relationships among racism, the SDOH, and health outcomes.

The Social Determinants of Health

Definitions and views of health have evolved considerably over the past few decades. The WHO's definition of health as "not just an absence of disease" has been refined and enriched to include determinants of health, including the social determinants of health (World Health Organization, 2003). The SDOH underscore the importance of using a more encompassing definition of health. Healthy environments, healthy child development, meaningful employment, and income security all play an important role in the health of individuals, families, communities, and nations. Although there are varying definitions of the SDOH, we base our discussion on a combination of the determinants cited by WHO (2003), and the Toronto Charter (Raphael, 2004). We expand on current definitions to include a broader scope of identity: such as race, social class, gender, ethnicity, culture, sexual orientation, age, (dis)ability, and spirituality as social determinants of health.

Historically, it has largely been assumed that differences in the health of people of colour were due to differences in biologic and genetic endowment—the biophysical attributes that are inherited from our parents or acquired throughout our lifespan. It is now well recognized that biologic and genetic endowment, although very important in determining health, are not the major determinants of the health of individuals, families, communities, and nations (Raphael, 2004). Rather, the social determinants of health play the major role in shaping health outcomes. Income inequality serves as a case in point. Differences in income levels demonstrate a continued primacy of material influences on health (Wilkinson & Pickett, 2005). Inadequate household income for securing healthy food creates nutritional deficits that greatly impact health and development across the lifespan. Thus, a broad definition of health underscores the complexity of achieving health and well-being, and the solid connections among health and well-being and the social and political context of people's lives. When families lack access to basic essentials such as food, education, and safe shelter, their health is compromised. Table 2.2 describes the social determinants of health, with a brief description using Canadian data.

The social determinants of health combine to amplify health concerns of people of colour. For example, the low-income rate among the most recent immigrants to Canada almost doubled from 1980 to 1995, before easing back during the last half of the 1990s (Statistics Canada, 2003). As a result, the gap in the low-income rate between recent immigrants and Canadian-born individuals widened significantly during the past two decades. In 1980, low-income rates among immigrants who had arrived between 1975 and 1980 were 1.4 times those of people born in Canada. In 1990, low-income rates among immigrants who arrived between 1985 and 1990 were 2.1 times those of Canadian-born adults. By 2000, low-income rates among recent immigrants were 2.5 times those of Canadian-born adults (Statistics Canada, 2003). Statistics Canada defined recent immigrants as those who arrived in Canada during the five years before the census in question. Immigrants of colour have the compounding burden of racism, which makes their incomes even less, on average, than the general population of immigrants in Canada. Figure 2.3 illustrates unemployment rates for immigrants, non-immigrants, and racialized groups in Canada in 2001.

The 2003 First Nations Regional Longitudinal Health Survey reported that over 50 percent of First Nations adults were not working for pay. Of the 48.8 percent of adults who were working for pay, the majority were working full-time. First Nations adults with post-secondary diplomas were almost twice as likely to be employed when compared with adults with less than a high school diploma. Overall, the proportion of First Nations adults living with a disability is over one and a half times greater than the general population (Assembly of First Nations, 2007).

Table 2.2: The Social Determinants of Health

Employment and working conditions *(e.g. meaningful employment; work safety; and dependable, consistent work):* Women with disabilities are twice as likely to be unemployed (Statistics Canada, 2005). Immigrant women face numerous stressors such as finding employment and establishing income, which can have a serious health impact (Meadows, Thurston & Melton, 2001).

Income and its equitable distribution *(e.g. adequate annual income and a family's capacity to meet basic needs):* Overall income of most Canadian families has steadily decreased since 1986 (Curry-Stevens, 2001). In some provinces, almost 30 percent of children in minority families live in poverty (Canadian Council on Social Development, 2000).

Food security *(e.g. a family's capacity to provide minimum nutritious food):* Food bank use doubled between 1989 and 2004. Forty-one percent of food bank users are children under 18 years (Raphael, Bryant & Curry-Stevens, 2004). Child hunger is an extreme example of family food insecurity (McIntyre, 2004). If you experience food insecurity, you are significantly more likely to have type 2 diabetes (Seligman, Bindman, Vittinghoff, Kanaya & Kushel, 2007).

Housing *(e.g. safe shelter, and green space for play):* As more Canadians spend more of their income on shelter, housing security is threatened. Canada's renter households have average incomes that are half that of homeowners (Shapcott, 2004). Damp housing further exacerbates health problems such as childhood asthma (Bryant, Chisholm & Crowe, 2002).

Early childhood development, education, and care *(e.g. nurturing and abuse-free environments): access to appropriate child-care supports and early childhood education:* Early childhood development is threatened due to continuing levels of family poverty (Raphael, 2004). There is a notable mismatch between known early childhood educational opportunities and public investment (McPherson, Popp & Lindstrom, 2006).

Education *(e.g. opportunity for post-secondary education):* Average yearly university tuition has tripled since 1991 (Statistics Canada, 2007). Health literacy is strongly related to the level of formal education, health outcomes, and access to care. Except for Nova Scotia, Atlantic provinces have lower literacy rates than the national average (Murray, Rudd, Kirsch, Yamamoto & Grenier, 2007).

Health services *(e.g. access to specialist and multidisciplinary services):* Rural people have less access to health services and have poorer health than urban people. Women living in the most rural areas are most likely to report fair or poor health (Canadian Institute for Health Information, 2006). Racism in health care is an important barrier in access to health services (Etowa, Weins, Bernard & Clow, 2007).

Social exclusion *(e.g. access to social supports and community participation):* Groups experiencing social exclusion tend to sustain higher health risks and lower health status. These include Indigenous peoples; immigrants; refugees; people of colour; people with disabilities; lone parents; children, youth in disadvantaged circumstances; women; the elderly; unpaid caregivers; gays, lesbians, bisexuals, transgendered people (Galabuzi, 2005).

Social safety nets *(e.g. access to income supplements and publicly funded home care support):* Maritime provinces have the lowest per-person spending on home care in

Canada (Coyte & McKeever, 2001). Home care has been left out of the national policy agenda, which has grave consequences for the health of many vulnerable populations, including elders, and chronically ill children (Shamian, 2007).

Identity *(e.g. gender, race, ethnicity, culture, age, social class, (dis)ability, sexual orientation, and age, to name a few, all determine health care access and health outcomes):* Gender and race have recently been added to earlier definitions of the SDOH. These definitions have been expanded to include the broader notion of identity as a SDOH (McGibbon, McPherson & Etowa, 2007).

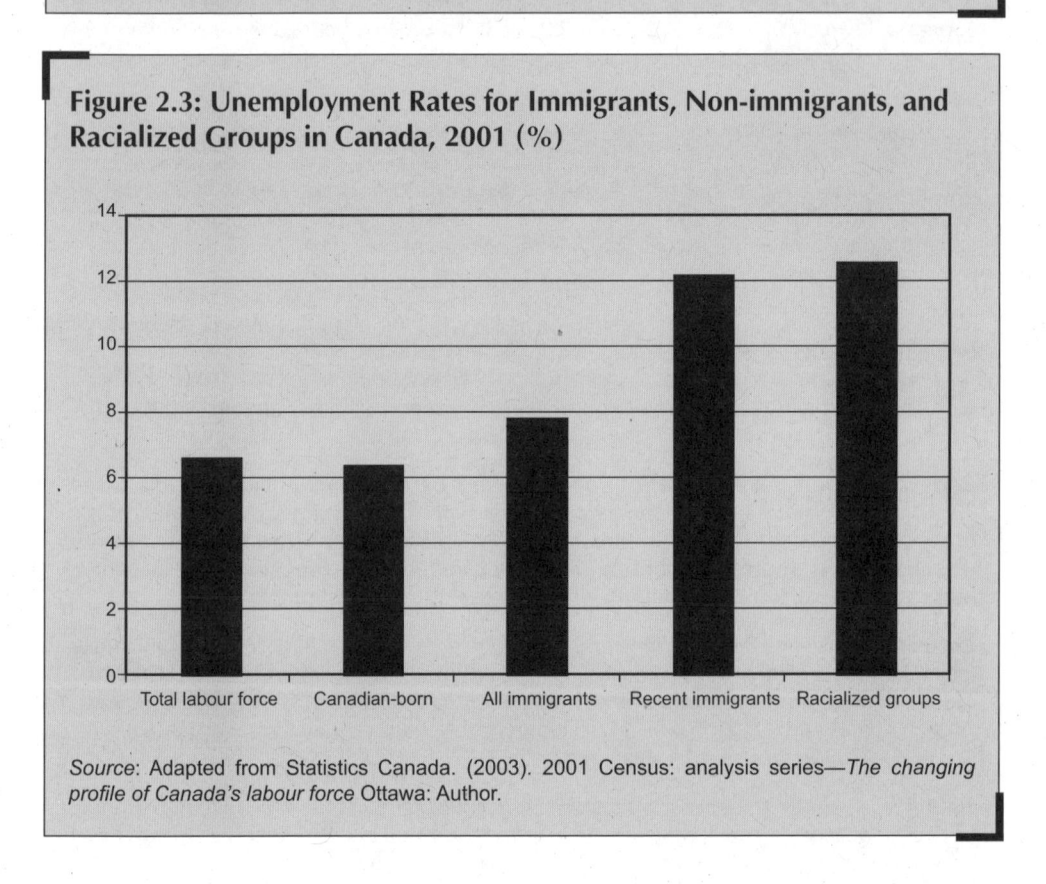

Figure 2.3: Unemployment Rates for Immigrants, Non-immigrants, and Racialized Groups in Canada, 2001 (%)

Category	Unemployment Rate (%)
Total labour force	~6.5
Canadian-born	~6.4
All immigrants	~7.8
Recent immigrants	~12.2
Racialized groups	~12.6

Source: Adapted from Statistics Canada. (2003). 2001 Census: analysis series—*The changing profile of Canada's labour force* Ottawa: Author.

Intersections of Social Determinants of Health, Identity, and Geography

Grace-Edward Galabuzi (2006) has written extensively about the interconnections among racism, social exclusion, unemployment, underemployment, individual and family income, and education. As Canada enters a new century, racialized peoples continue to experience stark inequities related to each of these social determinants of health. The income gap between racialized and non-racialized earners continues to be an important indicator of racial inequality in Canada as demonstrated by unemployment, labour-market participation, and employment income (Galabuzi, 2006). Galabuzi reported that employment income for racialized peoples is 15 percent lower than the national average; for racialized women, the inequity is even greater—average earnings in 1996 were $16,621 (CAD), compared to $23,635 for racialized men, $19,495 for other women, and $31,951 for other men.

In terms of education, the proportional numbers of racialized group members achieving post-secondary degrees is growing at a higher rate than in the general population, yet there has not been a corresponding increase in employment or income. So what factors cause this discrepancy? As Galabuzi (2006) pointed out, the discrepancy suggests an x, or unknown, factor: "We suggest that this 'x' factor is the devaluation of the human capital of racialized group members, resulting from racial discrimination in the labor market" (p. 111). Income is closely related to social determinants such as the chances of attaining an education and the ability to eat healthily. These social determinants also intersect with identity and geography to multiply disadvantage for racialized peoples.

The stark reality of racism as a SDOH is underscored by powerful intersections of the social determinants of health, identity, and geography. Intersectionality is a framework that recognizes the synergistic effects of various forms of oppression (McGibbon, 2008). Additive models, which view each oppression as "additive" rather than interlocking and synergistic, fail to stress the centrality of power and privilege (Collins, 1990). We discuss these ideas in detail in Chapter 5. The intersectionality framework has been used to describe the interwoven and synergistic influences of identities such as gender, race, and ethnicity on experiences of injustice. Feminist intersectionality frameworks emphasize "an understanding of the many circumstances that combine with discriminatory social practices to produce and sustain inequality and exclusion. Intersectional feminist frameworks look at how systems of discrimination such as colonialism and globalization can impact the combination of a person's social or economic status, race, class, gender, and sexuality" (Canadian Research Institute for the Advancement of Women, 2006, p. 7). Although there are differing definitions and understandings of intersectionality, we do not wish to engage in a debate about the meanings of these words. Rather, we focus on the synergistic, amplifying effects of the many forms of oppression. For example, gender is not an added oppression for women of colour. Sexism and racism are interlocked to compound oppression in numerous complex ways across the life course.

Some definitions of the SDOH have begun to include identities such as gender and race, that have been established as predictors of health outcomes. Evolving definitions notwithstanding, oppression may be usefully considered within an intersectionality framework that includes SDOH, identity, and geography. Figure 2.4 is an adaptation of McGibbon's (2008) intersectionality lens for identifying and addressing inequities in access to health care. The diagram depicts the intersections of the SDOH, identity as a SDOH, and geography. The lens is grounded in the interlocking, rather than additive, nature of the social determinants of health, identity as a SDOH, and geography.

For example, when individuals and families access health care, they arrive with more than their immediate physical and mental health concerns. The intersections of their identities (e.g. age, gender, race, social class) and intersections of their social determinants of health (e.g. early childhood development, employment)

Figure 2.4: Racism and Intersections of the SDOH, Identity as a SDOH, and Geography

SOCIAL DETERMINANTS OF HEALTH
- early childhood development
- employment and working conditions
- income and its equitable distribution
- food security
- health care shortages
- education
- social exclusion
- social safety nets

IDENTITY as a SDOH
- gender
- race
- ethnicity
- cutlure
- age
- (dis)ability
- social class
- sexual orientation
- spirituality ...

Racism as a SDOH

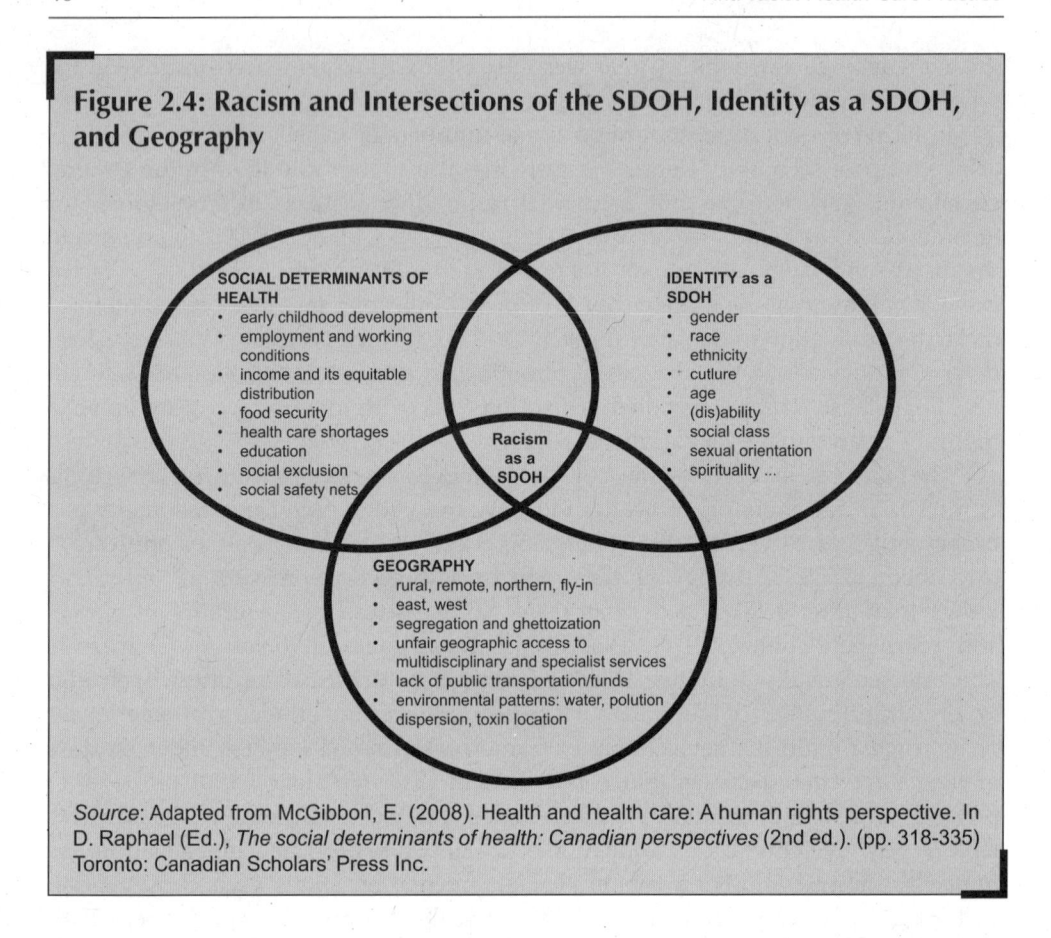

GEOGRAPHY
- rural, remote, northern, fly-in
- east, west
- segregation and ghettoization
- unfair geographic access to multidisciplinary and specialist services
- lack of public transportation/funds
- environmental patterns: water, polution dispersion, toxin location

Source: Adapted from McGibbon, E. (2008). Health and health care: A human rights perspective. In D. Raphael (Ed.), *The social determinants of health: Canadian perspectives* (2nd ed.). (pp. 318-335) Toronto: Canadian Scholars' Press Inc.

are inextricably linked to their health concerns. Statistics in the previous sections provided evidence of the direct and often devastating relationship among these intersectionalities and the life chances of people of colour. The vast majority of health care in Canada is provided with the assumption that individuals and families can afford costs currently considered as peripheral: transportation, prescription medications, over-the-counter antibiotics and anti-inflammatory drugs, orthopedic braces, time away from work, child care, and so on. Adequate employment and income thus become prerequisites for full health care access, particularly for rural, remote, and northern Canadians (McGibbon, 2008).

Health care then becomes a powerful determinant of health by virtue of its neutrality or presumptuousness about these hidden costs of full access, and its employment-neutral stance regarding which Canadians can or cannot afford access and health maintenance costs. When individuals and families cannot afford to follow up on recommended treatments due to lack of money, they are at risk for being labelled non-compliant, and thus having their health difficulties blamed on their lack of initiative (McGibbon, 2008). Lack of affordability is age, gender, race, and social class related. Canada now has 15.5 percent of children living in relative poverty, which is defined as households with income below 50 percent of the national median, thus ranking 17th out of 23 developed countries (United Nations International Children's Emergency Fund, 2005). Canadian women are less likely to be employed and earn an average of 62 percent less than men. The income of women aged 55 to 64 is barely over half that of men in their pre-retirement years (Statistics Canada, 2005).

Gender intersects with race to cause an even higher rate of unemployment among immigrant, Indigenous, and African-Canadian women (Galabuzi, 2006). Poverty has been directly linked to decreased access to health care and decreased health outcomes. Here the intersections of age, race, gender, and social determinants of health such as employment and income combine to limit health care access. Immigrant women of colour, who earn less than the Canadian average for women, face additional barriers related to geography since their extended families are often far away and many immigrant individuals and families lack the resources to maintain connections with their country of origin. Senior Canadians are at particular risk regardless of gender, race, or ethnicity since home care or family care is becoming medical support "on the cheap." Family members, usually women, have taken on the additional burden of home care. "Canada's health care system is becoming de-institutionalized but no less medicalized" (McDaniel & Chappell, 1999, p. 129).

Most women of colour experience all the major forms of oppression, including classism, racism, and sexism. The United States 1990 census revealed that 34 percent of Black women were living below the poverty line as compared to 11 percent of White women (Krieger, Rowley, Herman, Avery & Phillips, 1993). These figures mirror a recent Canadian study of Black women in rural communities where 62 percent of the 237 women surveyed earned annual incomes less than $15,000, and 28 percent earned less than $15,000 in annual household income, which is below both the national and provincial poverty lines (Bernard, Etowa, Clow & Oyinsan, 2007). Of all the 237 women in the study, 146 women (or 62 percent) earned less than $15,000 in average annual personal income, while 67 women (or 28 percent) earned less than $15,000 in annual household income.

As a proportion of Black women who responded to the income question, a significant 72 percent (146 women out of 202 women) earned less than $15,000 in average annual personal income, and 45 percent (67 women out of 149 women) earned less than $15,000 in average annual household income. These statistics revealed that a considerable proportion of Black families in these communities earn very low incomes. Income remains an important measure and integral determinant of socio-economic status of individuals and families, and there is a strong relationship between income, other health determinants, and health status. This inequity had a significant effect on the health status, health care delivery, and health services utilization among the Black women in the study. The family incomes of the women in the study showed a similar trend, with almost 30 percent of the women living in families with a combined annual income of less than $15,000 per year. Table 2.3 provides a statistical overview of the poverty experienced by rural Black women in Nova Scotia based on Etowa et al.'s 2007 study.

The intersection of gender and disability for Canadian women also shows a clear trend of disadvantage. Women with disabilities are twice as likely to be

Table 2.3: Black Women and Poverty in Rural Nova Scotia

Average Annual Personal Income	Total Sample		Digby Area		Yarmouth Area		Shelburne Area	
	No. of Women	% of Women	No. of Women	% of Women	No. of Women	% of Women	No. of Women	% of Women
Under $15,000	146	61	58	60	32	51	56	73
$15,000 but less than $25,000	30	13	17	18	8	13	5	6
$25,000 but less than $35,000	18	8	10	10	5	8	3	4
$35,000 but less than $45,000	5	2	1	1	1	2	3	4
$45,000 but less than $55,000	1	0	1	1	0	0	0	0
$55,000 but less than $65,000	2	1	1	1	1	2	0	0
$65,000 but less than $75,000	0	0	0	0	0	0	0	0
$75,000 but less than $85,000	0	0	0	0	0	0	0	0
$85,000 or more	0	0	0	0	0	0	0	0
No response	35	15	9	9	16	25	10	13
Total	237	100	97	100	63	100	77	100

Source: Etowa, J., Bernard, W.T., Clow, B. & Oyinsan, B. (2007). Participatory action research (PAR): Improving Black women's health in rural and remote communities. *International Journal of Transcultural Nursing*, 18, 349–359.

unemployed when compared to the Canadian average for women. In 2000, women with disabilities aged 15 and over had an average income from all sources of $17,200, almost $5,000 less than women without disabilities, and $9,700 less than men with disabilities (Statistics Canada, 2005). Low income has particular consequences for people with disabilities since there are many additional expenses associated with mental and physical health disabilities. When the already lower incomes for women of colour are compounded by the lower incomes of women with disabilities, the intersection of race, gender, and disability can form powerful barriers to full, meaningful employment.

Men in the poorest income groups have the highest rates of ischemic heart disease in Canada (Chronic Disease Prevention Alliance (CDPA), 2008). In 1996, 36.8 percent of women and 35 percent of men in racialized communities were low-income earners, compared to the Canadian average of 19.2 percent and 16 percent respectively. In 1995, the rate of children living in poverty in racialized communities was 45 percent — almost twice the overall Canadian rate of 26 percent (Galabuzi, 2006). For these children, age, race, social class, and family employment status intersect to create enormous barriers in access to health care. Family access to adequate full-time employment with benefits, and thus money and supports, is a powerful indicator of their capacity to successfully navigate the health care system.

Geography is increasingly cited as a determinant of health. Rural, remote and fly-in, northern, and urban locations all impact on health care access and on health outcomes. Eastern Canadians experience the poorest health outcomes in Canada when compared to the health of the general population. The Maritime region has one of the highest percentages of rural populations in Canada (Health Canada, 2003). Degree of rurality contributes to health indicators above and beyond socio-economic factors, and living in areas with low population density is associated with special health risks. Macro-economic changes, such as boom-and-bust economic cycles, which particularly impact rural communities, have an especially negative effect on the health of rural communities, particularly those with dependence on one industry for economic sustainability. Rural Canadians are more likely to report poorer socio-economic condition and lower educational attainment, and to have higher overall mortality rates (Canadian Institute for Health Information, 2006).

Women living in the most rural areas form the highest proportion of people reporting fair/poor health (Canadian Institute for Health Information, 2006). In 1996, infant mortality rates in rural areas were 30 percent higher than the national average (Ministerial Advisory Council on Rural Health, 2002). In terms of rural, remote, and northern health care, there is a lack of diagnostic services, poor access to emergency and acute care services, lack of non-acute health services, and underservicing of special needs groups, such as seniors and people with disabilities (McGibbon, 2008). Health care restructuring has centralized or reduced acute care services without community-based services being enhanced (Ministerial Advisory Council on Rural Health, 2002). Rural, remote, and northern geographic regions are home to over 50 percent of Canada's 1.4 million Indigenous peoples. The health status of rural Indigenous peoples follows the same pattern of decreased life expectancy and increased morbidity as Canada's Indigenous peoples as a whole.

The geography of segregation and its relationship to health care access and health outcomes has barely begun to be investigated in Canada. Current efforts to eliminate racial and ethnic disparities in health care treatment fail to address the effect of segregation—the physical separation of the races in residential contexts— on health disparities. Segregation causes racial disparities in health (Smith, 2005; Williams & Collins, 2001). Recent literature suggests a growing relationship between the clustering of certain visible minority groups in urban neighbourhoods and the spatial concentration of poverty in Canadian cities, raising the spectre of ghettoization (Galabuzi, 2006; Walks & Bourne, 2006). Since health care access is often dependent upon economic status (money for transportation, employment benefits, medications, etc.) and the cultural competence of service providers, segregation based on race has important implications for access to health care and the already evident racial disparities based on segregation. The unjust historical legacy of segregation of Canadian Indigenous peoples on reserves continues today.

Rural, remote, northern, eastern, western, urban, geographic segregation and ghettoization; weather patterns, especially in the North; and pollution-dispersion patterns all contribute to shape the health status of Canadians and their access to health care and other services. When one family experiences lack of access due to their rural location, and they are also located near a landfill, they will experience a multiplying of the effects of decreased access to health services as well as the health effects of their proximity to toxic substances. People living in geographies with high pollution rates have an unfair toxic burden that is not necessarily reflected in increased access to cancer and respiratory health care (McGibbon, 2008). Hazardous waste facilities, landfill sites, and incinerators are all disproportionately located near communities of colour, regardless of country or region (Cole & Foster, 2000). Geography thus acts as a foundation that underscores health system inequities. In all of these ways, the intersections of the social determinants of health, identity, and geography combine to compound health system inequity (McGibbon, 2008). The story in Box 2.3 clearly describes the many intersections of the social determinants of health, racism, and geography.

Of central importance to anti-racist practice is an understanding of how racism overlays all of these other health determinants for people of colour. So, for example, although rural women with disabilities are more likely to have a compromised health status, women of colour who have a disability and who also live in a rural area will face the powerful overlaying of racism in their encounters with the health care system. It is important to note that this discussion in no way minimizes the obstacles experienced by women with disabilities in general. The following section emphasizes racism as a social determinant of health. Although one's race is related to one's biologic and genetic endowment, it is racism that creates the wide disparities in health outcomes detailed below.

Racism and Health Outcomes: More Evidence for Racism as a SDOH

Racism has a profound impact on physical and mental health outcomes. Here, we build on the previous discussion about the social determinants of health by highlighting many of the well-researched, race-related inequities in health outcomes.

> **Box 2.3: Jason's Story: Intersections of the Social Determinants of Health, Identity, and Geography**
>
> Why is Jason in the hospital?
> Because he has a bad infection in his leg.
> But why does he have an infection?
> Because he has a cut on his leg and it got infected.
> But why does he have a cut on his leg?
> Because he was playing in the junk yard next to his apartment building and there was some sharp, jagged steel there that he fell on.
> But why was he playing in a junk yard?
> Because his neighborhood is kind of run down. A lot of kids play there and there is no one to supervise them.
> But why does he live in that neighborhood?
> Because his parents can't afford a nicer place to live.
> But why can't his parents afford a nicer place to live?
> Because his Dad is unemployed and his Mom is sick.
> But why is his Dad unemployed?
> Because he doesn't have much education and he can't find a job.
> But why ...?
>
> Jason's story suggests health is influenced by a number of factors. These factors interact with one another and affect individuals, communities, and even our nation's health. Health is closely tied to the environment around us—where we live, work, and play.
>
> Source: *Toward a healthy future: Second report on the health of Canadians*, Health Canada, (1999). Reproduced with the permission of the Minister of Public Works and Services Canada, 2008.

Although most available statistical and epidemiological research about racism and health outcomes is from the United States, we make the case that there is little reason to believe that these disparities are not present in Canada and elsewhere. There are many ways in which racism and other forms of social inequalities can affect health. These include interconnected factors of economic, environmental, psychosocial, and iatrogenic (caused by hospitals and clinicians) conditions (Krieger, 2003). Racism limits the socio-economic accomplishments of minority groups, and thus causes long-term consequences for their health.

Racial inequalities have been created and reinforced by limited access to educational and employment opportunities for minority groups through processes such as segregation (Collins & Williams, 1999). Racial difference in socio-economic status has been well documented in the literature, and health researchers examining the association between race and health routinely adjust for this variable (Krieger, 2003; Williams, 1999). Thus, socioeconomic status is not only considered an antecedent of racial differences in health, but "part of the causal pathways by which race affects health" (Williams, 1999, p. 177).

Race is therefore an antecedent and a determinant of socioeconomic status, and racial differences in SES are, to some degree, a reflection of implementation of discriminatory policies and practices premised on the inferiority of certain racial groups (Williams, 1999). Supporting this notion, Krieger (2003) asserted that "health is harmed not only by heinous crimes against humanity, such as slavery, lynching and genocide, but also by the grinding economic and social realities of what Essed (1991) has aptly termed "everyday racism" (p. 195). Furthermore, Krieger (1987) argues that the poorer health of Black people relative to the White population is the result of White privilege, enforced through slavery and other forms of racial discrimination, rather than innate inferiority.

Researchers have amply demonstrated that discrepancies in health are intimately associated with differences in social, economic, cultural, and political circumstances (Aday, 1993; Backlund, Sorlie & Johnson, 1996; Bloom, 2001; Brown, 1995; Chen & Fou, 2001; Rogers, 1997). Economic inequities, in particular, have been implicated in poor health. People with fewer economic resources are at much greater risk of illness and are much less likely to have timely access to health and social services (Hay 1994; Lynch, Kaplan & Shema, 1997; Lynch, 1996; Pappas, Queen, Hadden & Fisher, 1993; Poland, Coburn, Robertson, & Eakin, 1998). The impact of race and ethnicity on health has likewise attracted increasing attention. As with class and gender, race and ethnicity have been strongly correlated with poor health (Bolaria & Bolaria, 1994; Dana, 2002). For example, African Americans experience hypertension at earlier ages than White Americans, and are much more prone to dangerous complications, such as end-stage renal disease (American Heart Association, 2001).

African Americans are also twice as likely as White Americans to develop adult-onset diabetes, and to face serious sequelae of the disease, including amputation and blindness (Brancati et al., 2000). Although fewer Black than White women are diagnosed with breast cancer, they are more likely to be diagnosed at an advanced stage and to die from the disease (Miller, Kolonel, & Bernstein, 1996). Most vulnerable of all are people who experience intersecting disadvantages, including gender and ethnic discrimination as well as poverty. Women of colour routinely experience this "triple jeopardy" and its pernicious influence on their health (Bernard, 2001).

Socio-economic status as well as gender and ethnic identity also profoundly influence the quality of care available to Canadians. Cultural stereotypes sometimes translate into overt discrimination. For instance, sex trade workers, typically women, often find it difficult to access services or receive appropriate care when providers assume that "immoral" behaviour is at the root of ill health (Jackson, 2002). Blacks are similarly subjected to insensitive or inappropriate care when their illnesses are interpreted as the consequence of inherent predispositions to violence or sexual promiscuity (Bernard, 2001; Blake & Darling, 2000). Inappropriate and insensitive care may also arise from subtler assumptions embedded in the health care system, particularly the tendency to embrace White, middle-class, male experience as normative. For example, the health indicators assessed in the Apgar (newborn health scale) test are derived from studying White newborns. This narrow definition renders the test much less useful in the assessment of Indigenous and Black babies, to name a few (Enang, 2002).

Although there is substantive evidence for health inequities along racial lines, studies in the recent past have conclusively connected these inequities to racism, rather than to biological factors. For example, studies have compared hypertension rates of African Americans with West Africans, who are genetically quite similar because most slaves were taken from this part of the world less than 13 generations ago (Rotimi, Cooper & Ward, 1997). These studies showed that West Africans have very little incidence of hypertension when compared with their American counterparts. First Nations peoples in Canada have consistently poorer health outcomes on many important indicators. A 2003 study comparing First Nations self-reported health with the self-reported health of Canadians overall revealed that First Nations adults had higher prevalence rates in eight out of the 10 chronic conditions studied. Figure 2.5 illustrates these comparisons, with the first bar representing the general Canadian population, and the second bar representing First Nations.

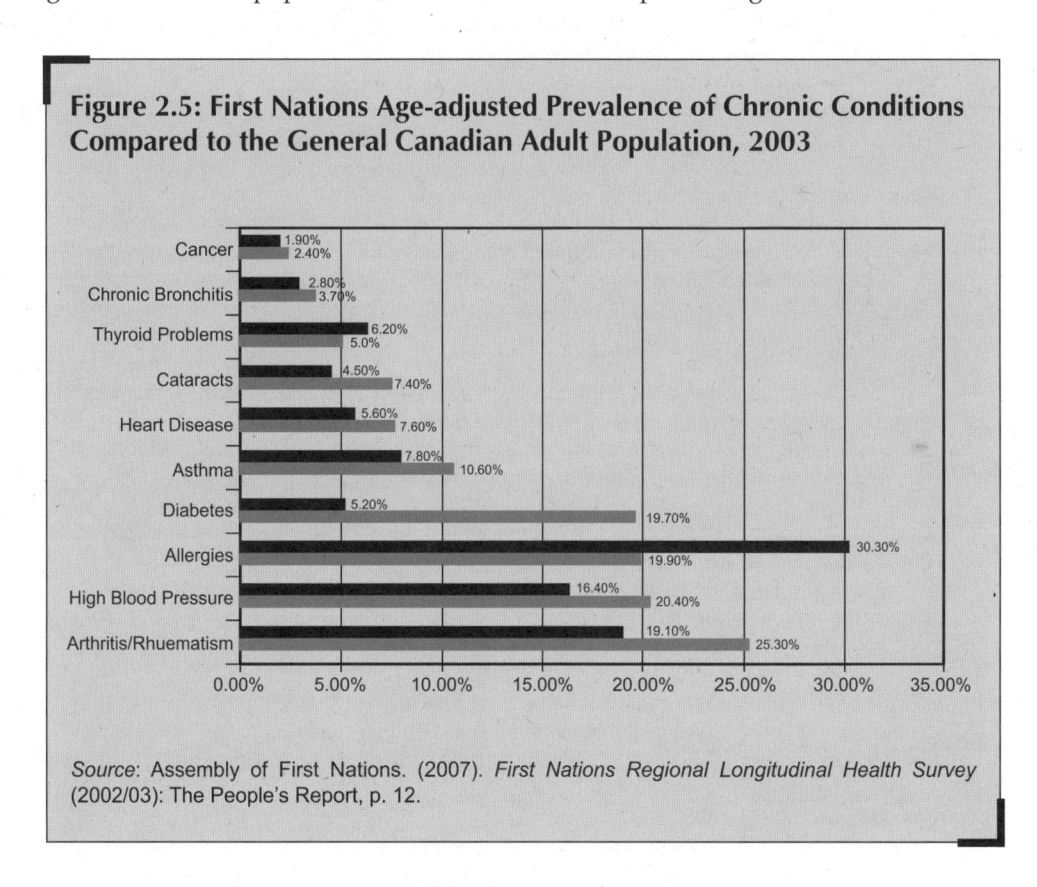

Figure 2.5: First Nations Age-adjusted Prevalence of Chronic Conditions Compared to the General Canadian Adult Population, 2003

Condition	General Canadian	First Nations
Cancer	1.90%	2.40%
Chronic Bronchitis	2.80%	3.70%
Thyroid Problems	6.20%	5.0%
Cataracts	4.50%	7.40%
Heart Disease	5.60%	7.60%
Asthma	7.80%	10.60%
Diabetes	5.20%	19.70%
Allergies	30.30%	19.90%
High Blood Pressure	16.40%	20.40%
Arthritis/Rhuematism	19.10%	25.30%

Source: Assembly of First Nations. (2007). *First Nations Regional Longitudinal Health Survey (2002/03): The People's Report*, p. 12.

Box 2.4 provides more evidence regarding racism as a determinant of health. The data underscores the disproportionate incidence of chronic health problems among racialized peoples, and the related racism in the health care system. The studies cited show that people of colour experience the burden of racism in their endeavours to seek adequate health care, and to receive timely diagnoses and diagnostic testing. The statistics reveal only the surface of pain and suffering caused by racism. Racist acts such as neglecting to diagnose or to refer for specialist assessment are inscribed on the bodies and minds of people of colour, despite health care clinicians' ethical

Box 2.4: Racism as a Social Determinant of Health

Please note: The information reported in this box uses the terms cited by the authors of the articles (i.e., Black, African American, Hispanic, Aboriginal, ethnic minority, visible minority, White, Caucasian, etc.).

Cancer: Breast and Cervical
- Ethnic minority women are diagnosed with more advanced disease and experience greater morbidity and mortality (Kim, Ashing-Giwa, Singer & Tejero, 2006).
- Black women are significantly less likely than White women to receive minimum expected therapy for breast cancer (Breen et al., 1999).
- Black women are less likely than White women to be screened or to present with asymptomatic disease (Merkin, Stevenson & Powe, 2002).

Cancer: Prostate
- African-American men have a much higher risk of prostate cancer, a higher-grade disease at diagnosis, and a higher mortality and morbidity than Caucasian men (Maliski et al., 2006).
- Population-based studies that use cancer registry data consistently show that African Americans with prostate cancer present with more advanced disease, and that they have poorer survival rates than do U.S. White men with the disease even when diagnosed at the same stage (Oakley-Girvan et al., 2003).

Cancer: Other
- First Nations adults in Canada have a 20.8 percent higher rate of cancer than the general Canadian population (Assembly of First Nations, 2007).
- African Americans are significantly less likely to receive major colorectal treatment for their cancer, follow-up treatment, or chemotherapy (Cooper et al., 2000; Schrag et al., 2001).
- Blacks are less likely to receive surgical treatment than Whites, and they are likely to die sooner than Whites (Bach et al., 1999).
- Members of visible minorities were less likely to have been admitted to hospital, tested for prostate-specific antigen, administered a mammogram, or given a Pap test; members of visible minorities were less likely than White people to have had a mammogram or Pap test (Quan et al., 2006).
- The rates of screening for most diseases are lower among Black patients than among White patients, and Black patients more often than White patients receive diagnoses when diseases are at a relatively advanced stage (Bach et al., 2005).

Cardiovascular
- First Nations adults in Canada have a 7.6 percent rate of heart disease compared with a 5.6 percent rate for the general population. High blood pressure is reported by 20.4 percent of First Nations adults compared with 16.4 percent for the general population (Assembly of First Nations, 2007).
- Black men, when compared to White men, were only half as likely to undergo arteriography and a third as likely to have coronary bypass surgery performed, despite a diagnostic imaging rate of 77 percent of that of White men (Ford et al., 1989).
- Among patients undergoing coronary artery bypass surgery in New York State, being African American or Asian/Pacific Islander is significantly associated with being treated by surgeons of poorer quality when quality is measured by risk-adjusted mortality rates (Rothenberg et al., 2004).

- In the United States, non-Whites are treated by lower-quality surgeons, quality being measured by risk-adjusted mortality rates (Mukamel et al., 2000).
- Cardiovascular diseases are the leading cause of death in Black people (Enang, 2002).
- As many as 30 percent of deaths of all Black men and 20 percent of deaths of all Black women are attributed to high blood pressure (American Heart Association, 2001).

Pain (Chronic and Acute)
- Minority patients were less likely than Whites to have pain recorded even after adjustment for language differences (Bernabei et al., 1998).
- African Americans were more likely than Whites to report that they felt discriminated against in their ability to obtain care or treatment for their pain because of race/ethnicity (Whites 9 percent, African Americans 15 percent, Hispanics 13 percent). This difference became far larger, however, when the focus was on males with low income (family incomes less than $25,000). In this subgroup, African Americans were almost three times as likely as Whites to feel that they have been discriminated against in their efforts to obtain treatment for pain (27 percent versus 10 percent, respectively) (Marisa, Ugarte, Fuller, Haas & Portenoy, 2005).
- In settings with predominantly racial and ethnic minority patients (i.e., African Americans and Hispanics), 62 percent of those patients were undertreated by WHO standards, and they were three times more likely to be undermedicated than patients seen in non-minority settings; African-American patients in nursing homes had a 63 percent greater probability of not receiving pain treatment than non-Hispanic White patients. African-American and Hispanic patients were less likely than non-Hispanic White patients to have pain reports documented in their charts (Green et al., 2003).

Palliative Care
- Aboriginal peoples are underrepresented in palliative care programs. Aboriginal peoples are more likely to die of acute illnesses such as cardiovascular diseases, and one might expect less need for palliative care. In fact, Aboriginal peoples are more likely to die of all causes, including cancer (Sullivan et al., 2003).

Diabetes
- First Nations adults have almost four times the rate of diabetes than the general population (Assembly of First Nations, 2007).
- Black women have more than twice the risk of developing adult-onset diabetes than White women. Black men have more than one and a half times the risk of developing diabetes (Brancati et al., 2000).

Sickle Cell Anemia
- Although sickle cell disease is not curable, early diagnosis would ensure appropriate management strategies, thereby reducing the number of deaths cause by the disease. Routine screening of Black newborns is an unrealized dream in Canada (Enang, 2002).

imperative to do no harm. Anti-racist care can begin with identifying these practices and refusing to participate in them or to condone them.

This evidence, when taken together, requires an understanding that includes considerations of biologic and genetic endowment. However, our gaze must be directed through the lens of racism. The psychological consequences of injustice have barely begun to be examined in the health fields. For example, we know that depression rates are higher among women, and even higher among women of colour. But what is the social significance of this statistical finding? What are the social, economic, and political paths that result in high depression rates? What may be fruitfully learned by *combining* what we know about the biophysical burden of racism-related stress with social scientific knowledge about oppressed peoples? According to Sheppard (2002), differences in depression rates are evidence of the significant psychological consequences of social injustice arising in both material and symbolic form. The spiritual and psychological sequelae of imperialism and colonialism are transmitted across generations. The savagery of slavery and the murderous treatment of Indigenous peoples most surely laid a template for struggle for many generations to come. Elders in Indigenous and Black communities across Canada have much to teach us about the near-loss of the old ways, and the spiritual renewal that is underway, despite the past. Anti-racist health care practice is a powerful way that white people can participate in the truth-telling and reconciliation that is so necessary in Canada. Box 2.5 provides an overview of some important evidence regarding race, racism, and mental health.

The following section builds on the evidence about racism as a SDOH and focuses specifically on health care design and delivery as a social determinant of health for racialized peoples.

Health Care Access as a Social Determinant of Health for Racialized Peoples

The previous sections focused on racism as a social determinant of health, including the impact of intersectionality. We would like to highlight health care access as a SDOH, including primary or preventive care and health services, which include hospitals and clinics. As the evidence above indicates, there is increasing evidence that health outcomes are related to health determinants such as race, social class, and gender. Although there are many variables associated with inequities in access, these inequities have been consistently linked to barriers in access to health services, particularly in rural areas (Vindigni et al., 2004). These barriers include: (1) geographic access to service variables, such as proximity to health care facilities and practitioners; (2) lack of cultural competence of health practitioners and lack of culturally congruent health services; (3) systemic racism at health service entry points and within the system; and (4) systemic racism in health and social policy (Krieger, 2003). Barriers such as these create significant inconsistencies in access to health care.

Studies investigating geographic access to service variables have shown that populations living in rural areas have decreased access to health services, especially specialist health services (Elliot & Larsen, 2004; Vindigni et. al., 2004). For example, according to Mainous and colleagues (2004), in a national survey of 11,775 African Americans and White Americans, "for diabetes and hypertension there is a double dose of risk for rural African Americans" (p. 5). The investigation of the relationship

Box 2.5: Racism and Mental Health

Please note: The information reported in this box uses the terms cited by the authors of the articles (i.e., Black, African American, Hispanic, Aboriginal, ethnic minority, visible minority, White, Caucasian, etc.).

Depression
- Off-reserve Aboriginal peoples are 1.5 times more likely than the non-Aboriginal population to experience a major depressive episode in the year before the survey (Statistics Canada, 2002).
- Among First Nations adults, 33.4 percent of women and 28.5 percent of men report that they have thought about suicide in their lifetime (Assembly of First Nations, 2007).
- Among First Nations peoples between the ages of 18 and 34, 21.3 percent of women and 14.8 percent of men reported that they attempted suicide in their lifetime (Assembly of First Nations, 2007).
- African Americans were substantially more likely to be untreated for depression (37.1 percent) than Hispanic (23.6 percent), White (22.4 percent), or Asian (13.8 percent) people. In logistic regression models adjusting for sex, state, long-term care status, and age group, African Americans with a primary diagnosis of depression were almost twice as likely as Whites not to receive an antidepressant (Strothers, Rust, Minor, Fresh, Druss & Satcher, 2004).
- When major depressive disorder affects African Americans and Caribbean Blacks, it is usually untreated and is more severe and disabling compared with that in non-Hispanic Whites (Williams et al., 2007).
- In the United States, members of racial or ethnic minority groups, including Blacks and Hispanics, are less likely than Whites to obtain treatment for depression (Goldstein et al., 2006).

Trauma (Post-traumatic Stress)
- Post-traumatic stress (PTSD) exists throughout Aboriginal communities in Canada, and is a result of the legacy of colonialism and Indian residential schools (Harry, 2008).
- African-American men and women are less likely to seek traditional mental health services, and are more likely to rely on existing support systems than Caucasian men and women (Bradley et al., 2005).
- PTSD was found to be a common yet underrecognized and undertreated source of psychiatric morbidity in an urban community of African Americans with low socio-economic status. Despite a high rate of trauma and PTSD, this population was not currently identified as being in need of treatment (Schwartz et al., 2005).

Dementia Care
- Even when formal services provide activities of daily living (ADL) care for those with dementia, African-American dementia caregivers report more unmet needs with care provision than do White dementia caregivers (Cloutterbuck & Feeney Mahoney, 2003).
- Negative, disrespectful health care provider attitudes and behaviour were encountered by African-American families during the process of obtaining a diagnosis of dementia for their loved ones. They described interactions with health care providers that consistently denigrated, devalued, and disrespected their observations and concerns about their demented loved ones. They reported feeling diminished when physicians glibly dismissed or did not take their concerns seriously. Many reported

being shuttled from one health care setting to another in search of a diagnosis. Most of the participants reported dissatisfaction with family caregiver–health care provider interactions during the process of obtaining a diagnosis for dementia (Cloutterbuck & Feeney Mahoney, 2003).

Mental Health –Additional Concerns
- Many Aboriginal peoples, because of their cultural background, face racism and discrimination on a day-to-day basis. Cultural discontinuity, including loss of Indigenous languages, has been associated with higher rates of depression, alcoholism, suicide, and violence, and as having a greater impact on youth (Health Council of Canada, 2005).
- Ethnic minorities who have symptoms or histories of mental disorders experience vastly different access and outcome histories when compared to their more socially accepted Caucasian counterparts. Psychiatric services are more often sought by Caucasians than by African-American, American Indian and Alaska Native, Asian-American, and Hispanic-American groups. Ethnic-minority people are at risk for not receiving adequate mental health care (Gary, 2005).
- Among those with perceived need, compared to Whites, African Americans were more likely to have no access to alcoholism, drug abuse, or mental health care (25.4 percent versus 12.5 percent), and Hispanics were more likely to have less care than needed or delayed care (22.7 percent versus 10.7 percent). Among those with need, Whites were more likely than Hispanics or African Americans to receive active alcoholism, drug abuse, or mental health treatment (37.6 percent versus 25.0 percent) (Wells et al., 2001).
- Disabled Aboriginal seniors are often discriminated against away from their reserves. To receive the care they need, many Aboriginal seniors are forced away from their communities and into unfamiliar, often urban facilities (Kuran, 2002).
- A history of racial discrimination, social exclusion, and poverty can combine with mistrust and fear to deter members of racialized groups and Aboriginal communities from accessing services and getting culturally appropriate care (Kafele, 2004).
- Although racialized groups and members of Aboriginal communities have mental health needs and issues that are extremely serious and warrant significant attention, few psychiatric services respond specifically with research, clinical support, programming, organizational change, health promotion, or community collaboration that indicate cultural competence, understanding, or awareness in a systemic manner (Kafele, 2004).
- Racial profiling, racist assumptions, and stereotyping in psychiatry are often believed to be strong determining factors in intake, assessment and diagnosis, and misdiagnosis. Misdiagnosis includes underdiagnosis and overdiagnosis, which can account for the non-delivery of appropriate treatments because of an erroneous diagnostic label. In some instances, this leads to a deferred intervention or, in some groups, help-seeking is delayed for unnecessarily long periods. Because of disparities and racial discrimination in mental health services, a disproportionate number of racialized groups and Aboriginal populations with mental illnesses do not fully benefit from, or contribute to, the opportunities and prosperity of our society (Kafele, 2004).

between racism and health, including racism in access to health care, is relatively recent, with the vast majority of empirical and theoretical literature appearing since 1980. Racism in health service delivery, at entry points and within the health care system, has been linked to decreased accessibility of health services for Aboriginal and African Canadians (Enang, 2002), African Americans (Williams, 1999), and Aboriginal peoples in Australia (Vindigni et. al., 2004). In Canada, there are relatively few empirical studies that link racism and health, or racism and access to health services.

However, there have been several literature reviews and syntheses regarding the health of Aboriginal and African Canadians. Of note are MacMillan and colleagues' (1996) review of the health of Canada's Native peoples; Enang's (2001) synthesis of health relevant to Black Nova Scotians; and Trumper's (2004) literature review of the health status and health needs of Aboriginal children and youth. There are no systematic literature reviews or scoping reviews in the area of access to health services for racialized peoples. McGibbon, Calliste, Arbuthnot, et al. (2008) completed a scoping review regarding barriers in access to health services for rural Aboriginal and African Canadians. Globally, current knowledge is fragmented and is primarily based in the United States and Australia. Although there is evidence that rural location, Indigenous origin, and African-Canadian origin are each related to disparate access to health services, there is a substantial gap in the nature and extent of current knowledge in this area.

Barriers in access to health care are an important cause of poorer health outcomes for racialized peoples. As the above evidence shows, lack of education and poverty are also disproportionately experienced by people of colour. These social and economic circumstances compound with racism-related barriers in the health care system to create substantial barriers in access to health care. In the United States inequitable access is often thought to be related to uninsured status or poverty, and thus lack of money to access care. However, even when education, income, and health insurance status are statistically controlled for, racialized peoples still have significant barriers in access to a broad variety of health care services. Box 2.6 describes barriers in access themes that originated from a Canadian Institutes for Health Research-funded workshop in June 2005.

The First Nations Regional Longitudinal Health Survey (Assembly of First Nations, 2007) reported that among First Nations adults living on reserve, there were five barriers to receiving health care: (1) the waiting list was too long (33.2 percent); (2) the services were not covered under the Non-Insured Health Benefits Program (NIHB) (20.0 percent); (3) a doctor or nurse was not available in their area (18.5 percent); (4) the health care provided was inadequate (16.9 percent); and (5) prior approval for services under the NIHB was denied (16.1 percent). Statistically significant differences were found between men and women for the following barriers: the waiting list was too long (37.3 percent of women versus 29.3 percent of men); a doctor or nurse was not available in their area (22.0 percent of women versus 15.1 percent of men); and prior approval for services under the NIHB was denied (19.4 percent of women versus 13.0 percent of men). One in three First Nations adults have trouble accessing health care because the service was not covered by the NIHB (Assembly of First Nations, 2007).

Box 2.6: Barriers in Access to Health Services for Rural Aboriginal and African Canadians

Barriers: Health Service Providers

Racial profiling in the health system: Aboriginal and Black people tend to be immediately treated differently and less competently. This is related to systemic racism, racist attitudes of providers, and White privilege.

Cultural literacy and health literacy: There is a lack of culturally appropriate health information, as well as a tendency for health workers to not care to give available information.

Resulting lack of safe services: People are not offered available care, not assessed in a timely manner when compared to White counterparts:
- There is a lack of personal attention from service providers; a habit of ignoring the concerns of Aboriginal and Black people; this leads to incompetent care, lack of assessment.

Lack of communication at entry point:
- Insulting questions based on stereotypes: "When was your last drink?"
- Attitudes that come from stereotyping.
- The language of service providers is not the same as the language of consumers; this creates a major barrier.

Insensitivity:
- Need cultural sensitivity/cultural competence education in the health system and in professional education of health providers, not just the learning of skills. Need to change values.
- This training is especially needed in rural areas where service providers

Barriers: The Agency, the System

Services are "streamlined": Economically efficient but still ineffective because they are too fragmented, i.e., when there are three doctors, yet no continuity of care (service providers not communicating with each other).

People and families are pushed into partnerships: Based on government department organization rather than the needs of the families; there is a lack of support from politicians in the advocacy process.

Lack of accountability throughout the system: "How can you hire a fox to look after the chickens?"
Power without accountability:
- Provincial professional organizations: How can they be held accountable for racist actions, forced to uphold a code of ethical conduct?
- Need more openly transparent professional organizations and governments; develop a process to hold people accountable. The current system does not provide a reliable method.
- In provincially funded health and social services, when something goes wrong in a person's care, there is a one-sided investigation of complaints, often with no offer of an explanation, no accountability, no compassion.

Barriers in the legal system: When people try to hold services responsible, lawyers may be in a conflict of interest due to their personal relationships with persons in the health and social services system.

> become very comfortable having the privilege of saying what they want.
> - Training needs to be anti-racist and human rights-oriented.
>
> **Communities used for experimentation in terms of treatments, including overprescription:** This needs to be addressed and changed. *Service provision is not reflective of the community:* In ways of health care provision and in lack of Aboriginal and Black providers.
>
> **The effects of the intersection of race, class, and gender need to be considered:** In terms of how service providers treat people and respond to their needs—to be a woman, a Black woman, and an ordinary Black woman. Service providers are unable or unwilling to provide proper, compassionate care unless you demonstrate some sort of privilege, such as being a professor.
>
> **Lack of accountability of professionals:** Due to systemic racism.
>
> **Long-term care options not available to First Nations persons on reserves:** Especially in the area of mental health.
>
> **Families are left to struggle on their own without resources when trying to navigate the system:** They may have a lack of knowledge about how the system works. There is a need to specifically make arrangements for advocates from the community.
>
> **Questioning people in power and authority is very difficult:** Takes much energy, resilience, and support, yet it is so important to do because you or your family members will die if you don't speak up. Obtaining safe care is very difficult and energy draining.
>
> **There is tremendous stress:** Associated with advocacy struggles and the process of overcoming these barriers; individuals and families are sometimes punished for bringing advocacy issues to light.
>
> **Fighting a system that is prone to retaliation:** There is a need to become more skilled in this area.
>
> *Source:* McGibbon, E., Calliste, A., Arbuthnot, E., Bassett, R., Cameron, C. Graham, H. & MacDonald, D. (2005). *Barriers in access to health services for rural Aboriginal and African Canadians: A scoping workshop* (pp. 149–150). Antigonish: St. Francis Xavier University.

The Links among Health Inequities, Racism, and Power Relations

The above qualitative and quantitative evidence indicates strong relationships among the social determinants of health and race. The pervasive power of systemic racism, sexism, and classism, determines health outcomes across a wide spectrum of physical and mental health struggles. The evidence that race is a determinant of health spans several decades and consistently points to race as central in the health and well-being of individuals, families, communities, and nations. While genetic factors are important, such as the higher incidence of sickle cell anemia in people of the African diaspora, health inequities of racialized peoples are rooted in systemic racism. For example, the poor health outcomes of Indigenous peoples in Canada can best be traced to brutal treatment at the hands of White colonial power, rather than deficits in lifestyle. Although lifestyle impacts on health outcomes, only systemic anti-racist social change will improve the health outcomes of Indigenous peoples (McGibbon, 2008). Health inequities have their origins in systemic power imbalances based in oppression. This is why an anti-racist approach to practice is necessary. Without explicit and ongoing attention to power (power over and lack of power), attempts at addressing racism in health care practice will be very slow and will produce limited results. Chapter 3 continues the discussion about power and extends the analysis to incorporate a critique of cultural competence and diversity models. While we acknowledge that these models were a first attempt at thinking about identities other than White in the health fields, we stress that the lack of attention to power and privilege severely limits their usefulness.

Conclusions

The sheer weight of qualitative and qualitative evidence indicates that racism is a social determinant of health. This evidence spans a very broad range of human experience, from the chance of receiving competent follow-up care for prostate cancer to the chance of receiving compassionate palliative care. Race, ethnicity, and culture all influence health outcomes far beyond causes that may be explained through differences in biological and genetic endowment. Practitioners in health and related fields most often view themselves and their profession as operating from a stance of caring that is grounded in the ethical treatment of everyone, regardless of identities such as race, social class, or gender. However, the evidence points to an urgent need to reflect on current professional and personal beliefs and practices. It is tempting to attribute racism to inaccuracies or inconsistencies in statistical measurement, or the supposed anecdotal nature of qualitative evidence. But the persistence of the evidence across time and geography points to an undeniable truth about racism in the health fields. This truth gives us a solid foundation to work for change.

CHAPTER 3

Beyond Cultural Competence
A Critique of Diversity and Multicultural Health Care Models

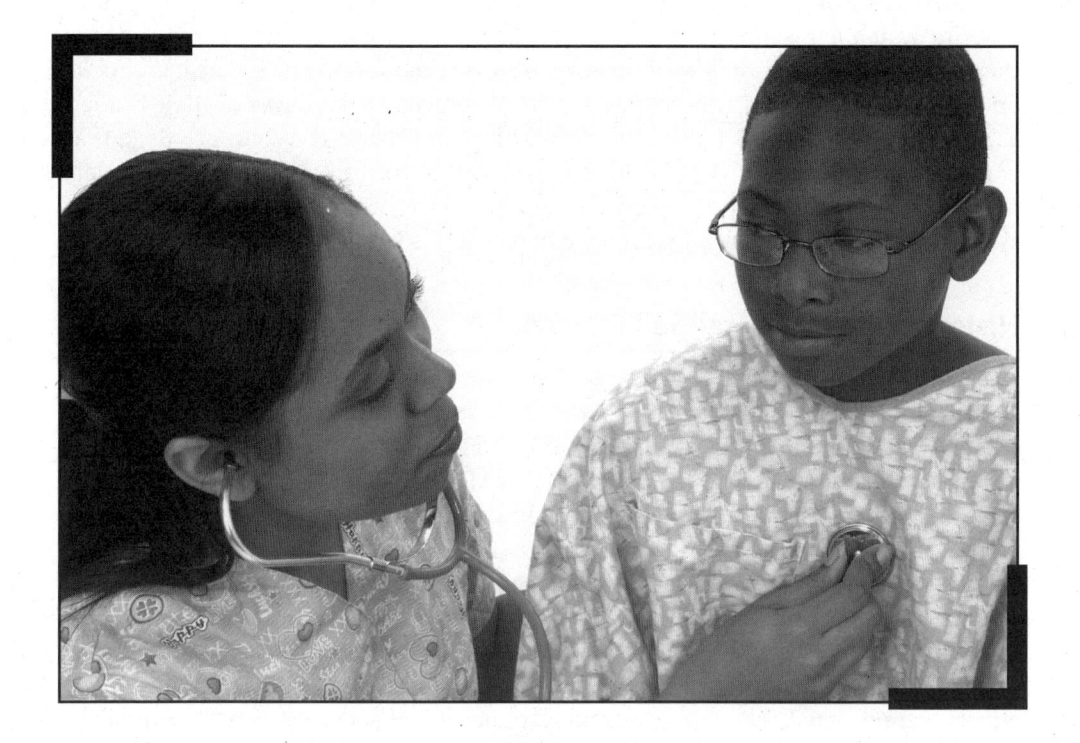

Multiculturalism in Canada is based on allowing cultural diversity to be maintained while, at least for certain groups of people — primarily Blacks, and many indigenous communities — marginalization, exclusion, poverty, disease, and humiliation describe their experience of living in multicultural Canada. (Frances Henry, 2002, p. 239)

Introduction

One of the main ways that the health fields have addressed the need to move beyond a Eurocentric model of care has been through the creation of cultural competence models. These models include ideas about culture, race, ethnicity, and religion. However, cultural competence is a limited framework to guide practice because it fails to analyze power in the therapeutic relationship, or the systemic power that overarches and impacts every health care encounter. We begin with an overview of the history of multiculturalism in Canada. The underpinnings of multiculturalism have very much influenced approaches to cultural competence. However, notions of acknowledging or celebrating diversity, recognizing difference, and working together obscure systemic racism, which is at the root of inequities. Cultural competence is then described using a review of several important models in current use. We focus on a critique of cultural competence models, particularly in terms of their hidden assumptions and overall failure to address the dominance of White privilege that is rooted in colonialism. We conclude with a call to move beyond current models of cultural competence and toward models that are rooted in acknowledgement of systemic racism and the White privilege that sustains it.

History of Multiculturalism in Canada

As discussed in Chapter 2, people from diverse ethnocultural backgrounds have come to Canada to farm the Prairies; to work in forests, factories, and mines; and to build the country since well before World War II. However, Canada and the rest of North America were already inhabited by Indigenous peoples and new generations of the European colonizers, so those with different cultural backgrounds were generally viewed as "foreigners" as a result of their racial and religious backgrounds and their skin colour. After World War II, there was a move toward assimilation as public policy pressured immigrants (and especially their children) to put aside ethnic traditions and integrate themselves into Canada. To ensure their success, these efforts were enacted through government policies and social services, teachings in schools and churches, and messages and images in the media. Although racism and discrimination existed, immigrants worked hard and carved a place for themselves in the new society. In the years that followed, Canada became home to waves of people from diverse backgrounds who fled their home countries in search of better lives for themselves, their children, and their extended families. Today, the diversity of the Canadian population is one of its distinctive features and many people of non-European descent have made Canada their home.

In 1971, in response to this diverse population, the Canadian government announced its multiculturalism policy. This policy not only had the goal of reversing earlier attempts to assimilate immigrants, it also recognized the reality of the population's multicultural nature. The introduction of this policy was influenced by a number of factors, including complaints from visible minority groups about their unfair and unjust treatment following World War II. Some Canadians did not support multiculturalism because they feared that it would divide Canadians rather than unite them. These Canadians also feared that multiculturalism would erode the rich British heritage of English-speaking Canada. Despite these worries, visible minorities themselves were much less disturbed about recognition of their heritage.

Many visible minorities saw the multiculturalism policy as a resource that would facilitate their ability to obtain employment, adequate housing, and education. The policy promoted cultural programs and services to support ethnocultural associations, and to help individuals address barriers that limited their full participation in Canadian society. The multicultural policy gained increased recognition when it became Section 27 of the Canadian Charter of Rights and Freedoms in 1982 (Canadian Heritage, 2008). The 1982 Charter also recognized and affirmed the treaty rights of Aboriginal peoples to protect their cultures, customs, traditions, and languages.

Multiculturalism policy, as envisaged in 1971, influenced some changes in health policies and practices, especially those related to ethnocultural diversity and the increasingly diverse Canadian population (Masi, Mensah & Macleod, 1993). These changes included the Canadian Council on Multicultural Health (CCMH) (founded in 1986), the 1988 Canadian Task Force on the Mental Health Issues affecting Immigrants and Refugees, and the 1991 Multicultural Health Curriculum Committee. These initiatives helped to identify and address multicultural issues, including increasing the cultural knowledge and skills of health care professionals through their educational programs. The main mechanism for addressing multicultural concerns in health care delivery is through the lens of cultural competence. However, as the following sections indicate, multiculturalism approaches tend to reinforce the invisibility of racism and White privilege.

Cultural Competence: An Overview

Culture is a complex construct with multiple, broad and often ambiguous definitions. Simply put, culture is a complex whole that includes knowledge, values, beliefs, and other capabilities and habits of people. Culture helps to provide group members with a set of ideas and possible actions through which they understand the world in which they live. The complexity of culture and the increasing diversity of Canadian society call for approaches to health care that reach well beyond dominant Eurocentric meanings of health and illness. Multiculturalism has influenced various health care professions and has led to the development of numerous cultural competence models and programs.

While cultural competence models have been used extensively in health care, the actual meaning of the concept is still debatable. Numerous authors have suggested a range of cultural competence definitions. In this chapter, we will highlight a few prominent examples of cultural competence models. Campinha-Bacote (2008) stated that cultural competence in health is necessary to improve the quality of services and outcomes; meet legislative, regulatory, and accreditation mandates; gain a competitive edge in the marketplace; and decrease the likelihood of liability and malpractice claims. Furthermore, the goal of culturally competent care is to create a health care system that is capable of efficiently addressing health disparities (Betancourt, Green, Carrillo & Park, 2005).

Meleis (1996) defined cultural competence as "care that takes into account issues related to diversity, marginalization, and vulnerability due to culture, race, gender and sexual orientation ... provided within the historical and 'dailiness' [everyday] context of clients" (p. 2). Cultural competence includes five essential elements that contribute to effective care from the level of the individual health practitioner to the health organization. They are: (1) valuing diversity; (2) conducting a cultural self-assessment; (3) recognizing and understanding the dynamics of differences; (4) acquiring cultural knowledge; and (5) adapting to diversity (Rounds, Weil & Bishop, 1994).

Valuing diversity involves acknowledging that cultural differences play a role in an individual's identity, and affirming that healthy family development and functioning is fundamental to culturally competent practice. Although racial, ethnic, and cultural differences among clients and staff make care more challenging and complex, they provide the best impetus and opportunity for culturally competent care. Rounds et al. (1994) stated that understanding how race, culture, and ethnicity contribute to the uniqueness of families, and recognizing the differences among and within various cultural groups, are basic to effective care of the culturally different family.

Conducting a cultural self-assessment involving awareness of one's own culture, and how it influences both personal and professional beliefs and behaviours, is critical to the provision of culturally competent care. Rounds et al. (1994) stated that "one's own culturally determined perceptual screen greatly influences the observation and assessment of clients' behaviours and beliefs" (p. 6). Further complicating this need for self-assessment is the fact that much of what professionals believe relies heavily on results of research carried out within Western culture, where the investigators, the participants, and the research questions are heavily influenced by that culture's values (Jackson, 1991). For example, some of Enang's (1999) childbirth experience study participants were frustrated when health professionals sent their visitors away so that they could "rest" because they did not share the belief that secluding them from family members would enable them to relax and rest. One may argue that such action on the part of health professionals is a result of socialization based on mainstream society's strong orientation to individuality and independence. This individual focus contrasts with clients' cultures, which may have a more inclusive perception of self as someone connected to family and community.

Although recognizing and understanding the dynamics of difference is a central feature of cultural competence, some of the differences in race and culture between individuals and families, and among care providers, may often appear subtle. The centrality of racism may also go unrecognized. According to Rounds et al. (1994), recognizing the ways in which racism and the current status of race relations affect the establishment of rapport between racially and ethnically different clients and practitioners is essential to effectively care for clients. For example, the racism experienced by successive generations of Black families may influence the level of trust, and the development of a collaborative relationship between a White perinatal nurse and a Black family. Acquiring cultural knowledge requires posing the right questions in an appropriate manner to the right people. Although general knowledge about cultural groups is necessary, it needs to be individualized to clients and families because variations within groups are often great. For example, it is best to always ask families during labour about their childbirth preferences in terms of diet, pain relief, and other coping strategies because there is a wealth of knowledge about different cultures among the families we care for, and the process of caring provides a wonderful opportunity to expand our knowledge about their socio-cultural world.

Cultural competence "does not mean knowing everything there is to know about another culture. It is instead, respect for the difference, eagerness to learn and a willingness to accept that there are many ways of viewing the world" (Dugas & Knor 1995, p. 298). It is also important to understand that cultural competence is not a goal but a journey, a continual process requiring constant learning, reflection, and self-assessment (Etowa & Adongo, 2007). The process of developing cultural competence, as illustrated in Figure 3.1, is essential for health care professionals seeking to effectively work across cultural boundaries.

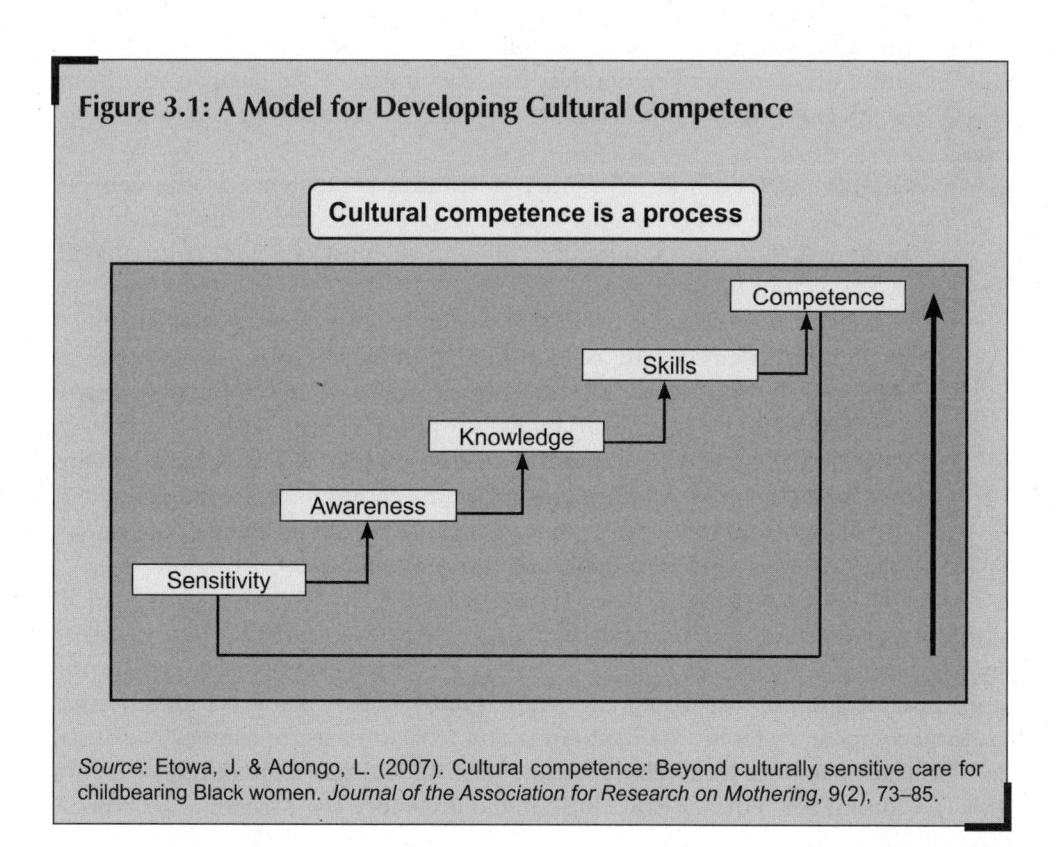

Figure 3.1: A Model for Developing Cultural Competence

Cultural competence is a process

Sensitivity → Awareness → Knowledge → Skills → Competence

Source: Etowa, J. & Adongo, L. (2007). Cultural competence: Beyond culturally sensitive care for childbearing Black women. *Journal of the Association for Research on Mothering*, 9(2), 73–85.

In Figure 3.1, cultural sensitivity is defined as a desire to work effectively across cultural boundaries and is positioned at the start of the continuum. Sensitivity precedes awareness, which involves recognition, leading to knowledge and more informed understanding of the influence that culture has on the behaviour of providers and recipients of care. This knowledge allows an acquisition of skills to improve self-assessment, and acceptance and adaptation to diversity, which are all essential components of cultural competence. However, competence in one area for a specific cultural group may not be transferable. Health professionals should be willing to engage in the process of developing cultural competence in a variety of health care settings for diverse cultural groups (Etowa & Adongo, 2007).

As society becomes increasingly diverse, so is the quest for health care professions to educate practitioners who can cater to the needs of a multicultural society. This quest has led to widespread development of various cultural competence tools. In addition to Etowa and Adongo's (2007) example described in Figure 3.1, some commonly used cultural competence tools include the following:

- Leininger's (1991) theory focused on culture, care, diversity, and universality. One of the earliest cultural competence models in the field of nursing, this theory explicated some of the factors that influence health care from an insider and outsider perspective in a given culture with a goal of providing culturally competent care.
- Kim-Godwin, Clarke, and Barton's (2001) model for the delivery of culturally competent community care encompassed the health care system, health outcomes, cultural sensitivity, cultural knowledge, cultural skills, and caring.
- Campinha-Bacote's (2002) model of cultural competence in the delivery of health care integrated the following five basic constructs: (1) cultural awareness, (2) cultural humility, (3) cultural knowledge, (4) cultural skill, and (5) cultural desire.
- Giger and Davidhizar's (2002) transcultural assessment model identified six cultural elements to be considered in health care assessment: (1) communication, (2) space, (3) social organization, (4) time, (5) environmental control, and (6) biological variations.
- Purnell's (2005) model of cultural competence integrated 12 cultural domains that should be used in health care, including communication (e.g., language and dialects), workforce (e.g., autonomy, acculturation, assimilation, gender roles), death rituals, nutrition, and high-risk behaviour.

The growth of cultural competence models has been accompanied by an increase in the development of instruments to measure cultural competence. As Kumas-Tan, Beagan, Loppie, MacLeod, and Frank (2007) noted, many commonly used cultural competence tools are quantitative and tend to measure competence at the individual practitioner level. These include the Multicultural Counseling Inventory (MCI), Cultural Self-Efficacy Scale (CSES), the Inventory for Assessing the Process of Cultural Competence (IAPCC), the Cross-cultural Adaptability Inventory (CCAI), and the Multicultural Awareness Knowledge and Skills Survey (MAKSS). It must be noted that despite the development of and wide use of these tools, a void remains regarding a full explication of what constitutes cultural competence and what the tools actually measure.

Although multicultural care approaches such as cultural competence models may be useful for individualized health care, a broader level intervention is needed to address population health and the complexity of a diverse society. This includes a sustained consideration of inequities in health outcomes and in the provision of health care. While we acknowledge cultural competence as an important aspect of the provision of health care across cultural boundaries, we also argue that issues affecting marginalized groups require broader socio-political and structural changes.

Cultural Competence: A Critique

This section provides a critique of cultural competence or multicultural care models. We focus on four central problems that underpin most efforts addressing the cultural competence of health care practitioners: (1) problems with measuring cultural competence; (2) the absence of attention to power relations; (3) problems with assessing the effectiveness of cultural competence; and (4) the promotion of stereotypes.

Overview: Getting outside the Goldfish Tank

Initiatives related to cultural competence have fostered cross-cultural health care and created a mutual ground to initiate a dialogue about issues of difference; however, a critical analysis of racism and an understanding of the macro-level workings of the health care system are necessary to design and implement policy changes to ensure truly accessible health services for racialized and marginalized peoples. Although health literature suggests that there is a need for health care professionals to understand and adapt to cultural diversity through culturally competent care, proponents of anti-racism have argued that health care professionals must challenge racism, and avoid opting for a politically soft option that embraces curricula issues that merely reify culture (Alleyne, Papadopoulos & Tilki, 1994). They further noted that such an approach denies the centrality or existence of racism and pays "superficial attention to cultural rites and rituals" (Alleyne et al., 1994, p. 583).

The very size of the problem and the deep social roots of multicultural dynamics embedded in the various systems and institutional structures create a major challenge for health care professionals. For example, the racism experienced by Indigenous peoples is not a simple issue of ethnicity, culture, and race; rather, it is a complex, pervasive social problem that arises from multiple sites, and as such it requires a critical lens for analysis. The complexity of these issues is reflected in the many ways in which they are manifested in the everyday health care experiences of non-mainstream people, as illustrated throughout this book.

Models of cultural competence fall short on a number of counts. Following years of efforts to implement cultural competence models in health care, there remains minimal evidence to demonstrate their effectiveness in improving health outcomes or reducing health inequities (Anderson, Scrimshaw, Fullilove, Fielding & Norman, 2003; Betancourt, Green, Carillo & Park, 2005; Capenter-Song, Schwaille & Longhofer, 2007). As Drevdahl, Canales, and Dorcy's (2008) goldfish tank analogy has illustrated, cultural competence is like a goldfish tank in the centre of the hospital waiting room. It improves the atmosphere and helps patients relax; however, it does not eliminate the actual problem that brought the patients into the hospital in the first place.

Problems with Measuring Cultural Competence

Although numerous cultural competence and multicultural care models have been created, and researchers have generated tools to evaluate their effectiveness, measuring cultural competence has proven to be a difficult task for a number of reasons. First, the reliability of cultural competence instruments has been questioned because most of these instruments are developed and tested on predominantly White, middle-class, well-educated people and with no input from patients (Boyle & Springer, 2001; Kumas-Tan, Beagan, Loppie, MacLeod & Frank, 2007). These instruments are also based on self-ratings, which make them susceptible to social-desirability effects. Social desirability refers to the phenomenon in which individuals filling out self-rating scales tend to answer according to what they perceive is more socially acceptable, and not necessarily what they actually feel or think.

Second, the utility of these measurement tools is problematic because existing tools are often too long and cumbersome, and may be of little relevance to those using them (Kumas-Tan et al. 2007). A recent review of instruments used in the health professions identified little uniformity in the tools, and a lack of rigour in the researchers' choice of measures, as some of the challenges confronting the establishment of an effective measure of cross-cultural health care. Third, there are concerns regarding the validity of existing instruments, including the argument that most of the instruments oversimplify both culture and cultural competence, including reducing its components to awareness, knowledge, and skill, and often focusing on race and ethnicity exclusively (Drevdahl, Canales & Dorcy, 2008; Kumas-Tan et al., 2007). Furthermore, the "cultural competence approach assumes that culture can be simplified and then managed as other kinds of content in curricula or practice—as a body of knowledge to be gained via lists of facts, and then applied to those who are defined as different" (Drevdahl et al., 2008, p. 20). This approach ignores the notion that culture is not a thing that can be found. Rather, culture is constructed in the process of doing something else (Drevdahl et al.).

In their analysis of available literature on cultural competence evaluation tools, Kumas-Tan and colleagues (2007) identified assumptions that are embedded in these instruments. Central to the hidden assumptions in cultural competence measuring tools is the notion of the Other. Culturally competent health care professionals are encouraged to increase knowledge about Others—other cultures, other customs, other ways of knowing. But who are these Others? The notion of the Other is rooted in centuries-old traditions of colonialism. It bears careful attention in any serious effort to engage in culturally competent care. The following is a brief description of the origins of the notion of the "Other."

The collective memory of colonization has been perpetuated through the multitude of images, writings, and narratives that were collected about Indigenous peoples—the "Others." These images were then represented to the West and then back to the Indigenous peoples themselves (Smith, 1999). Over the centuries, these meanings about Indigenous peoples became part of the collective memories of the colonizers, primarily the White peoples of Europe. Indeed, the colonizers' reflection back to Indigenous peoples on the various continents was that they were savage, unintelligent, and expendable. This process became a way to reinforce colonization. There was no room for the knowledge systems of the "Other" in the new colonies. In fact, as the history of Canada's Indian Act, enacted in 1876, demonstrates, the ways of knowing of Indigenous peoples were systematically excluded and, in some cases, lost forever.

So, similar to the legacy of colonization, the word Other is deeply embedded in modern societies, including Canada: "... we, Indigenous peoples, people 'of color', the Other, however we are named, have a presence in the Western imagination, in its fibre and texture, in its sense of self, in its language, in its silences and shadows, its margins and intersections" (Smith, 1999, p. 14). In contrast, White peoples' race is not noted. It does not mark them as being a particular colour. The word race, by its very meaning in health care practice and in modern society, signifies those who are not white-skinned. When we practise culturally competent care, which cultures require us to pay special attention to this competence? Even a cursory examination of the cultural competence literature indicated that Caucasian peoples such as the British and the Swedish are not of primary concern, or even particularly relevant to cultural competence. "Certainly, members of dominant cultural groups also have identities and worldviews that are re-shaped by culture and racism. Existing measures, however, rarely acknowledge or examine dominant cultures" (Kumas-Tan et al., 2007, p. 551). The focus is on the Other, the not-White. This is the crux of what is known as Othering, signifying an individual, a family, a whole people as the Other, the not-White, the people outside the boundaries of whiteness. As is the case with racism, Othering happens whether or not White people understand it, acknowledge it, or even see it.

Another assumption embedded in cultural competence measurement is that culture is a matter of ethnicity and race (Kumas-Tan et al., 2007). Although health care professionals recognize the significance of culture in the health care of service recipients, oversimplification of the concept of culture creates additional challenges. Culture is often made synonymous with race and ethnicity. For example, patients of a certain ethnicity and race, such as a "Nigerian patient," are assumed to have a certain core set of beliefs about illness based on fixed ethnic traits. Cultural competence becomes a veritable laundry list of do's and don'ts that dictate the kind of care provided to patients of a particular ethnoracial group (Kleinman & Benson, 2006). The tendency to equate culture with race and ethnicity limits culture to those identified as ethnoracial minorities. A narrow conceptualization of culture is contradictory to the understanding of culture as an inclusive broad range of human activities. This "Othering" makes it difficult for health care professionals to examine themselves within the context of the dominant White culture (Drevdahl et al., 2008; Giddings, 2005). Othering also makes it difficult to assess and determine meaningful approaches to evaluating a wide range of social differences.

The Absence of Power Relations

Historically, culture in health care encounters referred almost exclusively to the domain of the patient and her or his family. However, health care encounters are grounded in the world of the patient, the health care professional, the professional world of biomedicine and health institutions, and in broader systems of structural power. Cultural competence models often gloss over discussions about the ethnocultural background of health care professionals, and the Eurocentric nature of health care in the Western world. Advocates of cultural humility suggest that a starting point for cross-cultural care should be a careful consideration by health care professionals of the assumptions and beliefs that are embedded in their own understandings and the goals of health care interactions (Hunt, 2001). The focus of cultural competence education is on the "cultural" client and this often neglects due consideration of the health professional's world view, and the power relations that are part of every health care encounter.

An overemphasis on cultural differences, and a failure to recognize biomedicine as a cultural system itself, obscure structural power imbalances (Carpenter-Song, Schwaille & Longhofer, 2007). Culture is often seen as that which the Other has and the Other is often the owner of the problem since the dominant groups are not seen as having a culture (Kumas-Tan et al., 2007). An extensive review of cultural competence literature by Kumas-Tan et al. (2007) found that most cultural competence measures equate culture with the "ethnic and racialized Other" (p. 551). Othering in these measures creates a milieu where health care professionals learn little, if anything, about White privilege or the ways that institutional structures favour dominant groups. When cultural competence interventions focus on the Other as the problem, health care professionals identify the Other as an object of specialized knowledge that calls for providers to become experts in cultural minutiae involving dialects, diet, and dress.

Power imbalance may be a common problem in the patient-provider encounter, and miscommunication in health care encounters may be more about biomedical assumptions and less about the cultural background of the minority client (Carpenter-Song, Schwaille & Longhofer, 2007). Indeed, the culture of biomedicine and the resulting approach to health care is sometimes seen as a primary source for transmitting stigma, incorporating and maintaining racial bias in health institutions, and developing health inequities across minority groups (Keusch, Wilentz & Kleinman, 2006; Kleinman & Benson, 2006; Lee, Lee, Chiu & Kleinman, 2005; Wailoo, 2001). Historically, the models of cultural competence developed to address cultural diversity issues, including multicultural care and cultural competence, are from the perspective of dominant privileged individuals. Models that come from predominantly White hegemonic perspectives often ignore the history of colonization and the role of resistance toward colonial domination (Drevdahl et al., 2008). Thus, some of these models tend to recreate oppression and maintain the status quo in terms of the assumed neutrality of the scientific West to describe, label, and create descriptions of Others. These descriptions of Others are generally based on perceptions of how they differ from White societal norms.

The dominant view assumes that cultural groups have fixed identities and cultural needs that health care professionals must acknowledge, understand, and address (Culley, 2006; Drevdahl et al., 2008). This perspective ignores the fact that cultural and racial groups never exist permanently with fixed boundaries. Instead "culture is constantly made and re-made — ever changing, fluid and shifting" (Drevdahl et al., 2008, p. 21). As Kumas-Tan et al. (2007) stated, this approach to multicultural care sees culture as a confounding variable that confronts White health care professionals as they work with the Other. Thus, "cultural competence is achieved when practitioners acquire sufficient awareness and knowledge of the Other" (Kumas-Tan et al., 2007, p. 552), so culture is possessed by the Other. Similarly, cross-cultural health care is assumed to take the form of Caucasian practitioners working with ethnic and racialized groups. In this sense, cultural competence involves being confident in oneself and comfortable with others (Kumas-Tan et al., 2007).

Cultural incompetence is caused by practitioners' discriminatory attitudes toward the Other. "The understanding seems to be that if practitioners would only educate themselves about ethnocentrism and racism, and then free themselves of biased worldviews and prejudice, ethnocentrism and racism would no longer be a problem for either practitioner or patient" (Kumas-Tan et al., 2007, p. 554). These assumptions rely on dismissal of the importance of dominant power structures, and the pivotal role of Eurocentrism and White privilege in the perpetuation of racism in health care practice. In a related manner, the primary focus of cultural competence measures is whether or not the practitioner possesses sufficient knowledge about cultural differences, rather than on an analysis of racism. Therefore, most cultural competence models fall seriously short of addressing the oppression that is at the core of health inequities and barriers to competent care.

Table 3.1 summarizes Kumas-Tan et al.'s (2007) six assumptions embedded in cultural competence instruments.

Ineffectiveness of Cultural Competence Models

Although there is an overall consensus among health care professionals, policymakers, and academics that cultural competence has the potential to eliminate inequities in health and health care, there are very few cultural competence models that have been tested and proven to show positive results. Drevdahl et al. (2008) conducted an extensive literature review in the field of cultural competence and found only one study where the cultural competence of health care professionals showed a positive impact on health outcomes. Their study examined the health care needs of Orthodox Jews with a focus on changes made by a particular hospital to accommodate their dietary and places of worship needs within the hospital

> **Table 3.1: Assumptions Embedded in Cultural Competence Instruments**
>
> 1. Culture is a matter of ethnicity and race.
> 2. Culture is possessed by the "Other"; the "Other" is/has the problem.
> 3. Cross-cultural health care is when Caucasian practitioners work with patients from ethnic and racialized minority groups.
> 4. Cultural competence involves being confident in oneself and comfortable with the "Other."
> 5. Cultural incompetence is practitioners' discriminatory attitudes toward the "Other."
> 6. Cultural incompetence is lack of familiarity with, and knowledge about, the "Other."
>
> *Source:* Adapted from Kumas-Tan, Z., Beagan, B.M., Loppie, C., MacLeod, A. & Frank, B. (2007). Measures of cultural competence: Examining hidden assumptions. *Academic Medicine, 82*(6), 548–557.

setting (Foley & Wurmser, 2004). The study used Leininger and McFarland's (2002) transcultural care approach. The researchers could not clearly show the association between the hospital's culturally "responsive" initiative and improved maternal and infant health outcomes (Foley & Wurmser, 2004).

Additional studies regarding the prenatal breastfeeding education of Hispanic women have shown less success (Schlickau & Wilson, 2005). For example, although a pilot study was conducted to establish Hispanic women's breastfeeding attitudes, beliefs, and practices, the designed cultural competence interventions on those variables did not show significant differences between the intervention and control groups. Similarly, Anderson and colleagues (2003) conducted a synthesis of several studies that incorporated five commonly used cultural competence interventions in health care. These interventions included using cultural health interpreters, maintaining a diverse workforce, providing cultural competence training, creating cultural health education materials, and developing culturally specific health care institutions. The synthesis found very few studies that actually compared culturally competent care with routine health care. Studies that evaluated the impact of cultural competence interventions either showed no differences between the control and intervention group, or showed that patients in the intervention group reported a greater level of satisfaction with care. However, none of the studies reviewed actually measured or demonstrated improvement in clients' health outcomes. Furthermore, cultural competence models have been criticized for primarily focusing evaluation measures on providers' self-assessment of their own cultural competence (Drevdahl et al., 2008).

Researchers have also begun to examine cultural competence and its effectiveness in addressing health inequities. For example, Brach and Fraser (2000) researched the question: "Can cultural competence reduce racial and ethnic health disparities?" They reported that cultural competence interventions were not clearly associated with any measurable health outcomes. In addition, the inequities examined were not clearly identified, and the specific strategies used to reduce health inequities were inadequately described. Although, Brach and Fraser found cultural competence to be limited in terms of eliminating health inequities, they too created their own conceptual model that targeted health disparity reduction.

Betancourt, Green, Carrillo, and Ananeh-Firempong (2003) also developed a model for applying cultural competence measures to address racial and ethnic health disparities. Their model incorporated three aspects of socio-cultural barriers to health care for ethnoracial people: (1) organizational (the lack of minority people in the health care workforce, especially in leadership positions); (2) structural (the lack of health interpretation services and long wait times); and (3) clinical (the relationship between the health professional and the client). The goals of this model were to increase representation of minorities in the health workforce, to provide culturally relevant education for the health professionals, and to address cultural competence in health care institutions.

However, scholars such as Drevdahl et al. (2008) have critiqued these models for reducing health disparities, noting that they do not address broader level barriers such as poverty, systemic racism, violence, or health care insurance issues. In addition, Drevdahl et al.'s extensive literature review in this field showed that for the most part, "discussions of cultural competence interventions have been limited to the issues of language, particularly in terms of language access or interpreter support" (p. 18). They also noted that overall, clients' outcomes have been limited to process and survey tools, which are often targeted at clients' satisfaction or provider self-evaluation. While cultural competence models may be useful for individualized health care, unless they explicitly address individual and systemic racism, they will not ultimately help to ameliorate inequities in health outcomes and in health care provision.

Promotion of Stereotypes

Another concern with cultural competence models is their potential for unwittingly promoting stereotypes. According to Kleinman and Benson (2006), cultural competence interventions, like other interventions, have some unwanted effects. The most serious of these effects is that patients and their families can interpret the attention given to cultural difference as intrusive, and might even contribute to "a sense of being singled out and stigmatized" (p. 1675). The quest to promote cultural competence has also been criticized for emphasizing "cultural difference" and thus leading to a representation of culture as a decontextualized set of traits, providing a template for perceptions and behaviours of group members (Hunt, 2001).

In keeping with this way of thinking about culture, cultural diversity literature has provided extensive lists of traditional beliefs and practices that characterize certain ethnic groups. This approach also promotes the questionable notion that immigrants and certain ethnoracial groups are driven by traditions, while their mainstream counterparts have conventional beliefs that remain unnamed and unexamined. This misconception, common in practice settings, has some people treating culture as an explanatory variable, subject to prediction and control. As Hunt (2001) noted, such schools of thought represent cultures as a "codified body of characteristics that can be identified and then either modified or manipulated to facilitate clinical goals"

(p. 3). Ironically, the desire to encourage respect for cultural difference may instead promote stereotyping and bolster a sense of group boundaries between health care professionals and the "Others." It may also reinforce the notion that culture can be diagnosed and treated, or that unfamiliar beliefs and behaviours of already marginalized groups should be controlled and adjusted to resemble norms of the dominant group.

Carpenter-Song, Schwallie, and Longhofer (2007) suggested that the application of culture in clinical practice may unintentionally blame the client's culture for miscommunication and non-adherence to clinical recommendations, and other barriers to effective care. Similarly, in efforts to provide culturally competent care, there is a tension that may result in a contradictory understanding of culture (Santiago-Irizarry, 1996). This tension leads to culture being viewed as a source of problematic behaviour, and thus the cause of challenges encountered in clinical practice with marginalized populations. In addition to acknowledging the value of culturally appropriate care, Carpenter-Song et al. (2007) also identified the treatment of culture as static and as a variable in much of the cultural competence literature. This includes blaming clients' culture for their health care difficulties. The very idea that there are isolated cultures with shared meanings creates harmful stereotypes where entire ethnic groups can be described, for example, as "Africans believe this ...," "Mexicans believe that ...," "Chinese believe that ...," and so on. These kinds of assumptions espouse the notion that cultural groups have stable identities, and deny the everyday realities of systemic discrimination and other forms of social inequities.

Beyond Cultural Competence

Although health care professionals generally view culturally competent care as leading to improved health outcomes, patient satisfaction, and increased adherence to treatment protocols, they also admit that specific descriptions and measures of the nature of this kind of care are not readily available. In addition, the actual association between culturally competent care and client health outcomes is not yet established. While some cultural competence strategies appear promising and may have the potential to improve the quality of health care, the evidence in terms of reducing health inequities is very limited (Miranda et al., 2003). Although promotion of multicultural knowledge is central to cultural competence, the very notion of multiculturalism remains unproblematized.

Moreover, as anti-racism scholars such as Frances Henry (2002) stated, "multiculturalism has in fact failed to control racism against ethno-racial minorities" (p. 231) because even though cultural diversity programs are being maintained throughout the country, some groups such as people of African descent, Aboriginal peoples, and other marginalized groups continue to experience exclusion, poverty, and inequities in health and health care. Henry (2002) further suggested that diverse nations such as Canada require a stronger and more critical approach to diversity — one that espouses a restructuring and reconceptualization of the power relations among different cultural and racial groups. Communities and societies do not exist in isolation from one another and the lack of attention to power relations obscures the dominance of whiteness. A critical approach to cultural competence will lead to the much-needed ideological transformation that is necessary to address the root causes of racism and other forms of oppression. Box 3.1 provides a brief description of the genesis of Canada's first provincial guidelines for cultural competence in primary health care. The significance of the model includes its detailed and clear attention to racism and oppression. The description below focuses on the genesis of the guidelines.

Box 3.1: Cultural Competence, Diversity, and Social Inclusion in Primary Health Care

Our vision for primary health care is one in which communities can improve their health in a system that meets their needs. This means ensuring equitable access to those populations who have traditionally faced barriers.

In response to various recommendations, the Nova Scotia Department of Health's Primary Health Care Section developed the Diversity & Social Inclusion in Primary Health Care Initiative to begin to address the needs of culturally diverse populations.

A three-year initiative was established to raise awareness of diversity and social inclusion issues and to consult with primary health care stakeholders, District Health Authorities, Community Health Boards, providers, communities, and culturally diverse populations to develop policies for primary health care and guidelines for cultural competence.

The Primary Health Care Section launched the Initiative with a provincial Diversity & Social Inclusion Workshop, partnered with District Health Authorities to hold nine workshops across the province and linked with and supported provincial programs and chronic disease prevention efforts. A Cultural Competence Workshop targeting health professionals was held in partnership with the IWK Health Centre in June, 2005.

The result of this work was recommendations for culturally inclusive policies and the first, provincial guidelines for cultural competence in primary health care in Canada.

Cultural competence can work to reduce disparities in health services and increase detection of population-specific diseases and conditions.

It also addresses inequitable access to primary heath care and respectfully responds to Nova Scotia's existing and changing demographics. A culturally competent primary health care system can provide care to patients with diverse values, beliefs, and behaviors, including tailoring care to meet social, cultural and linguistic needs.

It requires and understanding of the communities being served and devises strategies to identify and address barriers to accessing quality, primary health care.

Source: Nova Scotia Department of Health

In order for health care professionals to recognize limitations in the care available to historically oppressed groups such as Indigenous peoples, Canadians of African descent, and visible minority immigrants, it is vital for them to understand the context of health inequities and the necessity for institutional and individual change. If health care professionals are to understand the complex ways in which racism interacts with other societal factors to determine health, then an anti-racist framework is necessary. Anti-racism explores the dynamics of discriminatory practices that structure many aspects of oppressed people's everyday lives. Racism influences both the patterns of health status and the utilization of health services by marginalized people. The dominant way of conceptualizing issues of race and health has many flaws that may obstruct the attainment of equitable health and health care in a multiracial society such as Canada (Culley, 1996). For example, inadequate education of health care professionals regarding racism may lead to a lack of understanding of institutionalized racism and discrimination within the health sector and in other societal structures in general. As Drevdahl and colleagues (2008) so clearly told us, increased knowledge about culture will make the fish tank more elaborate, but real change will require increased knowledge about oppression.

A United Kingdom study found a considerable deficit in the knowledge of racial issues among health care providers (Higham, 1988). Many nurses in this survey indicated that they received little or no information in their training for working in a multiracial society, and some of these nurses did not see the need for training that addressed attitudes and prejudice (Higham, 1988). Lack of knowledge of the dynamics of racial and cultural differences may lead to inadequate care. For example, it is not uncommon to find health care professionals who may be uncertain about how to recognize racism and how to respond to it. According to Culley (1996), a lack of understanding of difference may lead to value judgments placed on that difference as deviant, alien, and a problem. For example, not only can Indigenous, Black, and immigrant peoples be seen as different, but they can also be seen as inferior and subordinate. They are "Others" to the norm of White people.

As discussed in Chapter 2, like classism and sexism, racism is a form of discrimination. Boyd (1998) defined racism as "any action or institutional practice backed by institutional power that subordinates people because of their colour or ethnicity" (p. 9). She further noted that "those who hold the most power are the ones who keep the fires of racism burning. They do it by using their power to press their opinions and keep prejudice and stereotypes alive in the minds of others" (p. 9). It is widely acknowledged that while overt and blatant racism has become less socially acceptable across North America, racist values have not really changed. Rather, racism has largely become quiet, closeted, subtle, disguised, hidden, and covert (Naidoo & Edwards, 1991, p. 212). People of colour shoulder a heavy burden as targets of racism in Canada and in North America generally (Naidoo & Edwards, 1991).

The racism that lingers in Canadian society is still powerful enough to place people of colour under the pressure of always being on the watch for the hard edge of prejudice and discrimination (Naidoo & Edwards, 1991). While blatant racism occurred in the early part of the 20th century, systemic constraints still persist. Discriminatory immigration laws denied the entrance to Canada of Black people seeking escape from slavery in the United States. The excuse was that Black people were medically determined to be unable to adapt to the cold. In modern times, while Black Africans are not directly denied entrance into Canada on the basis of their cultural origin, many of them fail to meet the necessary immigration criteria of the modern-day institutionalized point system. Until the 1960s, Canada chose its immigrants on the basis of racial categorization. Northern Europeans, especially the British, were given priority, or more points, over categories such as the Black and Asiatic races. In the 1960s, a newly introduced point system attempted to eliminate racial reasons for denying entry to Canada. Although race officially ceased to be a factor, aspects of current policy continue to be reminiscent of the point system. For example: 1) refugees are required to produce identity documents, a near impossibility for many refugees. Women, youth, and rural refugees are even less likely to have identification; 2) The $975 Right of Landing Fee (ROLF), which all adult immigrants must pay in order to be granted permanent residence, represents almost a year's salary for some people in the global south, thus amounting to an extra tax for these people; and 3) in terms of the family immigration, requirements to produce official documents, such as marriage certificates, differentially affect people from countries where marriage, birth, and adoptions are not recorded in documents. Also, narrow definitions such as the nuclear family mean that countries whose definition of family includes the extended family are disadvantaged. The point system and its modern-day equivalent are evidence of xenophobia in Canada. Xenophobia is the deep dislike of foreigners (Canadian Council for Refugees, 2000).

Addressing institutional racism is a key element in ensuring genuinely equitable access to services for all clients and their families. This process can be difficult and may take a long time because people are often reluctant to see how their own actions may be unconsciously contributing to discrimination (Schott & Henley, 1996). To understand the complex meaning of racism in society, and to address it effectively, a critical examination of the many faces of the problem is needed. An anti-racist framework to guide practice is necessary to confront the complexity of racism and its impact on the health and health care of Canadian. As Spector (1996) pointed out, merely educating people about the cultural, racial, and/or ethnic differences that are embedded in values and beliefs of one another is not enough; "one must first confront competing ideals of truth" (p. 63) such as the power relations that form the backdrop to racism.

Conclusions

Although some would argue that multiculturalism and cultural competence models have encouraged society's openness toward people of diverse backgrounds, the universal experience of globalization and its impacts call for approaches that challenge the historical politics and dominance of mainstream culture. Health care professionals continue to develop more cultural competence tools and models and interventions; however, since cultural competence is not a skill that can be mastered, such as blood pressure reading, nor a problem-solving technique that can be learned, it is time to focus on the real problems facing marginalized people. The solution to health inequities cannot be found in "culturally competent interventions located within existing walls and halls of clinics, hospitals, nor through actions of individual practitioners and academics" (Drevdahl, 2008, p. 25). Concentration on individual practitioners or hospitals perpetuates avoidance of confronting the complexity of systemic oppression. This approach also makes people complicit with sustaining inequities in health and health care. Instead, power relationships among different racial and cultural groups must be restructured, and such an approach will see ethnoracial minority people as active and full participants in societal affairs.

Cultural competence models must acknowledge and name racism as a social determinant of health. There is a need to re-evaluate current cultural competence models since they have not been shown to positively impact health outcomes. Although there may be individual benefits to health interventions that acknowledge cultural difference, addressing health inequities needs to occur at the population health level, with explicit attention to societal power structures that perpetuate racism. Various stakeholders, including community people, health care providers, policy decision makers, and researchers, need to engage in critical dialogue and political action to address existing inequities in health and health care, and to create a more socially just health care system and society.

CHAPTER 4

Theoretical Foundations for an Anti-racist Framework

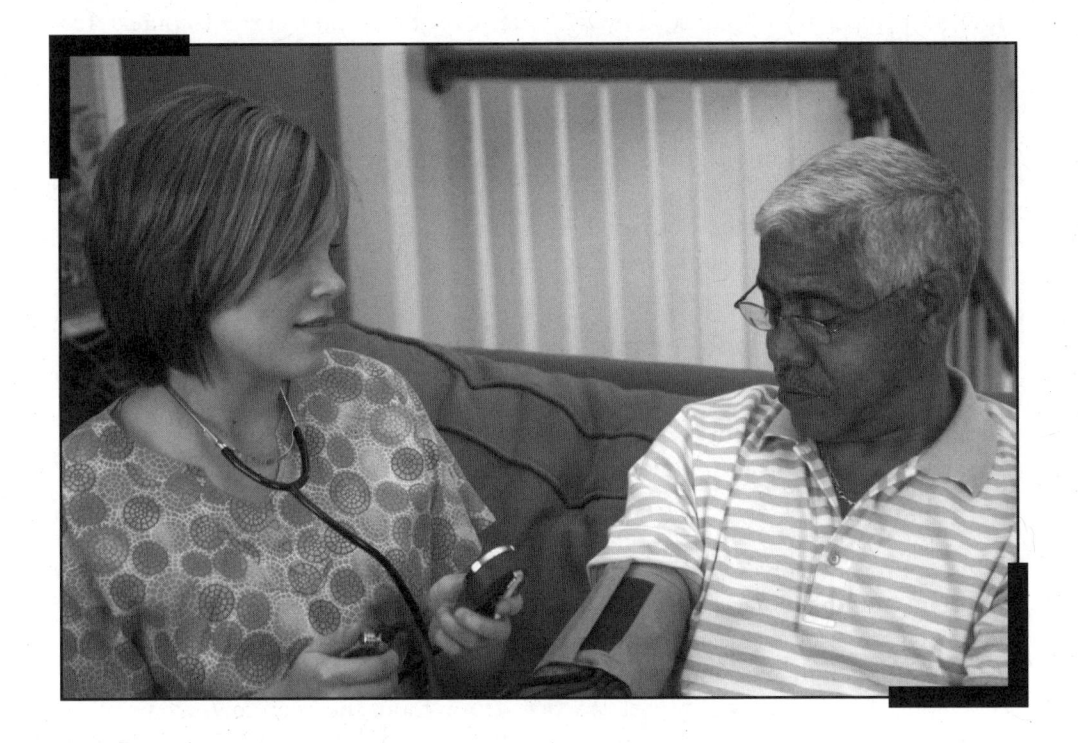

Although the encounter between colonizer and colonized changes in historically specific ways, and is always highly gendered, it remains a moment when powerful narratives turn oppressed peoples into objects, to be held in contempt, or to be saved from their fates by more civilized beings. (Sherene Razack, 1998, p. 3)

Introduction

This chapter lays a further foundation for our choice of an anti-racist approach to work for change in the area of health and health care. Anti-racist health care practice occurs within the current Canadian social and political context. Therefore, we begin with a discussion of important perspectives on health and health care based on Raphael's (2006) analytical categories. These perspectives are presented in terms of their relevance for health and health care, and in particular their relevance for anti-racist practice. We stress the importance of developing a core understanding of these perspectives because they provide a historical and current context for both the resistance to, and the promotion of, anti-racist practice. The relevance of biomedicine is discussed in terms of its dominance as a framework for health care delivery in Canada. Although the dominance of biomedicine has been discussed in detail elsewhere, its implications for racism in health system delivery and policy-making have not been fully examined. We draw attention to the importance of acknowledging biomedical knowledge, while at the same time encouraging a critique of the pitfalls of biomedical dominance.

Overview of Important Perspectives on Health and Health Care

There are several important perspectives on health and health care that are significant in terms of developing a core understanding of anti-racist practice: epidemiological, sociological, political economy, human rights, feminist, anti-racist, post-colonial, and anti-colonial perspectives. Our discussion provides an overview of these perspectives and is not meant to be a comprehensive representation of the works of the many important authors in each of the areas. The point is that these ideas have heavily influenced the way we view health in the Western world. Without a foundational understanding of the various perspectives, practitioners may find it very difficult to see avenues to work for anti-racist practice. Throughout the overview, we provide examples of how each of the perspectives influence our thinking about racism and health.

Although thinking in the health fields has, in some ways, moved beyond older sociological perspectives such as systems theory, the vestiges of this thinking remain and thus are important to consider. There has been recent incorporation of critical theory into some mainstream health care discussions in Canada, including public health. However, these efforts fall short of incorporating the rich critical perspectives that were developed after critical theory, such as feminism, anti-racism, and anti-colonialism. We stress the notion of critical perspectives, that have, as their foundations, an analysis of the creation and maintenance of societal power structures. Critical perspectives include critical theory, political economy, human rights, anti-racist, and post-colonial theories and practice. It is important to note that there are overlaps among the critical perspectives, all of which challenge dominant societal power structures. This overview will be beneficial for readers who have not had the opportunity to explore important theoretical underpinnings of anti-racist and anti-oppressive thinking and action.

Epidemiological Perspectives

Epidemiology concerns itself with disease etiology and prevalence. The field of epidemiology began in 1854 with John Snow's famous links between the incidence of cholera in a crowded London district and the location of wells. Snow discovered that the highest incidence of cholera occurred around several of the city wells that were found to be contaminated. The connection between disease incidence and causation, and hence treatment, was demonstrated dramatically. Snow's work also laid the foundation for the geographic study of disease incidence. An introductory epidemiology text for students in nursing, medicine, and pharmacy described the modern-day purpose of clinical epidemiology: "The purpose of clinical epidemiology is to foster methods of clinical observation and interpretation that lead to valid conclusions and better patient care. The most credible answers to clinical questions are based on a few basic principles" (Fletcher & Fletcher, 2005, p. 5). These principles include: clinical questions (i.e., How accurate are tests used to diagnose disease?); variables (i.e., independent, dependent, and extraneous variables); health outcomes (i.e., death, disease, discomfort, disability, dissatisfaction, distribution); numbers and probability (i.e., quantitative measurement of health outcomes); and additional quantitative principles such as population selection and samples. The latter includes standard quantitative concerns, including statistical bias and maximizing effectiveness of random sampling.

Thus, the foundations of epidemiology lie in the quantitative measure of human disease: its incidence, its etiology, its distribution, and its largely pharmacological treatment. Epidemiology has accomplished massive population health advances in the treatment of communicable diseases, most notably in the Western world. Although epidemiology has historically been central in some types of human disease management, its lack of attention to social factors is increasingly problematic. This is because the predictors of disease in Canada are now decidedly based in social factors that are beyond the traditional purview and capability of epidemiology. The work of social scientists such as Shaw, Dorling, Gordon, and Smith (1999) in the United Kingdom demonstrated the substantial contrast between conventional epidemiological perspectives on disease and the emerging social science of critical health studies. In their book *The Widening Gap: Health Inequalities and Policy in Britain*, these authors combined mortality and morbidity statistics across the lifespan and analyzed these statistics in the context of poverty, housing, and social policy.

This move to integrate social science with epidemiology is an increasing global trend with its genesis in concern and even alarm about the growing poverty rates in Western countries, including the so-called rich countries such as Canada and the United States. According to Krieger (2001), the term social epidemiology was first used in the *American Sociological Review* in 1950 in an article titled: "The relationship of fetal and infant mortality to residential segregation: an inquiry into social epidemiology" (Yankauer, 1950). According to Krieger, this topic is as timely now as it was in 1950, and the need to fully integrate social and biological origins of disease continues to be centrally relevant:

> Grappling with notions of causation, in turn, raises not only complex philosophical issues but also, in the case of social epidemiology, issues of accountability and agency: simply invoking abstract notions of "society" and disembodied "genes" will not suffice. Instead, the central question becomes: Who and what is responsible for population patterns of disease and well-being, as manifested in present, past and changing social inequalities in health? (p. 688)

Social epidemiology thus makes explicit the limited utility of conventional epidemiology in addressing inequities in health. Vincente Navarro (2002) stressed the importance of the relationship between social class and health, and called for a materialist epidemiology, which recognizes that the societal hierarchy of class relations "conditions most potently how other variables affect the population's health" (p. 21). Navarro's materialist epidemiology contrasts sharply with dominant views of epidemiology, especially with respect to its usefulness to inform anti-oppressive practice. Conventional epidemiology, with its very strong focus on quantitative analyses, leaves little room for incorporation of racism as a key factor in population health outcomes. Social epidemiology and materialist epidemiology hold great promise in their potential to provide richly contextualized evidence for policy change to fight racism.

Ultimately it is structural inequality that so powerfully determines the health of individuals, families, communities, and nations. Structural inequalities are caused by the systemic, institutionalized structures that create and maintain inequality. In modern capitalist societies these structures include the institutions of education, law, government and health care. Much of this book is dedicated to bringing these inequalities into plain view. Materialist epidemiology in particular seeks to discover the articulation of societal power structures with the everyday experience of inequality—lack of money for a good breakfast, school supplies or a raincoat; lack of the means for participation on sports teams; limited opportunity for post-secondary education; the near impossibility of having safe and dignified housing; and all of the other countless and persistent impacts of poverty on health.

As the field of epidemiology continues to draw from critical social science, the population health impact of racism will receive the serious attention it warrants. In fact, the integration of social science into the biomedically dominated field of epidemiology is echoed in several of the most important perspectives on health in the 20th century. These perspectives are described in the following sections.

Sociological Perspectives

Sociological perspectives help us to explore the historical influences of current thinking about social problems, health, and illness. When we understand some of the social influences on our behaviour and thinking, then we are usually in a better position to work for change. Sociological perspectives have been central in shaping the way we think about the world around us, including our thoughts about the nature of health, illness, and health care. Several overarching traditions in sociological thought are described below: structural functional, conflict theory, and symbolic interaction, and important new traditions such as critical theory, feminism, anti-racism, and post-colonialism. These traditions are briefly described in terms of their historical evolution and hence their influence on our current thinking. From the work of Erving Goffman (1961) and others, to the work of Marie Battiste (2000), Stuart Hall (Hall & duGay, 1996), Patricia Hill Collins (1990) and Dorothy Smith (1987), the evolving thread of critique of dominant societal structures has helped to form the foundation of anti-racist, post-colonial thinking and theory.

The work of Karl Marx (1991) is relevant to several of the perspectives discussed here. Many of the writings of Marx explored the labour process in capitalist societies, including the economic exploitation of workers, and the relationship between those who own and control the means of production of the goods and services of society, and those who do not. One of Marx's most enduring contributions was his analysis of social class as a central marker of oppression. His explanation of the causes and consequences of class-based economic inequality remains relevant for many modern-day analyses of the unequal distribution of poorer health outcomes around the globe.

Structural Functional or Systems Theory

Structural functionalism, also known as systems theory, analyzes social systems in a way that is analogous to biological and engineering models (Kelly & Field, 1998). Systems have parts and these parts function together to ensure the stability of the overall system. Component parts have their own function and they are functionally articulated to the larger system. For example, the liver is made up of cells that have their own structure and function. These cells function together to comprise the liver and all of its physiological functions. The liver in turn functions within the body to ensure dynamic equilibrium within the entire body as a system. Engineering analogies may be similarly described as a system that functions together with its constituent parts. Cables on a bridge are designed to function in dynamic equilibrium as their steel components expand or contract with daily temperature variations. The cables form a structural part of the rest of the bridge, which functions in a particular way to maintain its structural integrity. Structural functional sociology became increasingly based on these biological and engineering models, and society was viewed in terms of how individual and group social roles related, or articulated to, the functioning of society as a system.

Structural functional theory is based on several main assumptions, including: (1) society can be understood as a social system, which is relatively stable over time; (2) institutions, as regular and recurrent patterns of social roles, contribute to social stability, and therefore can be said to have functions; and (3) the social order is in a state of dynamic equilibrium in most societies (Garner, 2000). The application of structural functionalism to the field of medical sociology began with Talcott Parsons, who described in detail the function of the modern medical practice within society (Bourgeault, 2006). Parsons discussed elements of social relationships and described how they would change in the face of illness, and how equilibrium would be disturbed and then re-established when the illness was over (Kelly & Field, 1998) "In the Parsonian view of sickness, normal functioning is interrupted, ordinary responsibilities are relinquished, and a special relationship with medical professionals is established and negative moral connotations are not applied" (p. 222). For Parsons, it was essential to look for mechanisms that tend to protect order.

Systems theory has been very popular in the health fields, where undergraduate curricula in the 1970s and 1980s often used systems theory as a curricular frame in Western countries. This is no surprise, given the theory's links with the structure and function of biological systems. Today we still see the ongoing influence and use of systems theory in the health literature where it is used to describe concepts such as management. Structural functionalism or systems theory has been, and continues to be, critiqued for its mechanistic framework. A system has inputs, processes, and outputs. Dynamic equilibrium in society is maintained through consensus. Thus, systems theory assumes consensus and does not account for the particular modes of consensus building, or social sanctions that are imposed for lack of consensus building. Also, it clearly does not account for the complexity and synergy in complex adaptive systems such as the health care system (McPherson, 2008).

In terms of anti-racist practice, there are many problems with structural functionalism or systems theory, including the assumption of the possibility of attaining consensus (thus assuming that everyone has equal bargaining power at the decision-making tables, or even that people of colour have a seat at the table). Another strong shortcoming is the theory's ultimate failure to accommodate important philosophical questions in areas such as the centrality of social justice in health care.

Symbolic Interactionism or Interpretive Sociology

Symbolic interactionism, also known as interpretive sociology, was in some ways a rejection of structural functionalism with its large impersonal and mechanistic systems and its abstract detachment from actual social situations. For symbolic interactionists, behaviour is symbolic as people respond to their interpretation of the meaning of the actions of others. "The patterns of behaviour that people come to interpret as social roles are actively created and negotiated, sustained or abandoned, in on-going interaction. These patterns are constantly subject to reinterpretation by the role players involved as well as the onlookers" (Hale, 1990, p. 31). Thus, society and self are not fixed and well-defined concepts. Rather, they are open to ongoing interpretation, and these interpretations of social life may be as varied and different as those observing or experiencing them. Symbolic interactionists insisted that social theory should be based or grounded in everyday activities and behaviours, hence the term grounded theory. In this way, symbolic interaction became known as a micro-perspective due to its detailed attention to the nuances of human interaction.

Howard Becker and Erving Goffman were foremost symbolic interactionists in the 1950s to the 1970s. Howard Becker's (1963) famous work, *Outsiders*, described how perceptions of the world of jazz musicians and marijuana users were socially constructed. In keeping with symbolic interactionism's grounded focus in everyday life, Becker spent much time in the field. In the course of his work he also argued that difference and deviance were constructed social categories with inherent negative connotations, and that deviance in this case was "only deviant in the context of then current norms about race, drugs, and lifestyles" (Garner, 2000, p. 331). One of Goffman's (1961) most important contributions, *Asylums: Essays on the Social Situation of Mental Patients and Other Inmates*, provided a detailed critique of the social roles and controlling structures inherent in the daily operation of the "total institution."

Goffman's (1961) detailed ethnographic work in a large American mental hospital and his analysis of prisons had the chief aim of developing "a sociological version of the structure of the self" (p. xiii). Gofffman described how mental institutions worked to diminish and damage self-concept. This was accomplished through psychiatric labelling, the institutional placement of the physician as sole decision maker, and the systematic application and enforcement of institutional rules. Goffman and his contemporary Ivan Illich (1976) brought a sociological analysis to the largely taken-for-granted dominance and power of the medical profession and what Goffman described as "the medical model." These ideas are further explored in the discussion of biomedicine later in this chapter. Symbolic interactionism thus helped to open up the world of interrogating power in human relations and in human systems, a point that was to be taken up by all the critical perspectives that followed it.

Conflict Theory

Conflict theory emerged as a challenge to structural functionalism and the tendency for sociologists in general to seek theories that provided blanket explanations for all human behaviour. C. Wright Mills (1959), one of the most important conflict theorists, critiqued grand theories and sociology's attempt to legitimize these explanations through quantitative, usually survey, methods. He viewed these methods as an unfortunate tendency toward empirical studies of contemporary social facts and problems. In his 1959 book *The Sociological Imagination*, Mills took aim at the "grand theories" of Parsons and others, which had an embedded assumption of the legitimacy of power in societies.

> *In his [Parsons] scheme, we are required to read out of the picture the facts of power and indeed of all institutional structures, in particular, the economic, the political, the military. In this curious "general theory," such structures of domination have no place.... The idea of the normative order that is set forth, and the way it is handled by grand theorists, leads us to assume that all power is legitimated.... In these terms, the idea of conflict cannot be effectively formulated (Garner, 2000, p. 42).*

Mills argued that society is not a relatively harmonious system, and that conflict was inevitable. He stated that the basic problem of power lies in who is making the decisions about the rules and arrangements under which we live. This explicit attention to power distinguished conflict theory from structural functionalism and set the stage for critical analyses of social, political, and economic power.

These first writings in conflict theory drew upon North American political thought in the post-World War II era, especially the ideals of radical democracy and left-wing populism (Garner, 2000). Conflict theorists, although reluctant to call themselves Marxists, based their theory in acknowledgement of differential societal power, status, and wealth that results in inequities. Conflict theory holds that society is not a system and that it is formed by groups with opposing and competing interests. Mills's ideas about the limits of empiricism, the importance of examining power, and the need to study social problems within their historical institutional structures arguably established much of the foundation for critical social scientific thought in the latter half of the 20th century. Conflict theorists connected societal power with economic power and laid the groundwork for analyzing which groups of people had power, which ones did not, and how this situation came to be.

Critical Theory

As the three perspectives of structural functionalism, symbolic interactionism, and conflict theory began to lose their boundaries, sociologists such as Jurgen Habermas (1973) continued and refined the theoretical perspective known as critical theory (Bailey & Gayle, 2003; Garner, 2000). Here, the word critical is used in the philosophical sense of a close examination, which may or may not be negative. Among other important cultural and societal issues, Habermas critiqued common notions of the meaning of democracy. He argued that democracy was no longer about having a voice in collective decision making and self-determination. Rather, democracy became a means of distributing power among relatively few citizens. In his essay, *Formal Democracy*, Habermas (1973) stated: "This democracy makes possible *prosperity without freedom*. It is no longer tied to political equality in the sense of an equal distribution of political power, that is, of the chances to exercise power" (p. 123). The resulting political disenfranchisement meant that, for many, the tools for liberation remained elusive. The following principles were used by Patricia E. Stevens in 1992 to help public health nursing practitioners understand how critical social theory can be applied to front-line practice. They remain among the clearest applications of critical theory to everyday health care practice.

1. All research, theory, and practice are political because they are intimately affected by the social, economic, and political processes of the society.
2. Oppressive power relations are common in society and usually they operate without much notice and are taken for granted.
3. Scientific and practical ways of thinking and getting things done are open to systematic questioning and criticism.
4. Social, economic, and political conditions have a history.
5. One can better understand the changing conditions of society's health by studying the historical development of unsafe physical surroundings, oppressive social arrangements, economic inequities, and political disenfranchisement.
6. Liberation from oppressive environmental constraints is an indispensable part of any group's pursuit of well-being and integrity. (Stevens, 1992, p. 203)

Box 4.1 starts with an exercise about applying critical theory to practice, and provides examples of how critical theory applies to anti-racist practice.

Box 4.1: Applying Critical Social Theory to Practice

Directions:
1. Individually, or in groups, discuss each of Stevens's principles of critical social theory.
2. Using the examples below as a guide, discuss a health-related example. Incorporate the social determinants of health as much as possible.
3. Once you have thought of a general example, discuss more specific examples with: (a) children; (b) elders; (c) women; (d) families who live in persistent poverty; (e) lesbian, gay, bisexual, or transgendered people; and (f) people with disabilities.
4. Finally, pick a few of your examples and, if you have not done so already, discuss some of the ways in which race and ethnicity are important.

Critical Social Principle (Stevens, 1992)	Example
All research, theory, and practice are political because they are intimately affected by the social, economic, and political processes of the society.	Suicide is the leading cause of death for young people in Canada. Indigenous young people have an even higher suicide rate. The mental health of Indigenous peoples has been shown to be intimately connected with the historical trauma of colonialism.
Oppressive power relations are common in society; usually they operate without much notice and are taken for granted.	Have a look at any art history or philosophy text. Count the number of women artists and philosophers. Count the number of people of colour. Do the same procedure with today's local or national newspaper. Also discuss: When pictures of women and people of colour are represented, what is the context?
Scientific and practical ways of thinking and getting things done are open to systematic questioning and criticism.	The Apgar scale has been used for decades to assess the health of newborn babies. It is used for all babies regardless of skin tone. One of the criteria is pinkness of skin, which is not applicable to babies of colour. No adequate scale has been developed.
Social, economic, and political conditions have a history.	The Indian Act of 1876 is recognized as a key foundation of Indigenous peoples' struggles in Canada.
One can better understand the changing conditions of society's health by studying the historical development of unsafe physical surroundings, oppressive social arrangements, economic inequities, and political disenfranchisement.	Over the past 10 years, child poverty in Canada has been statistically proportional to federal and provincial cuts to social programs for families and children. Child poverty in Canada is higher than it has ever been.
Liberation from oppressive environmental constraints is an indispensable part of any group's pursuit of well-being and integrity.	Globally, birth rates are directly proportional to the level of education of a nation's women. Increased education results in lower birth rates. When women have the choice, around the world, they most often choose to have smaller families.

Feminism, Anti-racism, Post-colonialism, and Anti-colonialism

The critical perspectives discussed so far all address societal power structures. Although somewhat distinct in their origins, feminism, anti-racism, post-colonialism, and anti-colonialism share critical theory's focus on progressive social change that addresses societal power structures and societal oppression. For this reason they are described together. These areas of thought have important interconnections, based on the work of scholars of colour such as Joan Anderson, Himani Bannerji, Marie Battiste, Agnes Calliste, Patricia Hill Collins, Afua Cooper, George Sefa Dei, W.E.B. Dubois, Stuart Hall, Frances Henry, bell hooks, and Carl James. In terms of the interwoven nature of feminism, anti-racism, and post-colonialism, the early origins of modern-day feminism serve as a case in point. The term "feminism," in its historical and current meanings, is by no means cohesive or static. Feminism is most widely known as women's political activism on behalf of women for the continued advancement of women's rights. The centrality of patriarchal dominance is emphasized as a core area for social change. Although feminism is popularly viewed as some sort of homogeneous set of ideas, there are many feminisms, such as Black feminist thought, that focus on interrogating not only patriarchy, but also White privilege.

The first wave of feminism involved the fight for the right to vote and to be considered a person under the law. Suffragists such as Constance Litton and Susan B. Anthony were taken violently from quiet demonstrations in London and put in jail due to their insistence on women's right to vote. The movement to abolish slavery in the United States was also a concern for many of these early feminists, although it became apparent that this first wave of the women's movement was progressing at the exclusion of Black and Indigenous women. Sojourner Truth was a Black leader who was central in the fight for abolition. Her accomplishments were remarkable, given the brutal, overt racism she encountered in colonial America. In her speech at a Women's Rights Convention in Akron, Ohio in 1851, she brought the exclusion of Black women forward with her now famous question: "Ain't I a woman?"

Sojourner Truth's words still echo in the modern women's movement. Contemporary feminist scholars such as Patricia Hill Collins (2000), Agnes Calliste (2000), bell hooks (1994), and Himani Bannerji (2006) have emphasized the omission of women of colour in historical and contemporary feminist theorizing, echoing Sojourner Truth's words of over 150 years ago. Feminist theory has increasingly examined the intersections of race, gender, and social class as they compound to increase women's oppression. Bannerji's work, for example, builds on the Marxist notion of class to include gender and race. Black feminist scholars such as Collins, Calliste, and hooks have intertwined post-colonial and feminist theorizing, thus demonstrating the relationship between women's oppression and colonial oppression. Collins (2000) brings forward the "thrown away" intellectual work of African-American women over the centuries: "This painstaking process of collecting the ideas and actions of 'thrown away' Black women like Maria Stewart has revealed one important discovery. Black women intellectuals have laid a vital foundation for a distinctive standpoint on self, community, and society, and in doing so, created a multifaceted, African American women's intellectual tradition" (p. 319).

The exclusion of Black women's ideas in mainstream academic discourse and their marginalization in both feminist and Black social and political arenas demonstrates that Black women intellectuals have remained as "outsiders" within all three domains—they are known as the "Other." Collins (1990) noted that full membership in these three groups is assumed to be based on "Whiteness for feminist thought, maleness for Black social and political thought, and the combination for mainstream scholarship—all of which negate a Black female reality" (p. 12). As the "Other" within these areas of inquiry, Black women have continued to use the knowledge gained at the intersection of race, gender, and class oppression to provide a distinctive angle of vision on the theories generated in these areas of inquiry and the reality of Black women (Collins). From this perspective, feminist scholars strive to understand the differing roles of oppression that might undermine the "idea of sameness" of all women (Barbee, 1994). Box 4.2 provides a perspective on Black feminist thought from Patricia Hill Collins (1990).

Box 4.2: Patricia Hill Collins on Black Feminist Thought

Black feminist thought demonstrates Black women's emerging power as agents of knowledge. By portraying African-American women as self-defined, self-reliant individuals confronting race, gender, and class oppression, Afrocentric feminist thought speaks to the importance that oppression. Afrocentric feminist thought also speaks to the importance that knowledge plays in empowering oppressed people. One distinguishing feature of Black feminist thought is its insistence that both the changed consciousness of individuals and the social transformation of political and economic institutions constitute essential ingredients for social change. New knowledge is important for both dimensions to change.

Knowledge is a vitally important part of the social relations of domination and resistance. By objectifying African-American women and recasting our experiences to serve the interests of elite white men, much of the Eurocentric masculinist worldview fosters Black women's subordination. But placing Black women's experiences at the center of analysis offers fresh insights on the prevailing concepts, paradigms, and epistemologies of this worldview and on its feminist and Afrocentric critiques. Viewing the world through a "both/and" conceptual lens of the simultaneity of race, class, and gender oppression and of the need for a humanist vision of community creates new possibilities for an empowering Afrocentric feminist knowledge. Many Black feminist intellectuals have long thought about the world in this way because this is the way we experience the world.

Source: Collins, Patricia Hill. (1990). *Black feminist thought: Knowledge, consciousness, and the politics of empowerment (p. 221).* New York: Routledge.

Feminist theories, like any political philosophies, provide the intellectual tools to examine historical injustices and to build arguments to support action for social change. The core of feminist theory rests in the insistence that inequality is based in social oppression rather than individual misfortune (McCann & Kim, 2003). Simone de Beauvoir's *The Second Sex*, first published in France in 1949, was the first widely disseminated theorizing about women's inequality. It sold 2,000 copies in the first few weeks of its publication in France. Almost three decades later in the 1970s, de Beauvoir's book became a central force in galvanizing ideas about women's oppression and possible paths for working for equality. In 1976 Adrienne Rich's *Of Woman Born: Motherhood as Experience and Institution* provided a theoretical and personal analysis of the experience of motherhood from a feminist lens. "In order for all women to have real choices all along the line, we need fully to understand the power and powerlessness embodied in motherhood in patriarchal culture" (p. 23). Rich's (1980) "Compulsory Heterosexuality and Lesbian Existence" brought a feminist perspective to understanding lesbian experience.

Barbara Ehrenreich (1971) and Barbara Keddy (1996) helped to bring feminist thinking to the health fields with their critique of the manner in which women's bodies have been treated by the medical profession, and their call for a gender-based analysis of health and health care. These women linked patriarchy and oppression to women's poorer health outcomes. More recently women scholars in Canada have linked the even poorer health outcomes of women of colour with the oppression of racism (Etowa et al., 2007; Sharif, Dar & Amaratunga, 2002; Thomas Bernard, 2002). Their work continued the sociological interest in the body as a site of oppression, and in particular the body as a site of oppression of people of colour.

Feminist sociologists such as Dorothy Smith (1987) sought to develop a procedure for examining how local, everyday practices were articulated to extra-local relations of ruling. Relations of ruling were described as "a complex of organized practices, including government, law, business and financial management, professional organizations, and educational institutions as well as the discourses and texts that interpenetrate the multiple sites of power" (p. 3). Like Bannerji (2006), Smith drew from Marxian ideas about class structure and the transmission of power based on social class, and extended Marx's class analysis to include gender and patriarchy. Smith's method of institutional ethnography has been used to analyze power relations in a broad spectrum of areas in the health and human service fields. Smith provided one of the few critical research methods that brings forward the ways in which everyday clinical practice is articulated to societal power structures (Campbell, 1988, 1990; Cassin, 1990; Gregor, 1996; McGibbon, 2004; Smith, 1995).

In addition to examining women's work, Smith (1987, 1990a) provided an important feminist sociological analysis of mental illness. She explicitly linked the stress caused by oppressive social situations to the declaration of a mental illness and hence to the social control of psychiatry. Based on the work of Thomas Szasz (1961), R.D. Laing (1967), and others, Smith explored an alternative way of thinking about mental illness. Szasz, Laing, and Breggin (1991) began what was termed the anti-psychiatry movement in the 1960s and 1970s, so called for its explicit critique of psychiatry's lack of ability to incorporate sociological principles about power and oppression. Feminist psychologists such as Carol Gilligan and Judith Herman also solidified a feminist critique of dominant views of women's mental health. Carol Gilligan's (1993) book *In a Different Voice: Psychological Theory and Women's Development* proposed that women's psychological development could not be easily or accurately described by the dominant theories of Freud, Erikson, and Piaget, which used male psychology as the normative foundation.

The extent of the dominance of using male normative foundations for teaching is still evident in modern textbooks in fields such as nursing, medicine, and psychology, where Erikson's stages are still used as the gold standard to describe developmental stages across the lifespan, despite over three decades of voluminous feminist literature about women's psychological development. Heterosexuality is also presented as the normative sexuality throughout much of the 19th century and 20th century's prominent psychological writings. Feminists such as Adrienne Rich (1980) questioned "compulsory heterosexuality" and challenged the "erasure of lesbian existence from so much of scholarly feminist literature …" (p. 1).

Psychological theories, whether conventional or feminist, were developed largely with the exclusion of people of colour. Thus, Eurocentric norms have prevailed regarding concepts of optimal psychological development. The work of feminist scholars such as Calliste, Collins, and hooks incorporates ideas about women's oppression within the particulars of historical and current oppression of people of colour. Books such as Agnes Calliste and George Sefa Dei's (2000) *Anti-racist Feminism: Critical Race and Gender Studies* brought anti-racist and feminist thought together in the Canadian context. These authors continued a critical analysis of the interrelationships among gender, race, ethnicity, social class, and sexuality. In their book *The Color of Democracy: Racism in Canadian Society*, authors Frances Henry, Carol Tator, Winston Mattis, and Tim Rees (2000) described how racism operates in Canada. "Racist ideology provides the conceptual framework for the political, social, and cultural structures of inequality and systems of dominance based on race, as well as the processes of exclusion and marginalization of people of colour that characterize Canadian society" (p. 16). Anti-racism theory examines these systemic structures and corresponding mechanisms to counteract racism. Understanding the White privilege that sustains racism became an important feature of anti-racist education (Dei, 1996). According to Henry et al. (2000), a further important dimension of anti-racism is the critique of "liberal" notions such as individualism, equal opportunity, and colour-blindness.

Grace-Edward Galabuzi (2006), a Canadian anti-racist scholar, described the process of social exclusion of racialized peoples in *Canada's Economic Apartheid: The Social Exclusion of Racialized Groups in the New Century*. Galabuzi emphasized the restructuring of global and national economies and the resulting impact of market-oriented commodification of public goods and services, including health care services. Intensification of labour through longer hours, work fragmentation, individuals having multiple jobs, and increasing non-standard forms of work all disproportionately affect racialized peoples. Galabuzi's emphasis on the political and economic origins of inequality echoes elements of Navarro's political economy analysis. George Sefa Dei (2000) emphasized the teaching-learning context of anti-racism education and the need to rethink the role of Indigenous knowledges in academic settings such as universities. Dei (2000) described the process of transformative learning:

> ... education should be able to resist oppression and domination by strengthening the individual self and the collective souls to deal with the continued reproduction of colonial and re-colonial relations in the academy. It must also assist the learner to deal with pervasive effects of imperial structures of the academy on the processes of knowledge production and validation; the understanding of indigenity; and the pursuit of agency, resistance and politics for educational change. (p. 1)

Dei's emphasis on the relationships among anti-racist education, colonialism, and educating for change has been central in bringing an anti-racist discourse to education in Canada. According to Dei (1996), practice and experience should provide the context for the development of social and intellectual knowledge. This is an important distinction when we consider the context of the health fields, where scientific, observable facts form the basis for much of health care decision making. Although practice and experience do inform knowledge development, health field knowledge itself is generally required to originate in fact. This presents a dilemma for anti-racist health care practice. On the one hand, health care practice must be very much grounded in facts, such as the anatomical structures and physiological processes of the human body. The study of health inequities also relies, in part, on the collection and analysis of population health statistics. On the other hand, reliance on factual information will get us only so far in our pursuit of justice. As Dei points out, practice and experience must be central. However, scientific facts-based approaches are dominant in the health fields, regardless of the social problem being considered. Anti-racism has little room to flourish when biomedicine is the predominant approach because anti-racist practice must be grounded in the lived experience of oppression and its foundations in White privilege.

Carl James's (2003) focus on identity, the social construction of cultural identity, and racism, and his attention to stories of the lived experience of racism provided a close examination of notions of identity and difference. James's contribution included a critical analysis of the familial and social contexts of how we form our identities, and their relationship to psychological factors such as attitude, personality, motivation, and communication. James's work emphasized the complexities of bringing discussions about identity and difference into post-secondary classrooms, and how these discussions might inform social change. According to James, considering diversity in terms of race, ethnicity, racism, and difference is challenging because there are many schools of thought about how best to approach teaching and learning. For James, anti-racist education involves shifting our prisms of perception in such a way that new perspectives are opened up that help us to negotiate and renegotiate our identities.

> *Yet, consensus is not necessary or even desirable: our social, political and emotional investment in these issues differ, and we bring our subjective viewpoints to the interpretations and understandings we hold and articulate. So what happens when we explore issues of diversity related to race and ethnicity, and give students the opportunity to talk about such issues and concerns? What will they tell us? What knowledge will be forthcoming? (pp. 19 to 20)*

Sherene Razack (1998) provided detailed analyses of gender, race, and culture and the relationships among oppressors and the oppressed. Razack's emphasis on the roles of White people in the maintenance of colonial oppression provided clear links among the history of oppression in Canada and its modern-day perpetuation. "Although the encounter between colonizer and colonized changes in historically specific ways, and is always highly gendered, it remains a moment when powerful narratives turn oppressed peoples into objects, to be held in contempt, or to be saved from their fates by more civilized beings" (p. 3). Many Canadians still believe that colonialism is a thing of the past. The scant attention to colonialism in grade school and high school curriculum, if it was even called colonialism, did not help to educate White people regarding the enormity and longevity of oppression. Razack's attention to the ways in which racism is denied in Canada provided a direct gaze toward White people and the effective strategies used in contemporary Canada to muddy the issues of modern racism. Like Galabuzi (2006), James (2003), Calliste (2000), and Dei (2000), Razack brought forward a critical perspective on notions of multiculturalism, diversity, and tolerance, all terms that obscure the realities of unearned power, White privilege, and the perpetuation of claims that we are all equal in Canada.

Post-colonial perspectives explicitly name colonialism as a destructive and enduring societal force. In an anti-colonial perspective, explicit attention to the continued legacy of colonialism has led to sustained attention to the relationship between colonial oppression and racism. Oppression and racism thus form an overarching frame to understand the etiology and perpetuation of unjust treatment in the health care system and in society as a whole. Marie Battiste, a Mi'kmaq educator from the Potlo'tek First Nation in Nova Scotia, and a professor at the University of Saskatchewan, has spoken and written extensively about colonial oppression. Her book *Reclaiming Indigenous Voice and Vision* (2000) addressed four urgent issues: (1) mapping colonialism, (2) diagnosing colonialism, (3) healing colonized Indigenous peoples, and (4) imagining post-colonial visions of healing and well-being in more socially just societies. Battiste's work in some ways echoed the writings of Patricia Hill Collins (1990) regarding the significance of the oppressor's appropriation of voice and language. The material loss of homelands was accompanied by a strategic, systematic, and enduring attack on Indigenous culture and language. In this context, centuries of oppression in Canada cannot be ameliorated with state-based housing programs and "free" university tuition.

European colonization and cognitive imperialism have a five-centuries-old history on the planet. Cognitive imperialism involves the colonization of people's minds over many years and through all of the mechanisms of colonization. Systemic destruction of Indigenous ways of knowing, coupled with enduring replacement messages of savagery and laziness (perpetrated by systems such a government and education) have profoundly influenced the ways that Indigenous peoples think about themselves. However, as the new millennium unfolds, many voices and forums are coming together to form a new perspective on Indigenous knowledge (Battiste, 2000). These voices:

> ... represent the thoughts and experiences of the people of the earth whom Europeans have characterized as primitive, backward, and inferior – the colonized and dominated people of the last five centuries. The voices of these victims of the empire, once predominately silenced in the social sciences, have been not only resisting colonization in thought and in actions but also attempting to restore Indigenous knowledge and heritage. (p. xvi)

The centuries-old legacy of colonization is being increasingly brought forward by anti-colonialism scholars and practitioners. The groundbreaking work of Cynthia Wesley-Esquimaux and Maglalena Smolewski (2004) built on psychological trauma theory, including the work of Judith Herman (1972), to develop a critical analysis of the psychological transmission of oppression-based trauma in Aboriginal peoples. "Since the issue of repetitive and circular trauma never truly entered into Western perception, as it was never properly analyzed and never understood, no healing modality was designed to assist Aboriginal people to prepare for, or respond to, the demands associated with such a profound social and cultural loss" (Wesley-Esquimaux & Smolewski, 2004, p. 53). Research in the health fields is being transformed by critical and Indigenous methodologies, all of which address colonialism as a foundation for the struggles of Indigenous peoples.

Table 4.1 traces how each of the sociological perspectives discussed above might inform an analysis of a health care issue. Specifically, depression is described in terms of how the various perspectives would inform clinical approaches to intervention. It is important to note that some of the perspectives share similar ways of thinking. For example, it may very well be the case that feminist therapists use some of the principles of symbolic interactionism in their work with people experiencing depression. Anti-racism theory is consistent with the anti-oppressive principles of critical theory, and counseling with an adolescent experiencing depression could be informed by both of these perspectives. As Table 4.1 also illustrates, conflict theory laid the foundations for the critical perspectives that followed it such as critical theory and feminism. Interestingly, structure functionalism, also known as systems theory, still forms the foundation for much of modern psychiatry, where medication is usually the first choice of intervention for depression.

Table 4.1: How Sociological Perspectives Might View Depression

Sociological Perspective	View of Depression
Systems Theory	The body is a system. Intervention for depression will involve balancing various bodily systems (neurological, endocrine, etc.).
Symbolic Interactionism	Depression may be understood through a reflection of ongoing interpretation of a person's social contexts. Intervention for depression involves detailed attention to the nuances of human interaction. The context of psychiatric power must be analyzed.
Conflict Theory	Depression may be understood through an examination of differential societal power, status, and wealth that result in inequities. High depression and suicide rates in Indigenous youth originate in historical imbalance.
Critical Theory	Examination of oppressive conditions in a depressed person's life provides a social and political context for intervention. Action for social change to decrease oppression is a goal of clinical practice (advocating, lobbying, community development...)
Feminism	Women's depression is related to their position in a patriarchal society. Intervention will involve consciousness raising about oppressive personal and societal conditions. (Note that feminisms, such as anti-racist feminism, address many different oppressions.) Action for social change to decrease oppression is a goal of clinical practice (advocating, lobbying, community development...)
Anti-racism	Depression is related to the stress of individual and societal racism. Intervention will involve consciousness raising about the impact of individual and systemic racism. Action for social change to decrease oppression is a goal of clinical practice (advocating, lobbying, community development...)
Anti-colonialism	Depression is related to the racist legacy of colonialism, and the generational transmission of the traumatic experiences of ancestors. Intervention will involve consciousness raising about the ongoing impact of colonialism. Action for social change to decrease oppression is a goal of clinical practice (advocating, lobbying, community development...)

The above discussion about sociological perspectives demonstrates that many of them are not mutually exclusive. Differences in societal power, and related dominant societal power structures, are recognized for their creation of disadvantage that profoundly impacts health and well-being. Political economy perspectives also draw upon ideas about societal power and its inequitable distribution.

Political Economy Perspectives

Political economy perspectives on health and health care direct our attention to questions about why some groups of people have better health than others, and why some countries have different kinds of health care systems and correspondingly different health outcomes for their citizens. The focus is on the links among health and economic, political, and social life (Coburn, 2001). Political economy approaches echo Marx's focus on a critique of neo-liberalism and a call for a materialist analysis of health and health care. Although there is a growing field of knowledge regarding health inequities, an important area that has not received its due attention is the analysis of the social and political origins of ill health—the how and the why of ill health (Navarro, 2002). For example, the income inequality model acknowledges the relationship between income and health, but stops short of connecting the poor health of poor people to race and class inequality in capitalist societies (Muntaner et al., 2002). A political economy perspective is central to an understanding of the genesis of oppression-related health outcomes, such as those documented in Canada and elsewhere. People of colour have the poorest overall health outcomes in the country.

A political economy perspective links global policies such as those set by the International Monetary Fund and the World Bank with health outcomes in the global South and North. National, provincial, territorial, and local health and social policies are shown to be linked to population health outcomes. Even in the "rich" countries, such as Canada and the U.S., child poverty is relatively high, and in the case of the United States, is comparable to countries in the global South. Political economy perspectives on health focus on the "causes of the causes." While there is general agreement that the social determinants of health cause poorer health outcomes, we often fail to direct our attention squarely on what causes such differences in the SDOH in the first place. If we plan to achieve justice, there must be an awakening to the political economy of health inequities. Exactly which policies, which political parties and which ideas create the substrate for persistent poverty in Canada? A political economy perspective links public policy, the ideological foundations of political parties and governments, and the distribution of health and disease in citizens. These connections are further explored in Chapter 7. Political economy analyses of inequities in the social determinants of health, and related population health inequities, continue to play a central role in illuminating the unjust distribution of the goods and services of society. These injustices are increasingly being linked to human rights violations in Canada and around the globe.

Human Rights Perspectives

Human rights perspectives have provided an important foundation for discussion of inequities in health care access and in health outcomes. Locating health and health care within the scope of human rights provides a social justice framework for addressing health inequities and unfair access to health care. The word justice in everyday speech usually suggests fairness and ideas regarding decisions about what is owed to the members of a society. In the study of health inequity, distributive justice is emphasized because it encompasses the moral virtue of collective responsibility for the just distribution of the goods and services of society (Rawls, 1971). In this context, the measure of a society is how it treats its most vulnerable citizens. Rawls brought an examination of dominant social, economic, and political power structures to the philosophical examination of justice.

Although ethical principles such as informed consent and respect for autonomy are important in a social justice perspective, the focus, both nationally and internationally in the field of social justice and health, rests firmly on principles of distributive justice and social democracy (Bryant, Raphael & Rioux, 2006; Labonte, Schrecker & Gupta, 2005; McGibbon, 2008; Navarro, 2004). Social justice is related to human rights because human rights are legal mechanisms to promote or ensure social justice for the citizens of a country, and indeed for the global citizen, as is the case for United Nations Conventions that seek to protect the rights of women, children, and Aboriginal peoples.

A human rights and social justice perspective encourages questions such as: Why do certain groups of people consistently have poorer health outcomes, even when biologic and genetic makeup are taken into consideration? What is the additional cost of health care for rural families, and how does this cost affect health outcomes in families with children who have serious chronic illnesses? Why is there a higher suicide rate among lesbian-gay-bisexual-transgender (LGBT) adolescents (Kitts, 2005)? Through which policies, current and past, did racialized peoples come to have overall poorer health outcomes than White people? If Canadians all have the right to health care, as described in the Canada Health Act (1984), then why do inequities in access continue to persist across the country? These kinds of questions direct our attention to how societies make policy decisions about which citizens will be left out if everyone is treated equally rather than equitably (McGibbon, Etowa & McPherson, 2008).

The difference between equality and equity is central to social justice-based understanding and action regarding health care. If we treat everyone equally, we will not have such things as wheelchair ramps, health services tailored for homeless people, or health interpreters for immigrant families in the emergency department. Equity in health care occurs when all individuals, families, and communities have fair and universally comparable access to the goods and services of our health care system. Therefore, social justice in health refers to the fair, and hence equitable, distribution of the goods, services, and opportunities necessary for psychological, spiritual, and physical health and well-being. Explicit attention to societal power structures is fundamental to a social justice perspective because social injustice in health care systems has its roots in systemic power imbalance. Box 4.4 provides a summary of important historical milestones and global legal documents that have informed human rights perspectives on health.

> **Box 4.4: Health System Change through the Lens of Human Rights**
>
> The social movement to link health and human rights is relatively recent. The United Nations (UN) implemented the first worldwide public health and human rights strategy in the 1980s through its global program in AIDS. Further, World Health Organization (WHO) initiatives in the 1990s, based on the UN Charter of Rights and Freedoms, brought health and human rights together in international law (Gruskin, Mills & Tarantala, 2007). Decades earlier, in the challenge of the Jim Crow laws that legalized the dehumanization of African Americans, leaders in the civil rights movement in North America linked civil rights with the right to health care, based on the lack of access to basic health care for African-American people. The successful challenge of these laws led to the creation of a civil rights report card that detailed the results of human rights violations in the United States health care system (Smith, 2005). This direct link between human rights and health care remains one of the earliest strategies to address health inequities through legalization of equitable health care treatment. A human rights perspective on health care reframes healthy population outcomes as a legal entitlement, rather than a desired but not always achievable goal. The movement towards defining health as a human right requires a social injustice based analysis of the relationships among health and social policy decisions, health and social service expenditures, population health outcomes, and the social determinants of health.
>
> The Canadian Charter of Rights and Freedoms (1982), and a number of international human rights instruments that Canada has ratified, provide a legal and social policy basis for civil society pressure to remove barriers in access to health care. Relevant international documents include the United Nations Universal Declaration of Human Rights (1948), the International Covenant on Economic, Cultural and Social Rights (1966), and the Convention on the Elimination of all Forms of Discrimination against Women (1979). For example, the latter Convention obligates the state to uphold the right of rural women to: "have access to adequate health care facilities, including information, counseling and services in family planning ... to enjoy living conditions, particularly in relation to housing, sanitation, electricity and water supply, transport and communications" (1979). The Convention on the Rights of the Child (1989), Article 24, required that states "recognize the right of the child to the enjoyment of the highest attainable standard of health and to facilities for the treatment of illness and rehabilitations of health ... and strive to ensure that no child is deprived of his or her right of access to such health care services" (1989). Under Canada's Charter of Rights, Section 15, inequitable access to health care is unconstitutional.
>
> *Source:* McGibbon, E. (2008). Health and health care: A human rights perspective. In D. Raphael (Ed.), *The social determinants of health: Canadian perspectives* (2nd ed.) (p. 319). Toronto: Canadian Scholars' Press Inc.

Connecting Critical Perspectives to Clinical Health Practice

Thus far, the discussion has underscored the ways in which incorporation of sociological, feminist, anti-racist, post-colonial, anti-colonial, political economy, and human rights perspectives on health and health care have been instrumental in bringing a larger context to how we think about health. These critical perspectives inform anti-racist practice because they draw attention to the paths to oppression and the policies that create and sustain oppression. Critical perspectives also greatly help to illuminate the "why" of health inequity, and thus point to avenues for social change. Due to the works of authors such as Dennis Raphael (2004) and Ron Labonte (2004) in Canada, Richard Wilkinson (Wilkinson & Marmot, 1999) and Michael Marmot (Wilkinson & Marmot, 1999) in the U.K., and Krieger (2001) in the U.S., the social determinants of health (SDOH) have become an accepted and well-known framework for thinking critically about health.

Raphael's framework of the SDOH has been instrumental in bringing a critical perspective to health and health care in Canada. Consideration of the social determinants has become a significant indicator of the urgent need to reframe biomedical perspectives of human health. As the evidence in Chapter 2 demonstrates, poverty, race, and social class are strong and definitive indicators of health outcomes, and poverty is the most powerful determinant of health (Raphael, 2006). There have been great strides in acknowledging the SDOH in national and provincial health-related government websites and documents. The Public Health Agency of Canada, and Health Canada and its provincial counterparts all, to some extent, acknowledge the importance of sociological perspectives on health and health care through the SDOH. Literature in the health fields shows a similar attention to the SDOH in the past five years. Professional associations such as the Canadian Nurses Association have produced widely disseminated documents about the importance of the SDOH (Canadian Nurses Association, 2004).

This relatively recent explicit governmental and professional acknowledgement of SDOH is the first wave of systemic or state-based incorporation of the broader social, economic, and political context of health. Previous service provision and policy frameworks were based largely on biomedically defined aspects of health. Although considerations such as poverty and housing have certainly been accounted for in some services, there has not been a cohesive expectation that SDOH considerations be within the mandate of health delivery systems. There is, to a large extent, a corresponding lack of accountability in the health care system regarding SDOH aspects of human health. Our challenge now is to move more swiftly to the second wave of incorporation of sociological perspectives in health and health care. This second wave moves the focus from acknowledgement of the SDOH to explicit acknowledgement of the systemic oppression that causes differences in the SDOH and corresponding differences in health outcomes. In terms of solutions, attending to the creation and maintenance of oppressive social structures necessarily directs the focus to systemic points of intervention.

Attention to systemic power and social change are hallmarks of several of the critical perspectives on health described here, including critical theory, feminism, anti-racism, post-colonialism, political economy, and human rights. Application of these perspectives is in its infancy within the formal health care system in Canada. Acute care intervention remains largely based in biomedicine in most jurisdictions, despite words such as diversity and respecting difference in mission statements and codes of ethics. Biomedical dominance continues to be a central aspect of the resistance to critical perspectives in the health fields. However, it must be noted that the knowledge generated by some biomedical pursuits has resulted in the amelioration of much human suffering. Few of us have not benefited from detailed knowledge of the physiology, anatomy, and bodily processes that are the foundation of biomedicine. If one of our children suffers from a particular kind of severe headache, few of us would refuse to allow testing to rule out a brain tumour as the cause. If we are involved in a motor vehicle accident, few of us would refuse to be taken to an emergency department for assessment and intervention. Immunization against polio, diphtheria, tuberculosis (TB) has been so successful that many Canadians have no memory of the TB sanatoriums that once dotted Canada's geography. The problem with biomedical thinking isn't so much that it is not useful in many situations. Rather, its relentless dominance as a way of thinking in the health fields has meant that these fields are among the last to begin to understand and incorporate critical social scientific explanations for human suffering. There is evidence, mostly in non-profit community health centres, of how aspects of biomedical science may be interconnected with critical perspectives on health and health care. The following description of best practice guidelines within a critical perspective depicts what this process might look like, using the case example of a woman with a myocardial infarction (heart attack). In this book we argue that these perspectives are not necessarily mutually exclusive, as long as there is a consistent interrogation of biomedical dominance.

Best Practices Guidelines Within a Critical Perspective

The concept of best practices is used throughout health and other fields to indicate practices that are grounded in sound knowledge, and most likely to produce a desired result. "Activities, disciplines, and methods that are available to identify, implement and monitor the available evidence in health care are called 'best practice'" (Perleth, Jakubowski & Busse, 2001, p. 235). Although there are numerous definitions of best practices, the emphasis is usually on what is referred to as "evidence-based medicine" and clinical practice guidelines. The knowledge base is primarily quantitative, and evidence is presumed to be scientific evidence. As discussed in previous chapters, the notion of scientific evidence is always contestable due to the social construction of many ideas and claims in the health fields. In much the same way as cultural competence must be reframed, best practices must also be reframed within a critical perspective if they are to have any relevance for decreasing health inequities. Best practices within a critical perspective may be defined as optimal and ethical clinical practices, which are based on: (1) a broad foundation of experiential, practical, and Indigenous knowledge(s), as well as conventional scientific knowledge; (2) a critical social scientific analysis of the relationships among the biologic and genetic determinants of health and the social determinants of health, *and* the social, economic, and political contexts of local, national, and global health; and (3) a working knowledge of the theoretical and practical application of clear and well-articulated anti-oppressive principles, including intersectionality.

Although the notion of scientific knowledge is much debated, here we refer to knowledge such as optimal insulin levels for diabetics, optimal blood electrolyte levels, and so on, all of which we very much want when we arrive at the emergency department with blurred vision and nausea, regardless of our view on the objectivity of scientific knowledge. The problem with "scientific" knowledge is not so much this kind of knowledge in and of itself. Rather, the problem is the conflation of actual chemical, biological fact (such as the relationship of insulin with the pancreas) with socially constructed supposedly scientific fact (such as the claim that Black people were medically unable to withstand cold, so they were not permitted to immigrate to Canada to escape slavery). The following case study demonstrates a practical application of critical best practices in an institutional setting.

Case Study: Mrs. Upshaw and Cardiac Care

Ideally, intervention using critical best practices unfolds in continuously interconnected and nested layers, from point-of-care intervention to systemic action for progressive social change. Biomedical science is incorporated to ensure adherence to best-known treatment protocols for emergency health problems such as anaphylactic shock, lung collapse or spinal fracture. Individual and family intervention will account for the social determinants of health, identity, and geography. Finally, incorporation of critical perspectives on health and health care will address the creation and maintenance of societal power imbalances. In best-practices intervention, these areas of intervention will be integrated throughout the health care of individuals, families, and communities. This approach to care demonstrates the growing enrichment of health care that is possible through the lens of critical best practices. Figure 4.1 illustrates these nested layers of intervention, from point-of-care to systemic action.

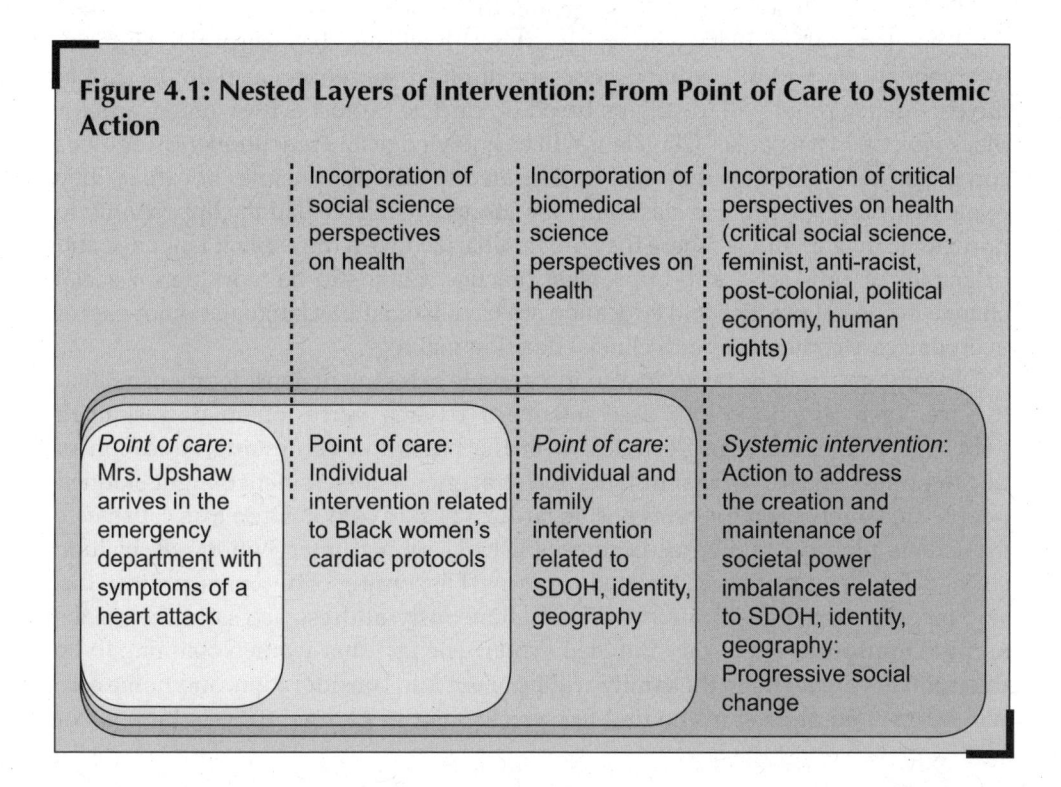

Figure 4.1: Nested Layers of Intervention: From Point of Care to Systemic Action

	Incorporation of social science perspectives on health	Incorporation of biomedical science perspectives on health	Incorporation of critical perspectives on health (critical social science, feminist, anti-racist, post-colonial, political economy, human rights)
Point of care: Mrs. Upshaw arrives in the emergency department with symptoms of a heart attack	*Point of care:* Individual intervention related to Black women's cardiac protocols	*Point of care:* Individual and family intervention related to SDOH, identity, geography	*Systemic intervention:* Action to address the creation and maintenance of societal power imbalances related to SDOH, identity, geography: Progressive social change

The following sections describe the nested layers of intervention that incorporate critical best practices. The scenario is an idealization of the enrichment that a critical social science perspective can bring to an analysis of clinical intervention.

Point of Care: Incorporation of Biomedical and Social Science Perspectives
Following the nested layers of intervention described in Figure 4.1, we start with Mrs. Upshaw's arrival at the emergency department of her local hospital. She has symptoms of a heart attack. Community emergency services are adequately funded so that paramedicine expertise is readily available, and the paramedics are paid commensurate with their pivotal position in the health care system. Since Mrs. Upshaw's geographic region adheres to the principles of the Canada Health Act, Mrs. Upshaw and her family will not receive a $500 bill for her trip from her home to the hospital.

When Mrs. Upshaw arrives at the emergency department, ideally her care is based on current best practices in cardiac care. The principles and practices of biomedical science will be applied to intervention strategies, and Mrs. Upshaw will be treated accordingly. Relatively recently, knowledge about cardiovascular problems has expanded to acknowledge that there are gender differences in clinical presentation. Until the 1980s, the treatment of cardiovascular disease was based entirely on knowledge about male physiology. It was assumed that treatment should be the same for women. Based on the foundation laid by feminist scholars and others, a critical analysis of disparities in health outcomes led to the recognition of gender differences in the pathophysiology of cardiovascular health problems. Best practices in cardiac care will account for these gender differences.

Knowledge about Black women's heart health will also be incorporated into the intervention plan. Mrs. Upshaw's assessment and intervention at point of care in the emergency room will ideally be based on cardiac protocols for women, and for Black women in particular. Clinicians will be knowledgeable practitioners in equities competent care, and thus they will be educated in ethical principles of care as they relate to racism, sexism, and classism. Practitioners will have had the opportunity to participate in workshops where they are familiarized with the explicit language and principles of anti-racist, anti-oppressive practice. Claims to be working for social change in clinical practice and education are trivialized if this language is not part of everyday case conferences and clinical decision making.

Ideally, care will be taken to also incorporate assessment considerations related to race, such as skin colour assessment for oxygen perfusion in dark-skinned people. This remains a neglected area in the basic and continuing education of health professionals, where standards and strategies for assessment of light-skinned people are largely used for everyone, regardless of skin colour. Once Mrs. Upshaw's immediate physical safety has been established, optimal intervention will include social determinants of health-related concerns. Dispensing of any prescriptions for, say, blood pressure medication, will simultaneously address access to the means and the transportation to buy the medication. The fact that women continue to be the primary caretakers in the family will be taken into consideration, and home care will be ensured at least in the first few weeks after discharge. If home care is not accounted for, it is likely that a recuperation period will not be possible, thus placing Mrs. Upshaw at higher risk for additional cardiac problems.

Systemic Intervention: Incorporation of Critical Perspectives on Health
Systemic intervention may then take the form of addressing the current state of home care in Canada, where funding has been consistently undermined over the last 10 years while post-operative and other forms of acute care have been steadily devolved to families and other community members (Shamian, 2007). Action to address Mrs. Upshaw's need for home care, as well as the related devolution of acute care into the community, brings intervention to the systemic realm. In order to work toward equity, addressing the creation and maintenance of societal power structures while simultaneously providing excellence at point of care, is central. This would mean that practitioners engage as much as possible in working for social change. There are already excellent examples across the country, particularly in non-profit community health centres, such as the North End Community Health Centre in Halifax, Nova Scotia (McGibbon, 2008). In tertiary care settings, managers at all levels and board members will partake in intensive and ongoing education in equities competence, including anti-racist practice.

This means that institutional policies will reflect responsibility and accountability for ethical care that incorporates equities competence in anti-racist practices. Educators of health and human service professionals will similarly involve equities competence and anti-racist training and continuing education so that they are positioned to engage in teaching this complex material. Systemic intervention requires an understanding of the political economy of inequality, and a shift from thinking about optimal health as a result of good intentions and adherence to a healthy lifestyle, to an acknowledgement of systemic oppression. Box 4.5 describes some of the common barriers to providing care from a critical perspective.

These barriers to providing care from a critical perspective are rooted, in part, to the overarching dominance of biomedical thinking. As evidenced in the case study about Mrs. Upshaw, although biomedical knowledge is an integral part of her care, its dominance must be consistently configured with a view to address oppression and work for social change. The following section discusses some of the main ideas to consider when thinking critically about biomedicine. Although biomedical dominance has been noted and debated for decades, this section explicitly links the significance of this dominance to anti-racist health care practice.

Biomedical Dominance and Anti-racist Practice

The centrality of biomedical dominance remains a core feature of the continued perpetuation of racism in the health fields. Although there are other important foundations that produce inequity in health and in access to health services, such as one's position in the structure of social class, the role of biomedicine also needs to be scrutinized. Two key aspects of biomedicine are germane to a discussion of

> **Box 4.5: Perceived Barriers to Providing Comprehensive Care from a Critical Perspective**
>
> The case study concerning Mrs. Upshaw may seem "unrealistic" because there is a great deal of historical and current resistance to anti-oppressive, anti-racist ideas in the health fields and in other professional fields as well. The following is a list of common points of resistance at point of care, in professional associations, and in academic teaching and research. We will further explore resistance to anti-racist, anti-oppressive practice in Chapter 5.
>
> - *Too expensive:* Resistance in this area runs along the lines of claims that all this "extra" accommodating cannot be accommodated in the budget. This thinking demonstrates a lack of understanding of the methods and principles of anti-oppressive education. The most effective and ethical strategy is to *integrate* a critical perspective into already-existing institutional structures. Everything from including a critical perspective when updating intake assessment forms to incorporating anti-oppressive education into already-existing staff development can be reframed to produce care provision that honours the needs of racialized peoples. It is not a case of budget restrictions; it is a case of restricted thinking.
> - *Too biased:* Since the health fields are immersed in the dominant culture of biomedicine, any glimpse into the world outside this dominance is commonly viewed as "biased." For example, introduction of critical perspectives such as feminism are often considered to be promoting bias. However, *not* addressing feminist ideas about patriarchy demonstrates bias; it is not viewed as such because neglecting to discuss patriarchy is the dominant norm in education.
> - *Too theoretical for practical application:* One of the core features of racism and all forms of oppression is that they are structural. In other words, they are embedded in societal institutional structures such as the health care system, the legal system, the education system, to name a few. In order to understand how racism operates, it is necessary to have at least a beginning foundation, as described in this chapter. Since health care professionals are already accustomed to learning complex theories and concepts of biomedical science, it does not make sense that they are not capable of learning core theoretical concepts necessary for anti-racist practice.

biomedical dominance and anti-racist practice: (1) the process of medicalization, and (2) the notion of scientific evidence as objective truth. As noted in this chapter, in 1974, Ivan Illich published *Limits to Medicine, Medical Nemesis: The Appropriation of Health*. Illich described the notion of iatrogenic, or medical treatment-induced, illness and argued that medicine was harmful in many ways. One of his chief contributions to the critique of biomedical dominance was his description of social iatrogenesis or medicalization—the rendering of life experiences as processes of health disorders that can be discussed exclusively in medical terms, and to which only medical solutions can be applied (Illich, 1976; Zola, 1972). Menopause and childbirth are notable examples of life experiences that have become largely subsumed under the domain of biomedical intervention, especially in the Western world.

A biomedical framework presents particular kinds of challenges for clinicians in the health field because in such a framework, scientific merit is predominantly measured in terms of objective truth. Historically, the biomedical framework has worked well in areas such as the detection of pathogens that cause infectious diseases. For example, in a biomedical frame, pneumonia is caused by pneumococcal bacteria, and can therefore be treated accordingly with antibiotic drugs. There is a direct, measurable, observable-under-a-microscope relationship among the signs and symptoms of the infection, the cause, and the treatment with drugs that eliminate the pathogen from the body. This direct relationship among disease, its cause, and its treatment is central to a biomedical approach that forms the foundation of modern epidemiology. Statistical correlations among pathogens, disease vectors, and human pathophysiology are some of the main foundations of biomedicine.

Controlling for extraneous or confounding factors such as gender, race, and socio-economic status is still an important underpinning of achieving valid results that are considered generalizable to the larger population. This model is still largely predominant in health research, and the gold standard of the randomized clinical trial is considered the most respected and is the most funded form of research in the health fields. It is clear that such a model is not consistent with incorporating concepts such as racism into an understanding of health. Race, along with gender, and age, far from being extraneous, are important predictors of health outcomes. Goffman's claims about medical psychiatric treatment in mental hospitals in 1961 are eerily similar in many ways to today's biomedical approach to mental health problems:

> *Whatever the patient's social circumstances, whatever the particular character of his "disorder," he can in this setting, be treated, if not dealt with, as someone whose problem can be approached, by applying a single technical-psychiatric view. That one patient differs from another in sex, age, race grouping, marital status, religion or social class is merely an item to be taken into consideration, to be corrected for, as it were, so that general psychiatric theory can be applied and universal themes can be detected behind the superficialities of outward differences in social life. Just as one in the social system can have an inflamed appendix, so anyone can manifest one of the basic psychiatric syndromes. (p. 351)*

In terms of spiritual and psychological distress associated with racism, if a biomedical framework is used to assess and intervene in the area of chronic stress for example, clinicians will ask well-developed assessment questions related to stress and anxiety. In many countries, they will most likely use the *Diagnostic and Statistical Manual of Mental Disorders* (DSM) or the International Classification of Diseases (World Health Organization, 2007) as a clinical checklist for assessment (American Psychiatric Association, 2004) While clinicians may exercise compassion and empathy during the therapeutic interview, the maintenance of clinical objectivity requires a dispassionate and scientific application of the assessment framework. There is little or no room for consideration of a complex topic such as racism-related stress. In the mental health system, stress and anxiety are almost always considered as an individual or personal problem with individual focused solutions. Although family assessment may be included in some areas, adult intervention rests primarily on the dispensing of medications. In Canada, a DSM psychiatric diagnosis, such as generalized anxiety disorder or dysphoria, is then coded with the patient's name into a provincial administrative health database.

The literature shows that the most likely intervention, whether in a mental health clinic or in the family doctor's office, is psychotropic medication such as an antidepressant, or an anxiolytic from the benzodiazepine drug group (Valium, Alprazolam, etc.). So, application of a biomedical framework to racism-related stress results in identification of the stress as an individual psychiatric disorder, with psychotropic medications as the primary mode of treatment. Despite the fact that drugs may be augmented with referrals for counselling or other assessments and interventions within the field of mental health, pharmacological intervention remains paramount. Although psychotropic medications may well be effective for some people, the absence of a social, economic, and political assessment context means that individual and systemic interventions based on racism are not considered. This is an example of the medicalization of oppression. Consistent with Illich's definition of medicalization, a social problem such as racism-related stress is reframed as an individual psychiatric problem that is amenable to psychotropic drug intervention. In this way the biomedical psychiatric model can be spiritually and psychologically damaging to oppressed peoples. Table 4.2 illustrates a comparison of biomedical and social science perspectives on health. The table serves as a summary of some of the important concepts related to the various perspectives on health and health care presented in this chapter.

Although medical approaches to health care have become more comprehensive, or social scientific, in the past two decades, assessment and treatment modalities in publicly funded health care continue to focus on individual pathophysiology. The dominance of this individual and biophysiological perspective makes it difficult to envision delivery of health care in a format other than the current one, where hospitals, professional schools' textbooks, and course descriptions are all organized around individual body systems and body parts. If there is any doubt, a glance at any hospital directory will confirm the body-part/body-system framework of health care delivery in the Western world. Although, social determinants of health-related concerns are sometimes considered, the point is that the body-part/body-system model is the foundational structure of the acute care system.

Much has been lost in the dismissal of Indigenous and African-Canadian knowledges, and the privileging of the biomedical model over all other forms of knowing about health in Canada. We begin to see what we have lost when we consider the sophistication of Indigenous healing patterns and rituals when compared to Western intervention for traumatic stress. Although storytelling has been given its newer, fancier title of narrative therapy, the use of stories as a way to make meaning of life is a centuries-old embedded tradition in Indigenous and African cultures. Over the past 25 years, the field of traumatic stress has moved substantially from the days when there was little acknowledgement of, and active resistance to, the relationship between traumatic stress and mental health difficulties. This resistance is still active in many ways. Clinicians in Canada are still far more likely to label post-trauma responses with the diagnosis of depression, anxiety, or

Table 4.2: Comparison of Biomedical and Social Science Perspectives on Human Health

	Biomedical Science Perspective	Social Science Perspective	Enhanced by a Critical Social Science Perspective
The nature of the body	The body consists of neurological, digestive, cardiovascular, and musculoskeletal parts and systems. Textbooks and chapters, hospital units, and professional schools' course descriptions are divided into categories based on these body parts and systems.	The body, in addition to the physical self, is intimately connected to a particular historical social context. Bodily health outcomes depend on social circumstances: political, economic, and educational—the social determinants of health (SDOH).	Bodily health outcomes also depend on social circumstances. Inequities in social circumstances, rooted in oppression, are "inscribed" on the body, and become evident in inequities in health outcomes. Societal power imbalance creates most ill health.
The nature of health and illness	Mental and physical health and illness are related to pathophysiology in various body parts and systems. Mental health is seen to have social and psychological aspects.	Mental and physical health are shaped by social context—the SDOH.	Mental and physical health are shaped by the SDOH, and the SDOH are solidly linked to inequities in societal power distribution and human rights violations. Mental health struggle is related to oppressive social structures.
The nature of assessment	Assessment protocols are largely based in the determination of abnormalities in body parts and systems.	Assessment systematically incorporates social context—the SDOH.	Assessment systematically incorporates human rights and SDOH inequities.

The nature of intervention	Intervention focuses largely on the amelioration of observable, measurable abnormalities in body parts and systems. Mental health intervention remains largely based in the biochemistry of psychotropic drugs.	Intervention systematically incorporates social context—the SDOH. Mental health places at least equal importance in SDOH-related action. In addition to biophysical concerns, physical and mental health intervention systematically incorporates the social context—the SDOH.	Intervention systematically incorporates balancing social power: addressing root causes of inequities in health related to human rights and the SDOH.
The nature of research	Gold standard: objective evidence generated by randomized clinical trials (RCT). Qualitative at the bottom of the research hierarchy: (1) RCT experiment (2) Statistical analyses (3) Survey (4) Qualitative research	Research incorporates social context through qualitative (i.e., ethnography, grounded theory, phenomenology) and quantitative approaches.	Qualitative and quantitative research attends to creation/maintenance of societal power. Participatory action research ethically involves oppressed peoples in the emancipation.

personality disorder. Traumatic stress can certainly result in depression and anxiety, but failure to acknowledge trauma is a political statement, especially in oppression-related trauma such as chronic racism. The concept of historical trauma transmission (Wesley-Esquimaux & Smolewski, 2004) has barely entered health care thinking in Canada.

Conclusions

Health care practitioners have, for the most part, had comparatively little exposure to the complexities of perspectives in health beyond the biomedical viewpoint. Although social, societal, and environmental considerations have always been fundamental aspects of health care practice, perspectives such as sociological, human rights, and political economy are only just beginning to be integrated into practice and policy. Moving forward for anti-racist health care practice means embracing these larger contexts and shaping ways to bring them into our everyday practice worlds, and into the policies that shape them.

CHAPTER 5

An Anti-racist Framework to Guide Practice

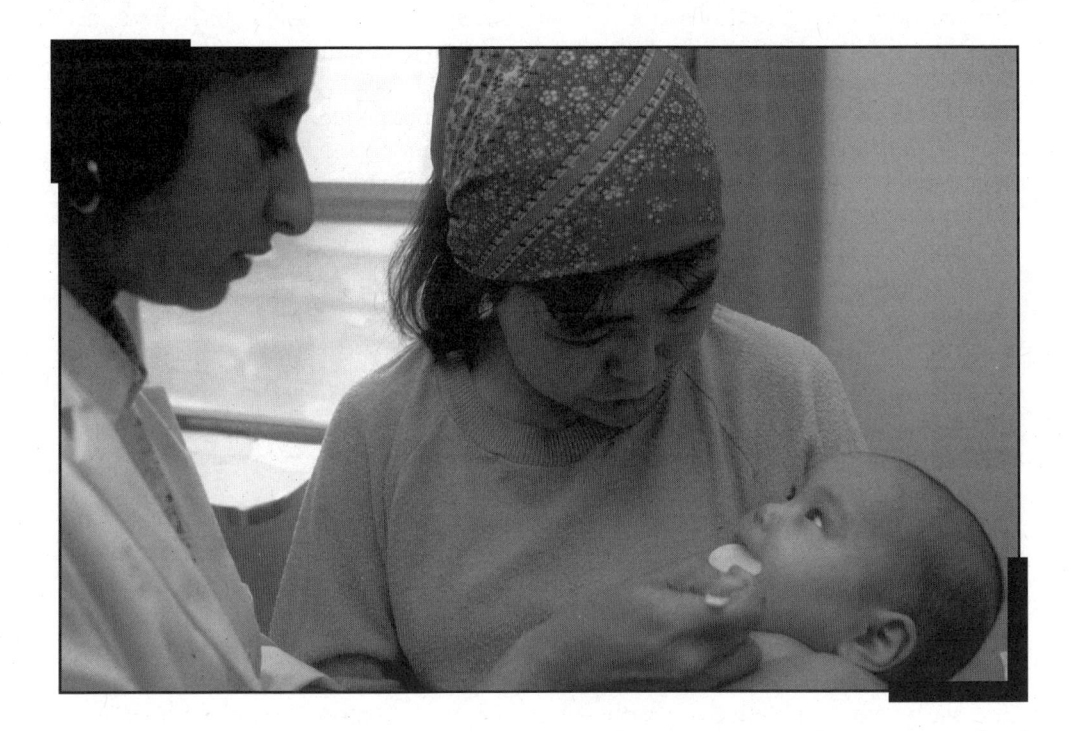

An anti-racism framework ... explicitly names the issues of race and social difference as issues of power and equity, rather than as matters of cultural and ethnic variety ... while the notion of culture(s) and cultural differences are relevant to anti-racism discourse, it stresses that a romanticized notion of culture, which fails to critically interrogate power, is severely limited in the understanding of social reality. (George Sefa Dei, 1996, pp. 25-27).

Introduction

In this chapter we define and describe terms and concepts that are central to developing a language to think about racism and engaging in anti-racist practice. Terms such as race, stereotype, bias, prejudice, discrimination, and oppression are discussed using examples from our practice and from the literature. Definitions are presented in an iterative way, so that the ideas build upon each other. The relationship between oppression and dominance is linked to disparities in health status and access to health care services. We ground our discussion in the social construction of race, and describe how any attempts to define and categorize race deny the fluidity of ideological constructs and their dependence on the subject's interpretive meanings.

The chapter uses our anti-racist health care practice framework, which illustrates the relationships among bias, stereotyping, discrimination, and oppression. We begin with a description of the paths from biased information and stereotyping to oppression. The many forms of racism are described, including individual, environmental, cultural, and systemic. White privilege is discussed, as well as the corresponding disadvantage that is experienced by people of colour. We conclude with a discussion of the concept of intersectionality and we emphasize its relevance for professional codes of ethics to guide practice.

An Anti-racist Framework to Guide Practice

Despite the sometimes overwhelming nature of racism, there are three overarching processes that can work in synergy to guide anti-racist practice: seeing the paths from stereotype to oppression; understanding and connecting paths of oppression to policy; and acting for social change. Figure 5.1 illustrates this anti-racist framework to guide practice. Racism is a complex system that is deeply embedded in centuries of history and in modern society. In order to stop the many forms of racism, we must first see and acknowledge the paths from stereotypes to oppression. This process involves a parallel and connected awakening about White privilege and how it operates to create and maintain racism. Understanding and connecting racism to the policy realm shows us how racism is sustained over time, whether in the education system, in government, or in everyday health care practice. We take up the relationships among racism, oppression, policy, and social change in Chapters 6 and 7. Acting for change is based in seeing the paths from stereotype to oppression, and understanding and connecting these paths to policy. The relationship is not linear, and action can happen at any point in the process.

Paths from Stereotype to Oppression

Systemic power is a core feature of oppression (Calliste, 2000). We all hold stereotypes about individuals and groups of people. These stereotypes are based on biased

An Anti-racist Framework to Guide Practice

Figure 5.1: Anti-racist Framework to Guide Practice: Seeing, Understanding and Connecting, Acting

SEEING the Paths from Stereotype to Oppression	UNDERSTANDING and CONNECTING Paths of Oppression to Policy	ACTING for Social Change
RACISM: • Individual • Internalized • Cultural • Environmental • Systemic **INTERSECTIONALITY:** Race, gender, social class… **WHITE PRIVILEGE**	**POLICIES:** • At point-of-care • In the classroom • In health care and educational institutions • In professional associations • In municipal, provincial, territorial, and federal governments	**ACTION:** • Educating self • Educating others • Supporting, encouraging others who speak up • Initiating, preventing: working to change individual and institutional actions and policies, and legislation

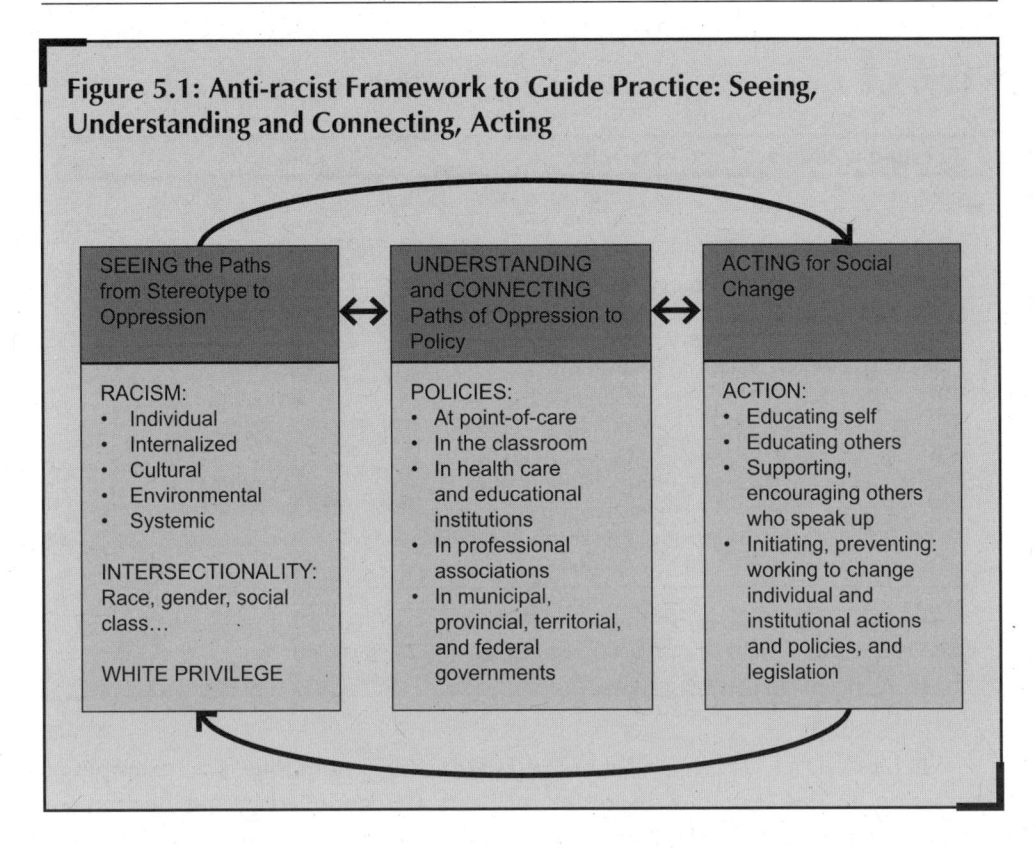

information. For example, the media's portrayal of people of colour in Canada and elsewhere is based on stereotypes. These stereotypes are powerful and enduring, and we are exposed to them on a regular basis from all forms of media, including television programs and advertisements, Facebook, YouTube, movies, and even health education pamphlets. "Contrary to myth, journalists, editors, broadcasters, and directors of media organizations are not always neutral, objective, impartial, or unbiased" (Henry, Tator, Mattis & Reese, 2000, p. 300). Table 5.1 illustrates common stereotypes of various groups of people of colour. These stereotypes are embedded in Canadian culture and are just as relevant today as they were in the days of cowboys and Indians television shows, although many people think that they are a thing of the past.

Stereotypes can lead to *thinking* in a particular way that is prejudiced. Prejudice is literally to "prejudge." In the health field, this prejudging or prejudice may, for example, be assuming that an Aboriginal man has a drinking problem when we assess him in the community health center. Or, in the education of professional clinicians, we may assume that Black students are not as intelligent as their White peers. When we *act* in a particular way based on our prejudice, we are participating in discrimination. For example, we may start our assessment of an Aboriginal man by asking him: "When was your last drink?" This occurrence has in fact been substantiated in workshops about barriers in access to health services for Aboriginal Canadians (McGibbon et al., 2006).

Table 5.1: Images of Various Groups of People of Colour

Aboriginal Peoples	Blacks	Asians
• Savages	• Drug addicts	• Untrustworthy
• Alcoholics	• Pimps	• Menacing
• Uncivilized	• Prostitutes	• Unscrupulous
• Uncultured	• Entertainers	• Subhuman
• Murderers	• Athletes	• Submissive
• Noble	• Drug dealers	• Maiming
• Needing a White saviour	• Murderers	• Quaint
• Victim	• Gangsters	• Gangsters
	• Butlers and maids	• Prostitutes
	• Simple minded	• Cooks
	• Inconsequential	• Store vendors
	• Savages	
	• Primitive	
	• Needing a White saviour	

Source: From HENRY. *The color of democracy: Racism in Canadian society.* Copyright 2006 Nelson Education Ltd. Reproduced by permission, www.cengage.com/permissions

When our *actions are supported* by the health care system, this is an example of oppression. In this case, our discriminatory acts are condoned by our health care institution, and the systemic power within the institution. For example, if clinicians hold the stereotype that all Aboriginal men have a drinking problem, they may provide less than optimal care because they believe that these men do not care about their health and there is no point in completing a proper assessment. When the health care institution condones this behaviour by overlooking or ignoring inadequate assessments, this is an example of oppression. Another way that this health care institution might participate in oppression would be failure to provide anti-racist-based cultural competence training.

Still another way that institutions promote racism is through the use of skin-tone prosthetic appliances and special burn-treatment bandages for all clients, regardless of race. The skin tone is assumed to be pink. If this practice is difficult to perceive as racist, try to imagine what would happen if hospitals used dark brown or black prosthetic appliances, and special bandages, *for everyone*. These are all examples of how oppression is discrimination backed up by systemic power. Figure 5.2 depicts this cycle of oppression. It is important to note that stereotyping, prejudice, discrimination, and oppression often happen without the perpetrator noticing or acknowledging the problem. On the other hand, those who experience these injustices are very much aware of their painful and sometimes devastating effects. In other words, it is not necessary for the perpetrators to notice or name their racism in order for racism to actually occur.

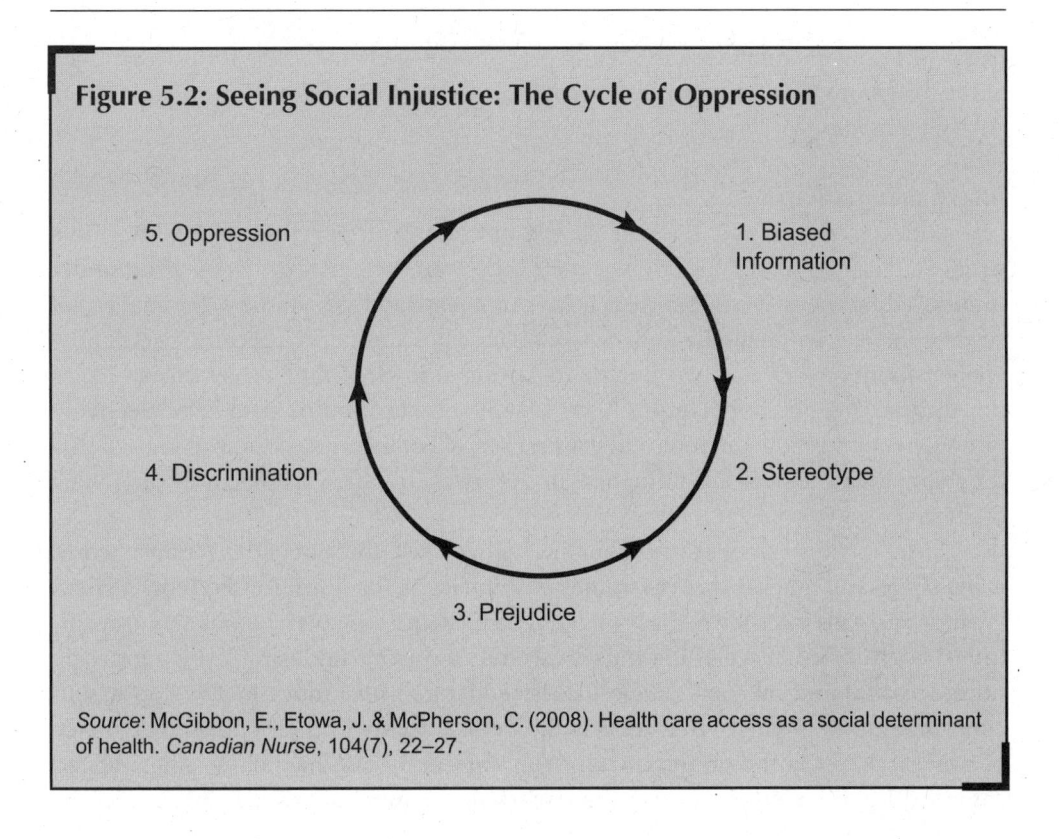

> **Figure 5.2: Seeing Social Injustice: The Cycle of Oppression**
>
> 5. Oppression
> 1. Biased Information
> 4. Discrimination
> 2. Stereotype
> 3. Prejudice
>
> *Source*: McGibbon, E., Etowa, J. & McPherson, C. (2008). Health care access as a social determinant of health. *Canadian Nurse*, 104(7), 22–27.

The Many Forms of Racism

Racism can operate in many ways and there are different kinds of racism. Some of the main forms of racism are described below. It is important to note that these forms of racism can overlap and interlock to create powerful barriers to full participation in society.

Individual Racism

Individual racism is practised at the individual, personal level. Individual racism takes the form of face-to-face stereotyping, prejudice, and discrimination. It involves discriminatory attitudes and resulting behaviours as previously described in the treatment of the Aboriginal man in the community health center. More specifically, individual racism involves thinking and acting based on the belief that one's own racial group has superior values, customs, and norms. In a related way, individual racism is based on the belief that other racial groups are inferior (Henry et al., 2000). Although individual racism is often seen as a personality flaw, it is intricately connected to the societal creation and maintenance of the stereotypes of people of colour. Individual racism is experienced in an everyday way by people of colour—at the grocery store, when hailing a cab, at the bus stop, when buying textbooks, when bringing family members to visit health practitioners, when waiting for prescriptions at the drugstore. The list is endless and it is also very difficult for White people to see or even to imagine.

Internalized Racism

Internalized racism happens when people of colour adopt or internalize negative racist stereotypes about themselves as if they were true. All of us are profoundly influenced by the way people treat us in our everyday lives, and by the images we see of ourselves in the media and all around us. These influences become part of how we feel about ourselves to varying degrees, depending on numerous factors such as our upbringing, our opportunity to critique images around us, and how positively or negatively we view ourselves in the first place. For example, it is well known that the media has a significant influence on the ways in which women and girls view themselves.

One of the most clear examples of internalized self-concept in the Western world is the successful marketing of extremes of thinness as the norm for the female body. Women and girls internalize these images and measure their own bodies against waif-thin models. Normal weight is thus viewed as ugly and undesirable by a growing number of adolescent girls. Hence, girls tend more and more to develop a self-concept regarding weight that reflects the undesirability of their bodies. The image of undesirability is thus internalized. Although this issue has many other related complexities, it nonetheless serves as a working example of how we internalize the external messages we receive on a daily basis.

Similarly, the relentless experiences of everyday racism and the thousands of racist messages associated with these experiences eventually start to influence the ways in which people of colour view themselves and their personal worth. Oppressive social structures reinforce racist messages in numerous important ways. Anne Bishop (2002) described how internalized racism became important in the creation of Indian residential schools in Canada. Indian residential schools are an example of "child abuse being used to force a people to internalize what their conquerors thought to be their rightful place in a racist, sexist, class-stratified society" (Bishop, p. 72).

Numerous stories of the consistent and ongoing physical, sexual, emotional, and spiritual abuse of Aboriginal children remind us of a powerful legacy of oppression at the hands of White people. These negative messages about the worth of Aboriginal children and the corresponding power of White people were reinforced and continue to this day. In our teaching work, some White students still believe that all that is over and that we are all equal now. Some students also believe that Aboriginal peoples are actually advantaged when compared to White people in Canada, citing free houses and free university tuition as examples of unfairness to White people. It is very difficult for these students to understand and to honour the context of historical oppression and the fact that centuries of systemic brutality and disenfranchisement cannot be ameliorated with efforts such as occasional assistance with housing.

Systemic Racism

Systemic racism is racism backed up by systemic power. At the core of racism is an unequal distribution of power. The results of this unequal distribution include decreased access to goods and services and a lack of access to basic human rights. For example, if we contrast the principles of the Canada Health Act (Health Canada, 2005), such as universality (health care is available to all citizens) and accessibility (health care is accessible to all citizens), with the statistics cited in Chapter 2, we see that limited access to health care is positively correlated to racial origin. According to the substantive field of research cited in Chapter 2, Aboriginal, Black, Hispanic and Latino peoples have decreased access to health care in a broad variety of settings and situations. Some may propose that this disparity exists due to other demographic or geographic constraints, or individual characteristics and preferences, such as not wanting to use services, or not following through on recommendations, and so on. This may indeed be true in some cases. However, the sheer enormity and variety of available statistics, and the consistency of findings from locations around the globe, direct our attention to unequal access and unequal treatment based in systemic racism.

Although many health practitioners' everyday practice involves working on a one-to-one basis with people and their families and communities, their practice unfolds within a larger context. This context includes social, political, and economic activities and patterns that intersect at local, national, and global levels. In this sense, systemic racism refers to racism that is entrenched in institutional systems such as the health care system, the education system, the legal system, and in professional associations. So, while individual hospitals may have promotion or arbitration policies that discriminate against, say, Black and Latino nurses, it is systemic racism in the health care system that enables people to actually carry out these discriminatory practices. For example, we know that Black nurses are less likely to be employed by health care institutions, and if they are employed, they are less likely to be promoted (Etowa, 2005). While individual hiring committee members may be practising individual racism in not hiring nurses of colour, the hospitals' sanction of persistent racism in employment practices is an example of systemic racism.

At the service delivery level in the area of organ transplantation, administrators, and physicians at individual hospitals make decisions about who will be transplant recipients. However, it is institutional racism in the health care system that coordinates and produces unequal allocation based on race. Although it may be argued that the various transplant decision makers and the individual hospitals are not engaging in racist acts, systemic institutional power gives them the sanction to legitimate racist decisions about organ allocation. In this way, racism is a complex interweaving of bias, prejudice, discrimination, and oppression that operates individually and systemically. According to Dei (1996), institutional structures have the power to provide a space for individuals in society to discriminate against one another. Systemic racism creates the space for the perpetuation of strategically created racist injustices such as the disproportionate number of women of colour and women who live in poverty who are incarcerated in Canadian prisons. Aboriginal peoples' experiences regarding the criminal justice system have been documented by the Canadian Criminal Justice Association (2000):

- Aboriginal peoples who are accused of a crime are more likely to be denied bail, and more likely to be charged with multiple offences, and often for crimes against the system.
- More time is spent in pretrial detention by Aboriginal peoples.
- Aboriginal peoples are more likely to not have legal representation at court proceedings.
- Aboriginal clients, especially in northern communities where the court party flies in the day of the hearing, spend less time with their lawyers.
- As court schedules in remote areas are poorly planned, judges may have limited time to spend in the community.
- Aboriginal offenders are more than twice as likely to be incarcerated than non-Aboriginal offenders.
- Aboriginal elders, who are also spiritual leaders, are not given the same status as prison priests and chaplains, in all institutions.
- Aboriginal peoples often plead guilty because they are intimidated by the court and simply want to get the proceedings over with.

The statistics regarding Aboriginal women and incarceration are a disturbing testimony of systemic racism and its colonial underpinnings. The increasing criminalization and incarceration of racialized women is a global phenomenon. The impact of economic restructuring and the dismantling of social safety nets has had a devastating impact on the lives of women, and especially racialized women (Pate & Neve, 2005). Figure 5.3 is a poster designed and distributed by the Canadian Association of Elizabeth Fry Societies (CAEFS). The association ensures substantive equality in the delivery and development of services and programs through public education, research, and legislative and administrative reform (Canadian Association of Elizabeth Fry Societies, 2008). The poster's aim is to bring attention to the plight of women in Canadian prisons, including the fact that 90 percent of Aboriginal women in prisons are survivors of incest, rape, or physical assault (Canadian Association of Elizabeth Fry Societies, 2008).

Environmental Racism

Environmental racism refers to the deliberate location of environmental toxins near the homes and communities of people of colour as well as the destruction, or attempted destruction of the environment around communities of colour. Hazardous waste facilities, landfill sites, and incinerators are all disproportionately located near communities of colour, regardless of country or region (Cole & Foster, 2000). For example:

- The 1983 study "Siting of Hazardous Waste Landfills and Their Correlation with Racial and Economic Status of Surrounding Communities" revealed that three out of four of the off-site, commercial hazardous waste landfills

An Anti-racist Framework to Guide Practice 119

Figure 5.3: Canadian Association of Elizabeth Fry Societies Educational Poster

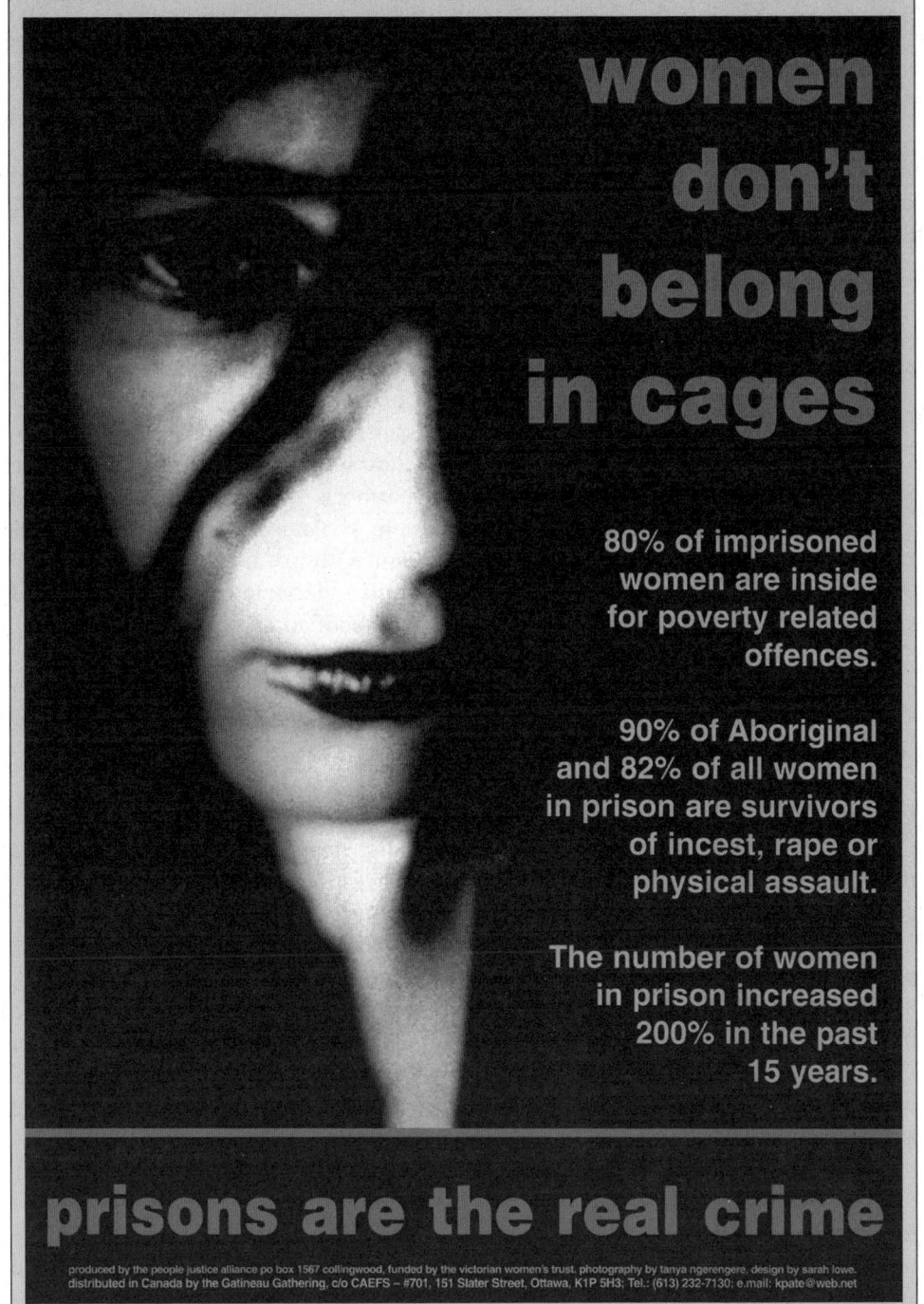

women don't belong in cages

80% of imprisoned women are inside for poverty related offences.

90% of Aboriginal and 82% of all women in prison are survivors of incest, rape or physical assault.

The number of women in prison increased 200% in the past 15 years.

prisons are the real crime

produced by the people justice alliance po box 1567 collingwood, funded by the victorian women's trust. photography by tanya ngerengere, design by sarah lowe. distributed in Canada by the Gatineau Gathering, c/o CAEFS – #701, 151 Slater Street, Ottawa, K1P 5H3; Tel.: (613) 232-7130; e.mail: kpate@web.net

Source: Reprinted with the permission of the Canadian Association of Elizabeth Fry Societies (2008).

in Region 4 (which comprises eight states in the South) happen to be located in predominantly African-American communities, although African Americans made up only 20 percent of the region's population; apartheid-type housing and development policies have resulted in limited mobility, reduced neighbourhood options, decreased environmental choices, and decreased job opportunities for African Americans. Numerous studies since this time have proven that environmental justice continues to be elusive in racialized and marginalized communities (Bullard, 2007).

- It is contended that the 1990 confrontation between the Canadian armed forces and the Mohawk communities in Oka, Quebec, Canada, should be interpreted as an act of environmental racism against the First Nations peoples. The Mohawks' form of self-government, and the Canadian government's attitudes toward the First Nations communities' governing systems have been linked to the environmental problems caused by the impending construction of a golf course in Oka, and the chronology of events that nearly culminated in armed confrontation. The notion of environmental racism was implicated because it was asserted that the proposed construction would have violated the Mohawk community's resources for meeting its material and spiritual needs. Furthermore, it is stressed that the local government's willingness to perpetuate ecological violence exemplifies the persistence of environmental racism within Canadian institutions. It is concluded that the Mohawk community's decision to take up arms and challenge the proposed construction was justified on environmental, legal, and moral grounds (Westra, 1999).

Box 5.1 includes an excerpt from a Canadian provincial newspaper describing several additional examples of environmental racism.

Cultural Racism

Cultural racism refers to the culturally embedded network of beliefs and values that encourage and justify discriminatory practices, including the belief that the cultural practices and beliefs of one's own racial group are superior (Henry et al., 2000). Cultural racism has its basis in ethnocentrism, which is "a tendency to view all peoples and cultures in terms of one's own cultural standards and values" (p. 57). Hospitals are excellent examples of how ethnocentrism operates. Approaches to family caregiving assume that the nuclear family is the dominant cultural mode of family coping during a health crisis. Although accommodation for extended family involvement is increasingly attempted, the very architecture of hospitals most often assumes limited extended family need for involvement.

The example regarding the assumption of pink skin tone illustrates another form of ethnocentrism. In this case it is the assumption that there is only a need for prosthesis that reflects the skin colour of White people. The dominance of the biomedical model is yet another example of ethnocentrism in the health care system. Aboriginal and African-Canadian cultural healing practices and rituals, based in centuries of successful implementation, are barely on the periphery of hospital care

> **Box 5.1: "Natives and Blacks—Always in Their Backyard": Environmental Racism in Nova Scotia**
>
> No community wants a landfill in its backyard—or a dump, either. Lincolnville, a small, predominantly Black community in Guysborough County, has both in its history. Residents held a Save Lincolnville march to make that point last month. When I started to look at the story, it seemed to get bigger and uglier. Bottom line: if you're Black or Native or poor in Nova Scotia, the view from your front window is pretty likely to include an old dump or landfill site. Lincolnville is just one example. About 60 people live in the town and its landfill, established in 2006, is state of-the-art. That means it's a hole in the ground with a liner and a system to collect runoff. A dump, like the one Lincolnville used to have, is just a hole in the ground. Lincolnville is in the middle of nowhere, which is the best place to put a landfill. That's what I figured, anyway, until I started to do some research.
>
> To begin with, Lincolnville, is in the middle of nowhere for a familiar reason in Nova Scotia. The original Lincolnville settlers, Black United Empire Loyalists, were promised better land in 1787. In the end, they were given the current Lincolnville lands and forced to settle far away from the ocean—or far by Nova Scotia standards, anyway. You've heard this before, probably, but it bears repeating—how Black Loyalists got to farm rocks and bogs while other United Empire Loyalists got to farm the Annapolis Valley. No mistaking the winners and losers in the British land grants in Nova Scotia, then, in the years after the American Revolution.
>
> Now, I'll be honest: I don't usually have much patience for this stuff. Get on with your lives, I say. But then I started talking to people at the Ecology Action Centre, which led me to a 1996 paper written by a Dalhousie University student. Lori Ann Fryzuk's thesis has a long title—*Environmental Justice in Canada: An Empirical Study and Analysis of the Demographics of Dumping in Nova Scotia*. It also includes lots of tough math and complex argument. But Fryzuk gets to the heart of the matter succinctly enough: "Blacks and natives only make up 1.2 per cent and 0.8 per cent of Nova Scotia's total population, respectively (but) 46 per cent of the waste sites have been located with EAs (enumeration areas) with Black and native populations exceeding these percentages." Fryzuk had to do some fancy calculating to get at those numbers.
>
> But you can't read her thesis and miss the point that we've located too many landfills and dumps where Black, native or just plain poor people live. She also notes, in passing, that Africville, the former Black community located on the shores of Bedford Basin, hosted enough toxic industry to suggest modern-day Beijing. The City of Halifax rezoned the community industrial in 1947, and it soon became host to "a fertilizer plant, a slaughterhouse, a tar factory, a prison, two infectious-disease hospitals, an open dump and an incinerator." Businessmen like to say this kind of past is a "sunk cost."
>
> Shakespeare said the "past is prologue," and his quote seems more apt. For the people of Lincolnville, their past dump, the site of a random collection of toxic gunk, was prologue to high cancer rates today. Just as their past land grant was a predictor of current poverty. There's no way to prove any of this. But Ecology Action Centre is right to suggest that Lincolnville deserves compensation. The white citizens of the Upper Sackville area got some financial compensation for hosting a landfill. Fairness dictates equal treatment for Lincolnville and other areas with landfills or old dumps. Any other resolution suggests that Nova Scotia is content to treat Lincolnville residents just as badly as the British Crown treated their ancestors in the 1770's. I don't like the word "racism"—it's too easy to hurl around. But it's the right one to describe what continues to take place in Lincolnville today.
>
> *Source:* Jim Meek (2008). The *Chronicle Herald*, Halifax, NS, Sunday, March 9, 2008. Republished with permission from the Halifax Herald Ltd

implementation. These examples also demonstrate a core feature of ethnocentrism: It is very difficult to notice unless it is brought forward with specific everyday examples. Table 5.2 provides definitions of important forms of racism discussed in this chapter, along with a health-related example.

Table 5.2: Definitions of Important Forms of Racism

Form of Racism	Health-Related Example
Individual racism takes the form of face-to-face stereotyping, prejudice, and discrimination. It involves discriminatory attitudes and resulting behaviours. More specifically, individual racism involves thinking and acting based in the belief that one's own racial group has superior values, customs, and norms. In a related way, individual racism is based in the belief that other racial groups are inferior (Henry, Tator, Mattis & Reese, 2000).	**Evidence shows that clinicians provide substandard care to people of colour**: The rates of screening for most diseases are lower among Black patients than among White patients, and Black patients more often than White patients receive diagnoses when diseases are at a relatively advanced stage (Bach et al., 2005).
Internalized racism happens when people of colour adopt or internalize negative racist stereotypes about themselves as if they were true. All of us are profoundly influenced by the way people treat us in our everyday lives, and by the images we see of ourselves in the media and all around us. These influences become part of how we feel about ourselves in varying degrees. The relentless experiences of everyday racism, and the thousands of racist messages associated with these experiences, eventually start to influence the ways in which people of colour view themselves and their personal worth. Oppressive social structures reinforce racist messages in numerous ways.	**Internalized racism became important in the creation of Indian residential schools in Canada** (Bishop, 2002). Indian residential schools are an example of "child abuse being used to force a people to internalize what their conquerors thought to be their rightful place in a racist, sexist, class-stratified society" (p. 72). High rates of suicide in Aboriginal young people have been linked to the enduring legacy of colonialism and its impact on the mental health of Aboriginal peoples.
Cultural racism refers to the culturally embedded network of beliefs and values that encourage and justify discriminatory practices, including the belief that the cultural practices and beliefs of one's own racial group are superior (Henry, Tator, Mattis & Reese, 2000). Cultural racism has its basis in ethnocentrism, which is "a tendency to view all peoples and cultures in terms of one's own cultural standards and values" (p. 57).	**Hospitals are excellent examples of how cultural racism and ethnocentrism operate.** For example, approaches to family caregiving assume that the nuclear family is the dominant mode of family coping during a health crisis. Although accommodation for extended family involvement is increasingly attempted, the very architecture of hospitals assumes limited extended family need for involvement.

Environmental racism refers to the deliberate location of environmental toxins near the homes and communities of people of colour, and the destruction, or attempted destruction of the environment around communities of colour.	**Hazardous waste facilities, landfill sites, and incinerators** are all disproportionately located near communities of colour, regardless of country or region (Cole & Foster, 2000). Health outcomes are negatively affected by environmental toxin exposure.
Systemic racism is racism backed up by systemic power. At the core of racism is an unequal distribution of power. According to Dei (1996), structures have the power to provide a space for individuals in society to discriminate against one another.	**Systemic racism in the health care system supports inequities in access.** If we contrast the principles of the Canada Health Act (Health Canada, 2005), such as universality (health care is available to all citizens) and accessibility (health care is accessible to all citizens), with the statistics cited in Chapter 2, we see that limited access to health care is positively correlated with race.

White Privilege

Oppression is an endemic feature of societal structures. It often occurs without our notice. Peggy MacIntosh's (1990) now-famous work about White privilege brought oppression related to race into the view of White people in a way that was clear and practical. MacIntosh showed that White people:

> ... can turn on the television or open the front page of the newspaper and see people of my race widely represented.... I can be sure that my children will be given curricular materials that testify to the existence of their race.... Whether I use checks, credit cards or cash, I can count on my skin color not to work against the appearance of financial reliability.... I can be pretty sure that if I ask to talk to the "person in charge," I will be facing a person of my race.... (MacIntosh, 1990, p. 32).

Privilege is a special right or benefit granted to a person or groups of people. White privilege is the rights and benefits granted to white people by virtue of their skin colour. According to MacIntosh (1990), White privilege is "an invisible package of unearned assets that [White people] can count on cashing in each day ... White privilege is an invisible weightless knapsack of special provisions, maps, passports, visas, clothes, tools and blank cheques"(p. 24). Many of us are not aware of this kind of privilege and for health care professionals, White privilege remains elusive. As the list in Chapter 1 showed us, White privilege applies in countless areas in the health fields, from the lack of people of colour on boards and other decision-making bodies all the way to decreased chances of promotion. White privilege is fundamental to the perpetuation of injustice based on race. An understanding of the ways in which White privilege operates in an everyday way is central to undertaking anti-racist practice.

However, White privilege is difficult to bring forward for consideration, in part due to its invisibility for White people. A comparison with gender stereotyping often helps in understanding why White privilege is difficult for White people to perceive. In her explanation of the embeddedness of gender, Judith Lorber (1982) likened people noticing how gender operates to fish noticing water. Since we are surrounded by gender stereotyping in television shows, advertisements on TV, in magazines, and on billboards; in the electronic world; and in our everyday lives, it is very difficult to actually see how gender stereotyping is created and perpetuated.

A powerful strategy that we have used for helping students learn about stereotyping involves systematically examining the images all around them in popular culture. Over the years, in their experiences of recognizing gender stereotyping, students' responses clustered around several themes: (1) students are usually aware of gender stereotyping in general, but have not had the opportunity to actually analyze, in detail, what it means for women and men, girls and boys; (2) the connections between gender stereotyping in the mass media and social issues such as family violence rates have rarely been explored in the students' previous learning, except in cases where students took a related elective course (i.e., it is not a part of their core education in the professions); (3) the students found that after their experience in analyzing the images, they were no longer able to see advertisements without seeing gender in an analytical manner; and (4) the students recognized that the differential positing of men and women in these images literally and figuratively reflected male dominance in society in areas such as educational achievement, job mobility, and physical safety in the family home.

This last theme often generated the most lively debate. Moving from seeing gender to seeing the societal implications of the *dominance of one gender over the other* was more fraught with difficulty. In our community and academic teaching and learning work over the years, no matter what the topic of discussion, whether it was gender, race, social class, and so on, when the discussion moves to the means of dominance of one group over another, there is a natural shift in the tone of the discussion. This is because as soon as one talks about *dominance*, the corresponding notion of *privilege* comes into play in the discussion. The muddled middle (Hagey & McKay, 2000), where everyone is pretty much equal and we are all just trying to get along, get our work done, treat everyone the same, and mind our own business, is no longer possible. This is the way dominance works because dominant ways of seeing the world are just that—they dominate the media in all its forms; the curricular choices in schools and university departments; the health and social policy documents of municipal, provincial, and national governments; to name a few.

Although there are key differences in seeing gender and seeing White privilege, there are many parallels. White people may acknowledge the existence of racism, but attending to the other side of the coin—White privilege—is much more difficult. Ideas in popular culture, academic literatures, and policies that reflect government

> **Box 5.2: Ask Yourself These Questions**
>
> How did it come to be that the words "race," "culture," and "ethnicity" are associated primarily, and in some cases only, with people of colour?
> In descriptions of the various races, how did it come to be that White is not considered a colour?

decision making, all reflect dominant views. Kirby and McKenna (1989) noted that we live in a world where knowledge is used to maintain oppressive relations. Information is presented and interpreted in a way that presents the views of a small group of people as objective knowledge seekers or producers, while women, people of colour, and all other oppressed people are on the margins of the production of knowledge. When we cite statistics about inequities in income and employment status based on race, it is important to note the White privilege side of the coin. People of colour occupy a structured position subordinate to White people in the Canadian labour market, and in society (Galabuzi, 2006).

On closer examination, theories that were developed as being universally applicable to all people become greatly limited by the White, middle-class origins of their proponents (Collins, 1990). In her critique of the concept of double jeopardy (racism and sexism) and triple jeopardy (racism, sexism, and classism), King (1988) noted that because each of these concepts presumes a direct independent effect on status, neither is able to deal with the interactive effects of sexism, racism, and classism. Women of colour are subjected to these oppressions simultaneously. As Barbee (1994) reminded us, women's experiences of patriarchal oppression are defined by race, class, and culture, so by viewing the experiences of women of colour through White female lenses, their lived experiences are diminished or trivialized.

Much of the thinking that health professionals bring into a health care interaction is heavily based on White middle-class perspectives that are considered rational and scientific. For example, while knowledge in the health fields is thought to be research-based, it is usually based upon White eurocentric cultural norms. Consequently, there is a tendency for many professionals to assume that ethnocultural minority groups are irrational, primitive, and less than scientific. The embeddedness of racism also means that professionals may not consciously notice their assumptions These views of minority groups stem, in part, from Darwin's theory of evolution of species, which gave a scientific basis to the idea that "some groups of people are cultured while others remain 'closer to nature' and hence uncultured. It was assumed that European civilization represented the pinnacle of evolutionary success, the end of the long road from darkest Africa through numerous primitive and barbaric groupings to the high 'white' culture of Europe, and eventually, North America" (Lock, 1993, p. 144).

It is little wonder that some health care professionals think that they know what is best for clients and coerce them into complying with their professional values. Learning and attitudinal change involves interaction between the learner's present understanding of the world and their acquisition of new knowledge. Thus, when care providers are educated in a society that identifies the values of one group — Whites — to be superior to others, they take on the same values and tend to maintain the status quo. This process contributes to their inability to recognize that a large number of the health problems encountered by marginalized groups, such as Indigenous, African-Canadian, and immigrant peoples, have socio-political and economic components and cannot be simply cured. As Toumishey (1995) pointed out, "professional health practitioners must recognize that it is not sufficient to base ethical considerations only on the values that they personally hold. This is particularly relevant in that the present North American monolithic view of human nature and culture can lead to bio-ethnical considerations which are inadequate when caring for multicultural clientele" (p. 120).

In its most subtle, everyday form, racism is a razor within the psyche, slicing into self-confidence and self-love, an inner wound that is constantly being reopened by covert and sometimes overt messages that people of colour are inferior to the dominant White race. White people often view racism as an issue experienced by people of colour who are poor. However, racism cuts across all social classes, regardless of income and education. The racism that people of colour experience is not related to any individual lack of effort. Rather, racism is related to race, social class, and gender dominance. The interlocking hierarchies of Canadian society reinforce White male dominance and allow those who are advantaged not to be held accountable for their privilege.

As MacIntosh (1998) noted, as a White woman, she was taught to see racism only in individual acts of meanness, not in invisible systems conferring dominance on her group. This process supports and maintains a racist societal view where one group of people are made confident and comfortable while others are alienated and stripped of confidence and comfort. The cumulative effects of so much hostility, frustration, endless chipping away at one's confidence, and being exiled to the margins of society create a sense of hopelessness at times so great that the fight for one's dignity and the dignity of one's culture seems an impossible task.

Given that minority people are seen as inferior, it is not surprising that health care policies and services are implemented from the perspective of White people. For example, in the Apgar test, the normal colour of a newborn is described as pink, connoting that Black newborns, who are usually not pink at birth, are abnormal. This is a reflection of White dominant values of society revealed through the health care system. "Mainstream society is depicted as at the centre of a community, and those excluded from power and resources are at the periphery" (Hall et al., 1994, p. 26). In Western societies, the centre of the community is the seat of hierarchical power and the conceptual location of White people, while marginalized groups are relegated to the outside. They are not expected to speak as equals to their superiors at the centre, and their language is usually not in public and written discourse. For example, there are no clinical words to describe the colour of a healthy Black newborn. Further complicating the problem is the fact that most historic records to which people of colour have been exposed have been written from a White or Eurocentric perspective (Boyd, 1998).

Although health institutions in Canada do not have formal barriers based on race, informal barriers exist within their professional bodies, where non-White people are regarded as being inferior, or "if you're not white, you're not smart" (Boyd, 1998, p. 39). Systemic racism and invisible White privilege are pervasive in our everyday encounters. They are often reflected in the faces one can see on television, skin-care products at the store, and in health care providers. This is quite troubling in a society that professes to value all human life equally, and in health care professions that are governed by ethical codes that emphasize their humanitarian duties. Michele Fine (2004) explained some of the seemingly elusive nature of whiteness:

> *I find myself trying to understand the micromoves by which whiteness accrues privilege and status within schools; how whiteness grows surrounded by protective pillows of resources and second chances; how whiteness — of the middle class and elite variety in particular — provokes assumption of, and then insurance for being seen as "smart."* (p. 244)

The unearned gains that privilege bestows on White people carry with them a logic of disadvantaging others, thus creating a duality of dominance/subordination, freedom/restriction, access to correct means/lacking access to correct means, and order/disorder (Hagey & McKay, 2000). Consider the parallel mirror of privilege that exists along with some of the racism-related statistics listed in Chapter 2:

- White people are over twice as likely to have access to health care treatment for alcoholism, drug abuse, or mental health concerns than African Americans (Wells et al., 2001).
- White women are significantly more likely than Black women to receive expected therapy for breast cancer (Breen et al., 1999).
- White patients were more likely than minority patients to have pain recorded, even after adjustment for language differences (Bernabei et al., 1998).

It is important to note that White people who are women or elders, who live in poverty, have a disability, or who are lesbian or gay, also have decreased access to health care when compared to other White people. The point here is not to diminish the importance of these inequities. They are also very powerful. Rather, people of colour also experience inequities that are a result of racism in its many forms and the White privilege that sustains it.

The Other Side of White Privilege: Disadvantaging People of Colour

Based on her experience as a Black woman living in American society, Elaine Tassy, a writer and journalist, created a list of the ways in which White people are unfairly advantaged and Black people unfairly disadvantaged in various walks of life. Tassy (2006) defined unearned Black disadvantage as:

- A set of traps, slights, dismissals, denigrations, judgment, obstacles and setbacks white people will visit on me openly or aversively throughout the course of everyday in America, based solely on my race;
- A set of circumstances I am expected to react to in the presence of white people as if they are normal, and as if I am unaware of the inherent unfairness of them;
- A set of hurdles I took no part in erecting and fires I took no part in lighting, which I can expect to remain fairly constant and can anticipate and prepare for; and
- A set of experiences that I can expect will be reacted to defensively if I bring them to the attention of more than half the white people I know (Tassy, 2006).

Although this list may not be a representation of the experiences of all Black people, nonetheless, it is a catalyst for discussion about unearned White privilege within the context of underserved Black disadvantage, especially in educational settings. It may also be a tool for White people to begin the process of deconstructing White privilege in a contemporary and challenging way. Box 5.3 lists Tassy's questions about unearned White privilege in the context of Black disadvantage. These questions can help White people recognize privileges that are normally taken for granted.

The previous sections described core features of the anti-racist framework to guide practice. The discussion underscores the complexity of anti-racist practice, from understanding the cycle of oppression to understanding White privilege and its corresponding disadvantaging of people of colour. The following section describes how oppressions intersect to cause poorer health outcomes. Intersections of the social determinants of health, identity as a social determinant of health, and geography were described in Chapter 2. Here, intersectionality is revisited in order to underscore how oppressions such as racism and sexism can have a compounding and synergistic impact on health. Understanding intersectionality is a core feature of achieving anti-racist health care practice.

Intersections of Oppression and Poorer Health Outcomes

As the discussion and the qualitative and statistical evidence thus far has demonstrated, oppression related to race carries with it a set of profound and systemic consequences for people of colour in terms of their mental, physical, and spiritual health. The *intersections* of many forms of oppression are also central to understanding the how and the why of poorer health outcomes for people of colour. Intersections of oppression means that oppressions such as racism and sexism are not simply added to produce twice as much oppression. Rather, oppressions have a powerful

Box 5.3: Unpacking the Empty Duffel Bag: Unearned White Privilege in the Context of Unearned Black Disadvantage
by Elaine Tassy

Law Enforcement
- Can you name three people in your race that police officers of another race have shot, beaten, or sodomized?
- When you hear that a police officer has killed an unarmed suspect, do you assume the officer will not be of your race, but that the suspect will?
- Can you think of more than one example where a person of another race was convicted of a violent crime, then set free, pending an appeal?
- If a person of your race is assaulted by a person of another race, do you expect the police work to be affected by the race difference?

Employment and the Workplace
- If you send your resumé to a recruiter, can you expect your trendy or nontraditional first name to interfere with your chances of getting an interview?
- If you hear an offensive, non-religious, non-nationality-based joke concerning someone of your race, can you complain about it risk free to your opposite-race superior?
- If your opposite-race administrative assistant performs your assignments sloppily, do you ask yourself if it is because of your race?
- Is the expected earnings potential of people of your race lower than that of people of other races?
- In your place of work, have you been the only person of your race present to answer questions or give perspective on issues concerning your race?
- Can you think of at least three employment fields it would not be worth it for you to try to find a job in, based solely on your race?

Education
- Are you reasonably sure most tenured professors you study with will be of your race?
- Are you reasonably sure that most people deciding what books constitute literature are of your race?
- Can a child of your race audition for a play in an integrated school and reasonably expect a chance of getting a leading race-neutral role?
- If you skip a class held in a large lecture hall at a liberal arts college, will the colour of your skin tip the professor off to the fact that you decided not to show up?

Relationships
- Do you notice that many well-educated, professional, and/or well-paid men of your race get a social boost when they marry women of another race?
- Can you buy condoms, cervical caps, diaphragms or stick-on contraceptive patches that match your skin colour?
- Have single women of your race expressed concern that the shortage of available men of their race is connected in part to the fact that they are marrying women of other races?
- Does your race prompt your friends of other races to tell you, "When I look at you, I don't see colour"?

Beauty
- Do the promises shampoos and conditioners make on TV commercials about detangling, strengthening or otherwise improving the health and appearance of hair apply to people of your race?

- When you've sunbathed, do people of other races ask you what your purpose is for doing so?
- When you go to a dermatologist to treat acne or another topical skin condition, can you confidently anticipate that he or she will have expertise treating the skin of people of your race?
- For powerful members of society to consider your beauty marketable (for example, to be a model or anchorperson), do you have to have, adapt or simulate physical features similar to those of people of another race?
- Are any of your physical characteristics associated with beauty (size of lips, feet, buttocks, weight, genitals, shape of eyes, or nose, or texture of hair) considered out of the ordinary in society?

Popular Culture
- Is it assumed that a character in a book is of your race, if not explicitly stated?
- On the top three TV networks, do you regularly see characters of your race depicted as powerful heads of households and as love interests?
- Do people tell you you'll like a certain book or movie, only because the author or actors are of your race?
- Can you be pretty sure that lawyers, consultants and psychologists of your race will regularly be esteemed as experts worthy of interviews about race-neutral affairs on mainstream news magazine shows?
- Do you see contestants of your race winning dating reality shows?
- Can you count on regularly hearing the voice of someone who sounds like he or she is of your race in a voice-over for a movie trailer or TV commercial at least once a day?
- Can you imagine being denied the chance to audition for a part in a play because a casting director might tell you, "We don't do non-traditional casting"?

Community
- Can you go an entire day without thinking your race might bring about an experience that will lessen the quality of your day as you do errands in your community?
- Can you be pretty sure you'll find a doctor, lawyer, teacher, minister, and hairdresser of your race in any town in the country?
- Can you feel sure that if you call about a vacant apartment, the person renting it will show it to you when you arrive?
- If an empty cab you flag down in your community doesn't stop, do you wonder if it was because of your race?

Dining Out
- If you want a well-placed table in an upscale restaurant, would you consider sending someone of another race in first to secure one?
- If you don't leave a tip in a restaurant where the service was poor, do you think the server will factor in your race in reacting to being stiffed?
- If you wait longer than other diners for a table, service, or the arrival of your meal, do you wonder if race has anything to do with the length of your wait?

Source: Tassy, Elaine. "Unpacking the visible duffel bag: Teaching about White privilege to Philadelphia-area Community College Students." March 2008, Comparative and International Education Society Teachers College, Columbia University, New York.

synergy and together they interact to greatly disadvantage people of colour. For example, although we know that racism is a social determinant of health, we also know that sexism is a social determinant of health. This intersection leads us to ask how race and gender intersect in a compounding way to affect health. A case in point is the study of menopause. The medicalization of women's natural life events such as childbirth, menstruation (premenstrual dysphoric disorder, American Psychiatric Association, 1994), and menopause has meant that women are a major target market for the multinational pharmaceutical industry. The prescription of hormone-replacement therapy (HRT) to post-menopausal women serves as a recent example of how gender-based oppression of women has significant negative health consequences.

During several decades, HRT was the only long-term treatment used by millions of women without any trial (Rozenbaum, 2004). This means that HRT was prescribed to, and taken by, millions of women before an extensive, broad-based, and long-term study about its safety had been undertaken. Subsequent studies were then conducted, most notably the Women's Health Initiative (WHI). The WHI was the largest preventive study of its kind, and was launched by the National Institutes of Health (NIH) in 1993 in the United States. Its goal was to focus on defining the risks and benefits of strategies that could potentially reduce the incidence of heart disease, breast and colorectal cancer, and fractures in post-menopausal women. The study also examined HRT and found that various combinations of HRT increased the risk of dementia, breast cancer, and cardiovascular disease, with a significantly increased incidence of coronary events, such as heart attacks and stroke. Thus, HRT is no longer promoted in the same way as it was 20 years ago. The driving force for the use of HRT was not women themselves, but the billions of dollars of profit that were realized by the multinational pharmaceutical industry.

Thus, millions of post-menopausal women, regardless of colour, were placed at risk for serious health consequences. What happens when we consider the added burden for women of colour? While all women experience the process of menopause, our attitudes and feelings regarding the biological process of menopause do not evolve in a vacuum. History, culture, geography, social class, race, ethnicity, age, and personal experiences shape the way women feel and thinking about menopause. The perspectives of women from diverse ethnic and cultural backgrounds are often not represented and the lifelong constraints of living in a racist society are neglected, which adds to the burdens of dealing with physical changes of mid-life. In these ways, analysis of the social context of menopause demonstrates the deeper meaning that can be understood through considerations of the intersections of gender and race. Although all women were subjected to prescription of HRT despite the lack of research about its safety, women of colour experienced the compounding burden of racism.

This example of menopause demonstrates how consideration of intersectionality expands our thinking to be able to overlay and intersect two or more identities *at the same time.* Consideration of gender and race enriches our understanding of the menopausal experiences of women of colour. As this example shows, oppressive forces of sexism and racism combine to create a doubly jeopardy for these women. Just as identities can intersect to compound oppression, the other social determinants of health, as well as geography, can intersect. To further clarify this important concept, we return to our discussion about the intersections of the social determinants of health, identity as a social determinant of health, and geography. These areas may also be fruitfully examined in terms of their relationship with oppression.

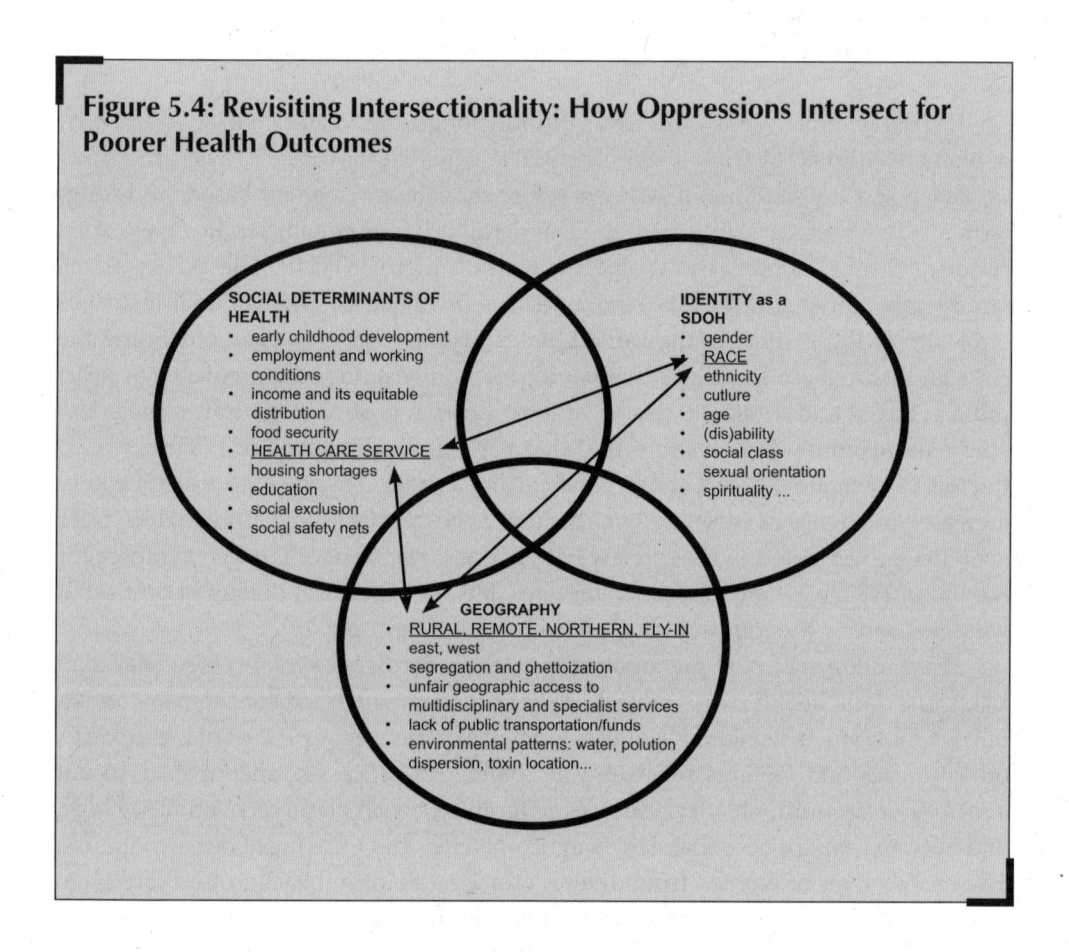

Figure 5.4: Revisiting Intersectionality: How Oppressions Intersect for Poorer Health Outcomes

SOCIAL DETERMINANTS OF HEALTH
- early childhood development
- employment and working conditions
- income and its equitable distribution
- food security
- HEALTH CARE SERVICE
- housing shortages
- education
- social exclusion
- social safety nets

IDENTITY as a SDOH
- gender
- RACE
- ethnicity
- culture
- age
- (dis)ability
- social class
- sexual orientation
- spirituality ...

GEOGRAPHY
- RURAL, REMOTE, NORTHERN, FLY-IN
- east, west
- segregation and ghettoization
- unfair geographic access to multidisciplinary and specialist services
- lack of public transportation/funds
- environmental patterns: water, polution dispersion, toxin location...

While intersections of gender and race, are experienced by women of colour, other intersections such as those related to geography are also at work. Consider the intersections of race, access to health services, and rural location, depicted in Figure 5.4. As discussed in Chapter 2, rural people have less access to health services and have poorer health than urban people. Women living in the most rural areas are most likely to report fair/poor health (Canadian Institute for Health Information, 2006). In 1996, infant mortality rates in rural areas were 30 percent higher than the national average (Minsterial Advisory Council on Rural Health, 2002). The evidence for racism as a determinant of health was detailed in Chapter 2. When we consider the intersections of health care access, rural location, and race, it becomes clear that there is a complex and synergistic relationship among these areas. This synergy creates a compounding or multiplying of disadvantage that changes over the lifespan. Box 5.4 describes an exercise to help practitioners understand how oppressions can intersect to cause poorer mental and physical health outcomes.

Connecting Intersectionality to Professional Practice Codes of Ethics

This final section brings together many of the ideas in the anti-racist framework to guide practice. We focus specifically on several codes of professional ethics in Canada. These codes provide clear avenues to discuss anti-racism in the world of everyday practice. It is through codes of ethics that practitioners may be held accountable, yet professional codes of ethics vary widely in their commitment to social justice, including racial justice. With the exception of a few of the codes of ethics, justice remains a nebulous concept and as such is very difficult for practitioners to embrace.

An understanding of the ways in which intersectionality shapes mental and physical health and well-being is fundamental to ethical practice. It is one of the most important clinical tools in the health and human service professions. It is just as important as learning diabetes protocols, the biochemistry of stress, and the legal complexities of child welfare. As the evidence demonstrates, lack of knowledge about intersectionality can be just as lethal as lack of knowledge about more conventionally accepted clinical knowledge. We need both of these knowledges. Without the capacity to understand and apply intersectionality principles in clinical practice, it is very difficult to provide ethical care. The following discussion offers an overview of selected codes of professional ethics in Canada. We direct specific attention to any elements of the codes that either state directly, or allude to, principles of social justice.

Although all the codes of ethics included basic ethical principles, we examined them for explicit language related to oppression and justice. It is certainly true that principles of justice could be *inferred* in ethical principles such as dignity, advocacy, and choice. However, we do not believe that inferential reference represents adequate or valid inclusion of principles of social justice in professional codes of ethics. We then propose important additions to codes of ethics that add accountability measures regarding social justice. We argue that omission of these accountability measures renders professional practice complicit in the profound injustice of morbidity and mortality that is the result of the intersectionalities of oppression in Canada.

Overview of Current Status of Selected Professional Codes of Ethics in Canada

Codes of ethics for professional associations, including the Canadian Nurses Association (2002), the Canadian Association of Occupational Therapists (2007), the Canadian Medical Association (2004), the Canadian Association of Social Workers

Figure 5.4: Revisiting Intersectionality: How Oppressions Intersect for Poorer Health Outcomes

Goal
To identify how the social determinants of health (SDOH), identity and geography intersect to produce compounding oppressions, and thus poorer health outcomes. The emphasis is on everyday examples that bring theoretical concepts of oppression into plain view.

Instructions
1. In small groups or collectively as a large group, think of various different combinations of the SDOH, identity as a SDOH, and geography. Start by choosing one element from each of the three circles (i.e., early childhood development, race, lack of public transportation and social safety nets, sexual orientation, and ghettoization).
2. Once you have worked through several examples using one element for each of the circles, brainstorm examples that include any combination from the three circles (e.g. social exclusion, education, male gender, race, lack of public transportation). We have provided an example in #1 below (health care services, race, rural). Use the space provided in 2, 3, 4 to detail your examples.

Questions for Personal Reflection, Discussion/Debate, and Action
1. How does an intersectionality lens help to illuminate the ways in which oppression operates in everyday life?
2. What are some of the barriers to thinking about oppression in this way?
3. What might be some of the reasons why the intersections of oppression are not widely discussed in the curriculum of health professionals or in their continuing professional education after they enter the workforce?
4. What are some paths for action? Individual (i.e., your own study or practice), institutional (i.e., within institutions such as universities and hospitals), and systemic or structural (i.e., public policies and government decision making).

Social Determinant of Health (SDOH)	Identity as a SDOH	Geography	Example of Intersection	Oppressions at Work in Your Example
1. Health Care Services	Race	Rural	Rural Indigenous peoples have decreased access to health care.	Racism in the health care system intersects with systemic policies that disadvantage rural people in terms of access to health services. Therefore, health outcomes are doubly jeopardized.
2.				
3.				
4.				

(2005), and the Canadian Psychological Association (2000), are based on principles such as respect, dignity, choice, confidentiality, and accountability. Some codes of ethics explicitly include items relevant to an anti-oppressive framework, although they are not identified as such. The concept of justice is a central feature of two of the codes of ethics: the Canadian Nurses Association and the Canadian Association of Social Workers. These will be further discussed in terms of their contribution to anti-racist practice.

The Canadian Medical Association Code of Ethics includes one statement under the heading "Initiating and Dissolving a Patient-Physician Relationship": "In providing medical service, do not discriminate against any patient on such grounds as age, gender, marital status, medical condition, national or ethnic origin, physical or mental disability, political affiliation, race, religion, sexual orientation or socioeconomic status. This does not abrogate the physician's right to refuse to accept a patient for legitimate reasons" (Canadian Medical Association, 1996, p. 1176a). Under the heading "Responsibility to Society," the code states: "Recognize the responsibility of physicians to promote fair access to health care services; Refuse to participate in or support practices that violate basic human rights" (p. 1176b). There are no further statements in the code that use the language of social justice.

The Canadian Nurses Association Code of Ethics (2008) specifically holds justice as a core ethical principle: "Nurses uphold principles of equity and fairness to assist persons in receiving a share of health services and resources proportionate to their needs and promoting social justice" (p. 17). The following is a summary of practice requirements specified.

1. When providing care nurses do not discriminate on the basis of a person's race, ethnicity, culture and spiritual beliefs, social or marital status, gender, sexual orientation, age, heath status, place of origin, lifestyle, mental or physical ability, or socio-economic status, or any other attribute.
2. Nurses refrain from judging, demeaning, stigmatizing, and humiliating behaviours towards persons receiving care, other health care professionals and each other.
3. Nurses do not engage in any form of lying, punishment or torture or any form of treatment or action that is inhumane or degrading. They refuse to be complicit in such behaviours. They intervene and they report such behaviours.
4. Nurses make fair decisions about the resources under their control, based on the needs of persons, groups, or communities to whom they are proving care. They advocate for fair treatment and for fair distribution of resources for those in their care.
5. Nurses support a climate of trust that sponsors openness, encourages questioning the status quo and supports those who speak out to address concerns in good faith (i.e. whistle blowing) (Canadian Nurses Association, p. 17).

Unfortunately, the following stronger, policy-based and social change language of the 2002 CNA Code was deleted in the formulation of the 2008 Code: "Should promote ethical care at the organizational/agency level by developing and implementing ongoing review of policies designed to provide the best care with the best available resources; should advocate for fairness and inclusiveness in health resource allocation, including policies and programs addressing determinants of health; should be aware of broader health concerns such as environmental pollution, violations of human rights, world hunger, homelessness, violence, etc and are encouraged to the extent possible to work individually as citizens or collectively for policies to bring about social change" (CNA, 2002, p. 15).

The Canadian Psychological Association (CPA) Code of Ethics includes explicit reference to discrimination and a clause regarding not practising, condoning, or collaborating with unjust discrimination, and a statement that all people have the right to have their innate worth as human beings appreciated, and that "this worth is not dependent on their culture, nationality, ethnicity, color, race, religion, sex, gender, marital status, sexual orientation, physical or mental abilities, age, socio-economic status, or any other preference or personal characteristic, condition or status" (Canadian Psychological Association, 2000, p. 8). Unjust discrimination is defined as activities that are prejudicial or promote prejudice to people because of their culture or nationality as listed above. The code leaves open the possibility of "just" discrimination, which could be an oversight, but still remains problematic due to the possible interpretation that there are situations where discrimination is justified. The Canadian Psychological Association (CPA) Code of Ethics thus devotes explicit attention to the language of social justice—prejudice and discrimination (albeit with the caveat above).

The Canadian Association of Social Workers Code of Ethics (2005) specifically holds "pursuit of social justice as a core ethical principle: "…Social workers promote fairness and the equitable distribution of resources, and act to reduce barriers and expand choices for all persons, with special regard for those who are marginalized, disadvantaged, vulnerable, and/or have exceptional needs. Social workers oppose prejudice and discrimination against any person, or group of persons on any grounds, and specifically challenge views and actions that stereotype particular persons or groups" (p. 5). The following is a summary of principles specified:

Social workers:

1. Uphold the right of people to have access to resources to meet basic human needs;
2. Advocate for fair and equitable access to public services and benefits;
3. Advocate for equal treatment and protection under the law, and challenge injustices, especially injustices that affect the vulnerable and the disadvantaged;
4. Promote social development and environmental management in the interests of all people (Canadian Association of Social Workers, p. 5).

CHAPTER 6

Engaging in Everyday Anti-racist Health Care Practice

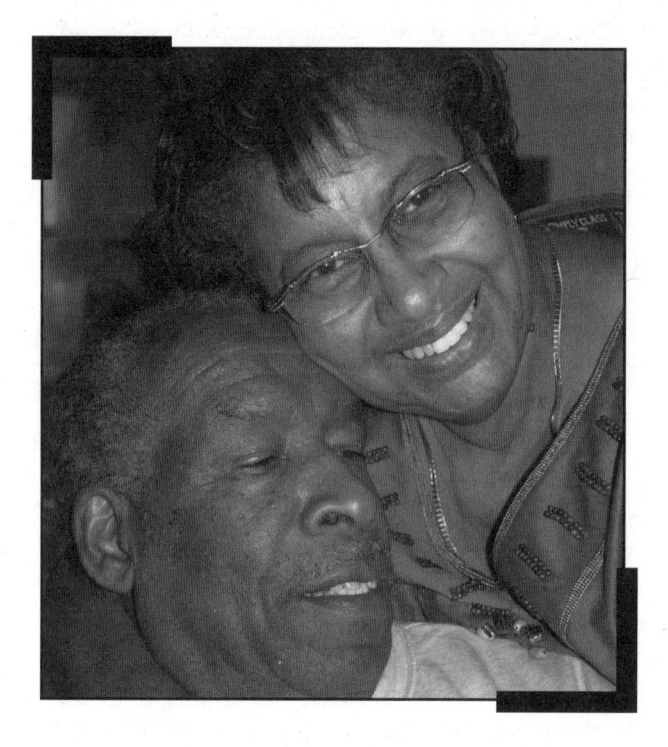

My commitment to engaged pedagogy is an expression of political activism. Given that our educational institutions are so deeply invested in a banking system [of learning], teachers are more rewarded for when we do not teach against the grain. The choice to work against the grain, to challenge the status quo, often has negative consequences. And that is part of what makes the choice one that is not politically neutral. (bell hooks, 1994, p. 203)

Introduction

In this chapter we draw upon many sources to describe a way forward for anti-racist health care practice. There has been relatively little practical application of anti-racist theory to health care practice. However, there has been a great deal of work in the area of anti-racist education. Our aim in this chapter is to bring these two worlds together in a form that serves as a useful springboard for change. We begin with a description of guiding principles for anti-racist practice, including the centrality of power, oppression, and confronting whiteness. The concept of situated practice is described with particular attention to power in the therapeutic relationship. We broaden the context of therapeutic power to include the systemic power that overlays all therapeutic encounters. Confronting the myth of neutrality in therapeutic work is emphasized. We call for the creation of a new meaning for critical thinking in the health fields that involves integration of ideas from the field of critical social science. The chapter would not be complete without a discussion of working with everyday resistance to anti-racist practice. We conclude with a description and discussion of the action continuum for social change.

Anti-racist Health Care Practice: Guiding Principles and Their Application

Anti-racist health care practice happens when practitioners actively engage in confronting racism in all its forms, with the understanding that racism is grounded in unequal and oppressive power relations and in White privilege. We build on Dei's (1996) work in the development of central principles, as well as some of our earlier work. Central principles of anti-racist health care practice are: (1) understanding and addressing the centrality of power; (2) understanding and addressing the facts of oppression; (3) confronting whiteness; (4) engaging in situated practice; (5) confronting the myth of neutrality; and (6) creating a new meaning for critical thinking in the health fields. These six principles are grounded in our anti-racist framework. As such, they provide a cohesive way to describe the philosophical underpinnings of the framework. The following sections describe each of these principles.

1. Understanding and Addressing the Centrality of Power
In order to engage in anti-racist practice, it is necessary to tackle the centrality of power. It is not sufficient to view oneself as good or trying hard or meaning well or dedicated. Whenever "race" enters the health care practice realm, power, and power imbalances in particular, are also present. In clinical practice there are a multitude of important facts to continually understand, synthesize, and apply. Each area of practice in the human services has unique and complex challenges. In the health fields, one of the most important challenges is the seeming contradiction between the relatively linear memorization of lists of facts, and the decidedly non-linear

process of actually applying these facts in the care of a vulnerable human being. In her book *Teaching to Transgress: Education as the Practice of Freedom*, bell hooks (1994) discusses the banking system of education: "The banking system of education (based on the assumption that memorizing information and regurgitating it represented knowledge that could be deposited, stored, and used at a later date) did not interest me. I wanted to become a critical thinker" (1994, p. 5). When we decide to incorporate anti-racist, anti-oppressive principles into our education and practice, we transgress the usual modes of learning and working—we move to illuminate our work with an understanding of the centrality of power, and a commitment to be part of social change in small and large ways. When we transgress, we challenge usual ways of getting things done and we question taken-for-granted ideas and claims.

Personal change is at the heart of learning anti-racist health care practice. If teaching and learning are to be transformative, then they will involve an engagement in how we as clinicians are located in our practice. Differences in location will be central to understanding where we are situated in our practice. As the discussions and exercises in Chapter 4 indicated, for White people this location is tied to membership in the dominant group. It is important to recognize the social aspects of race, including its socially constructed meanings. This understanding cannot happen without explicitly attending to intersections of oppression, such as race, gender, sexuality, and social class. According to Dei (1996), understanding race, even with its changing and socially constructed meaning, is a key to anti-racist education: "The concept of race is central to an anti-racism discourse as a tool for community and academic organizing for social change. There are powerful social meanings to race which are anchored, particularly, in the lived experience of minority groups in white-dominated societies" (p. 27). The power and privilege of whiteness is a necessary entry point for members of dominant groups in society to join the anti-racism debate.

2. Understanding and Addressing the Facts of Oppression

Action for change is based in developing a critical awareness of injustice and health. We must listen to the stories and learn the facts of racial discrimination, and how it operates in everyday practice. It is very difficult to grasp the scope and depth of discrimination and oppression without an active interest, and hence awareness, of the everyday facts of oppression. The social determinants of health have been pivotal in helping people make the links between oppressive societal structures and poor health. These facts will continue to be important in working for change—numbers talk. The field of health inequity statistics is in its infancy in Canada, and there is a growing desire to bring these numbers forward for policy intervention. Ethical concerns about data are also being discussed and debated with people of colour holding a meaningful place at the table.

The importance of lived experience will also be central for moving forward. Qualitative research has the potential to inform policy intervention far more than is currently recognized by policy-makers in North America (Denzin & Lincoln, 2007). More first-person testaments about the lived experience of oppression need to be heard by health practitioners. When the stories of oppression are told by oppressed peoples themselves, in their own languages and ways of communicating, it is much more difficult to deny the brutal realities of oppression. This is human nature—we are more likely to respond in a spiritual and emotional way when we hear first-person stories. Rather than being a threat to our professional objectivity, these stories are the essence of human survival and connection.

Statistical data that does not address health inequities continues to be the norm for policy evidence. Critical mixed-methods research also has great potential to bring the worlds of quantitative research and qualitative research together to paint a clearer picture of inequity and injustice. Health geomatics—the use of geographic information systems to study health—has proven to be pivotal in the study of health inequities in the United States. (Krieger, Chen, Waterman, Rehkopf & Subramanian, 2005). Bringing forward stories and numbers about the facts and experiences of oppression is a key feature of understanding oppression and discovering paths for change.

When we have the lens of anti-oppressive practice, we develop the capacity to continue to learn how oppression operates in our everyday lives. In health education materials, not only do the depictions of white-skinned people far outnumber people of colour, the contexts of representations of the latter are often steeped in racist stereotypes. Over a decade ago, we presented a paper at a national nursing conference that detailed this phenomenon. We demonstrated our points with routinely available health education pamphlets and posters. Among the few representations of people of colour were a Black basketball player in a diabetes pamphlet, and a Black woman in a "Don't drink alcohol when you are pregnant" poster. In many ways, this has changed very little in the first decade of the 21st century. This is not surprising since racism is built on centuries of oppression. Dorothy Smith (1999) called this the textual mediation of societal power. Textual mediation refers to the process of using textual representations to mediate or reinforce ideas and ways of thinking. Most of us are familiar with the way that sexism is mediated by textual images in magazines, textbooks, billboards, advertisements of all kinds, television, and the Internet. These are all avenues to mediate the perpetuation of sexism.

Critical examination of textual materials (and these include everything from actual textbooks, to course descriptions, advertisements in all their various forms, and policy and procedure documents) is a much neglected area of analysis in anti-oppressive work. This is increasingly worrisome because popular culture bombards all of us with an unprecedented barrage of images, and the electronic age has created numerous complex and often unnoticed ways of influencing our thinking. Throughout her work, Dorothy Smith (1987, 1990b, 1999) emphasized the importance of the textual mediation of social relations. For example, when we examine social relations of power, the way that textual materials reinforce dominant

> **Box 6.1: Case Example**
>
> **The Texts of Racism: Health Education Materials and the Perpetuation of Racism**
> Recently, while waiting for an appointment at a doctor's office, we took a sample of every health education pamphlet from the various racks and promotional displays in the waiting room. There were 29 pamphlets in total, with 220 pictures of human faces and bodies. One hundred and ninety pictures were of White people, and 32 pictures were of people of colour. This disparity is further accentuated by the fact that 11 of the 32 pictures of people of colour were from a Foster Parents Plan pamphlet. The other 21 depictions of people of colour were pamphlets about being overweight ("Start losing weight today"); baby feeding ("Good food habits mean a lifetime of good health"); breast cancer ("Cook-for-the-cure fundraising campaign"); the importance of immunization ("Don't hesitate to vaccinate"); meningitis in Africa ("Meningitis can be found all over the world"); and osteoporosis.
> There is much to be said about the lack of people of colour in the pamphlets as well as their relationship to content choices (infectious diseases; the need for foster parents, cooking, and the need to lose weight). We have little doubt that a much larger and methodologically sound study would produce similar findings. Pictorial representations in journals, textbooks, and so on reveal a similar pattern. These textual representations are articulated to systemic racism in the health care system, in multinational drug and food companies, in the educational system and in systems of government, to mention a few. The texts become part of how health professionals participate in racism by *not noticing* the astounding amount of racism in these materials, and by *remaining silent* about it.

power structures is very important to consider. The case example in Box 6.1 shows how health-promotion pamphlets serve to reinforce the dominance of whiteness and the inferiority of people of colour. This is textually mediated racism. As Kinsman (1995) claimed, textual mediation is a crucial aspect of the contemporary social organization of maintaining power hierarchies.

3. Confronting Whiteness

The third anti-racist principle is based on work by Anne Bishop (2002, 2005). *Becoming an Ally: Breaking the Cycle of Oppression* laid an important foundation for understanding the positioning of White people in the struggle to end racism. We build on Bishop's years of work as a White person facilitating anti-oppressive practice. Allies work for change through an acknowledgement of their own roots, their grasp of the concept of social structures and collective responsibility, their knowledge and sense of history, their acceptance of the anti-racist struggle, and their understanding that good intentions do not matter if there is no action against oppression (Bishop, 2002). Allies "take responsibility for helping to solve problems of historical injustice without taking on individual guilt. Most look for what they can do, with others, in a strategic way, and try to accept their limitations beyond that" (p. 110). Wijeyesinghe, Griffin, and Love (1997) also added that allies are willing to be confronted about their own behaviour. Bishop (2002, p. 22) described the following six steps in working for change. The steps are illustrated with health care examples.

1. *Understanding oppression, how it came about, how it is held in place, and how it stamps its pattern on the individuals and institutions that continually recreate it.*
   This step is analogous to seeing the paths of racist oppression in our individual selves as White people; in our culture; in the choices we make about where to site landfills and toxic dumps; and in the systemic, policy-based decisions that demonstrate our difficulty in acknowledging and addressing disadvantage in the school system. In health care practice, unequal access to services comes about through discrimination when clinicians treat people of colour unfairly. It is held in place when hospitals permit such things as substandard assessments. Oppression stamps its pattern on institutions as these substandard assessments of people of colour are not challenged.
2. *Understanding different oppressions, how they are similar, how they differ, how they reinforce one another.*
   This step is about intersectionality—understanding how the intersections such as those of race, gender, and social class will compound and multiply each other to increase disadvantage. Racism, classism, and sexism all operate in similar ways. The cycle of oppression is set in motion and bias leads to discrimination based on race, social class, and gender. Each of these *-isms* also have their own history and ways of operating in societies around the globe. For example, in health care, systemic racism is demonstrated by the dearth of Indigenous and Black health care practitioners throughout Canada. Systemic classism is demonstrated in the preferential treatment of people who have the money to navigate the health system for the best care. The health care system operates on the assumption that families have the cash for cars, buses, and taxis to get to an appointment, even if the specialist appointment is hundreds of miles away from home. Systemic sexism is demonstrated by the predominance of male decision-makers. Look at the pictures of the board of directors of any health care institution. There are increasingly more (White) women, but the boards are still dominated by (White) men. If we put all these instances of racism, classism, and sexism together, we see that the intersections of several oppressions create a synergy of disadvantage.
3. *Engaging in consciousness-raising and healing.*
   First, resist the urge to skip this discussion. This step speaks to the need for personal connection to our work. This might seem self-evident, especially for health field workers since we often find ourselves amid the mental and physical health struggles of the people for whom we care. This is the nature of our work. However, many of us spend relatively little time reflecting on how we might become more conscious of injustice. Consciousness refers to raising the knowledge of oppression in our consciousness—becoming deliberately conscious of the various forms of oppression. Consciousness can grow through personal practices such as journal writing, reflection, conversation, counselling, research, observation, and analysis. The process of consciousness raising often creates psychic pain as we come to know some of the depth of injustice that oppressed peoples experience. This pain

is, in many ways, evidence of our connection to the collective consciousness of all human beings. It is what keeps us moving to work for change. As Bishop (2002) noted, pain is part of consciousness raising. Bishop also linked consciousness raising to the importance of healing. Collective healing can happen in well-facilitated group discussions, and in many other ways such as public grieving rituals, informal gatherings, or in emotional expression with trusted people in the context of therapy or through the arts.

4. *Becoming a worker for your own liberation.*

Bishop (2002) emphasizes that in order to be an effective ally, one must be a worker for one's own liberation. For White women, this might mean working to understand sexism, and to educate our children about sexism. One of the ways that I [Elizabeth] became acutely aware of sexism was in the birthing and subsequent nurturing of my two daughters. I learned to connect the relentless stereotyping of little girls as sweet and nice to their diminished chances for earning and promotion in the workplace. In 1976 when I entered nursing school, one of my housemates brought home a poster that talked explicitly about gender discrimination. It detailed girls' decreased chances for making as much as their male playmates, or for achieving advanced education. Current statistics are pretty much the same as they were in the 1970s. The poster is still as relevant today as it was then.

5. *Becoming an ally.*

Becoming an ally involves learning about yourself as a member of particular oppressive groups. As the discussion about White privilege in Chapter 4 demonstrated, it is embedded and systemic. It is not only difficult for White people to perceive, it may evoke considerable anger for White people, especially since denial of oppressive tactics means that many White people remain ignorant of their privilege. Here are some reflections on being an ally [Elizabeth]:

- *The challenge of vicarious anger from other White people:* Allies become targets of other White people's anger. The anger that White people often have toward people of colour who speak up about racism is transferable to other White people who speak up. These kinds of anger are very different and have different consequences for the recipient. In my experience, anger from other White people is remarkably consistent and enduring over time. I can only attempt to imagine what every day must be like for people of colour who speak up about racism. The once-removed resistance from other White people can be very draining in clinical practice and in academia.
- *Is it possible?:* Sometimes I am struck by the near-impossible project of White people's ability to have a constructive role in ending racism. Even the language we use is the language of European colonizers. Part of the process of oppression was and is to diminish or destroy the languages of people of colour. Our privilege is so taken for granted that we can only ever attempt to stay one step ahead of

actively oppressing people of colour. We, as White people, step into the easy comfort of knowing how to move the agenda forward by including words such as "marginalization" and "discrimination" in policy documents and in provincial and national research funding agency calls for proposals, all the while making it next to impossible to obtain funding from the general pots of money if the words of anti-racist practice are included in the proposal. This also includes examples such as blocking a research proposal due to issues such as the survey term "Black" is not properly defined, even though the one-drop rule has been meticulously explained in the proposal. It is difficult to imagine a situation where a White research participant would have to prove her or his whiteness before being allowed to participate in a survey.

I am reminded of the first time anyone explained White privilege to me. It was at a workshop almost 20 years ago. I was fascinated by this analysis, and I agreed with everything the presenters said. They were Black and White people. They demonstrated how all the people on soap boxes and diaper packages, etc., are White: White babies; White plastic people on the tops of wedding cakes; and White people posing as Jesus, Mary, and Joseph on Christmas cards (a historical impossibility). After the presentation I approached one of the Black women and asked how I could help. She said, in a gentle but directive tone, "You have to do your own work around whiteness." She was right.

- *On White navel-gazing:* It is important to think about whiteness, but whiteness is relevant only insofar as the thinking is consistently connected to power, privilege, and social change. In many ways the situation is so urgent that White involvement in the struggle is useful only if it is part of a clear and strong move for educating White people for the purposes of social change. I was at an academic conference several years ago where I had a paper abstract accepted in a session titled "Interrogating Whiteness." My paper was about many of the concerns in this list of reflections about being an ally. The audience consisted of an intercontinental mixed-race group with a broad background in anti-racist work. I was the last presenter. The White people presenting before me talked about whiteness: what it is, what it means, how it makes them uncomfortable in certain situations, and how they are jealous of the sensuousness that dark-skinned people seem to innately have. I was disgusted. I do not mean to imply that I was operating on some sort of enlightened plane that was above these other White people. I was barely able to understand the implications that I knew some of the people in the audience were fully grasping. I lost all interest in presenting, but I slogged on anyway. Sessions like these seem like clear, real-time examples of claims about how White people will adjust to anti-racist rhetoric as needed and still appropriate the voices of racialized peoples.

6. *Maintaining hope.*
   There is an ebb and flow to maintaining the hope and energy needed to continue. The key is surrounding yourself as much as possible with justice-minded people, regardless of their race, age, gender, social class, sexuality, and so on. Then you will not be exhausted with the continual energy of having to justify what to you has become perfectly obvious. Hope is related to consciousness raising and healing. It is tough to do this kind of work without a repertoire of personal reflective practices of some sort, such as writing or meditation.

4. Engaging in Situated Practice

The fourth principle of anti-racist health care practice is engaging in situated practice. Situated practice must be our starting point for anti-racist health care practice: explicitly identifying our own positioning on an ongoing basis. Moving forward happens through individual and collective reflective questioning of our own location in the creation and maintenance of societal power imbalance. Situated practice means that we consciously locate ourselves in terms of our own social locations vis-à-vis our social determinants of health, our identity, and our geography. Situated practice happens when practitioners engage in ongoing reflection of where their own identity is situated in relation to the dominant groups. "The notion that clinicians and clients may have different experiences of social class, gender, and racial dominance has scarcely been addressed by helpers in the health fields, and the implications of the social class, gender, and race of the helper have barely been mentioned" (McGibbon, 2000, p. 185). Although situated practice begins with reflecting on one's own identity, the foundation of situated practice has to do with applying an understanding of power and power over in the context of the therapeutic relationship.

There are informative documents that can help us to understand power and power over in the therapeutic context. *Power, Paternalism, and Partnerships* (Canadian Mental Health Association, 2007) discussed the connections among power, patriarchy, power over, and professional practice. The association stressed attention to the power imbalances inherent in therapeutic relationships. Documents such as this can usefully be applied to anti-racist practice: How does racism influence the power dynamics in our interpersonal therapeutic relationships with individuals, families and communities of people from marginalized or racialized groups? If we are members of the dominant groups, such as White women and men, and people on the upper end of the socio-economic scale, how does this dominance reflect our position of power in our therapeutic work?

These core ideas regarding power and interpersonal dynamics in the therapeutic relationship are a useful starting point to further discuss situated practice. A post-colonial, anti-racist perspective also directs our attention to the continued and profound legacy of colonialism. If practitioners find themselves angry about all the things we have 'given' to Native peoples in Canada, this attitude will be a significant barrier in their ability to work competently and compassionately with Indigenous peoples. Figure 6.1 illustrates the relationship between power in the local (person-to-person) context of therapeutic work, and the overlay of the systemic power context within which all therapeutic work takes place. Understanding power imbalances related to oppression enriches clinical practice and provides a therapeutic milieu that is more likely to be physically, emotionally, and spiritually safe. As practitioners, we have a professional and ethical responsibility to be mindful of how we are in a position of power already by virtue of the nature of therapeutic work.

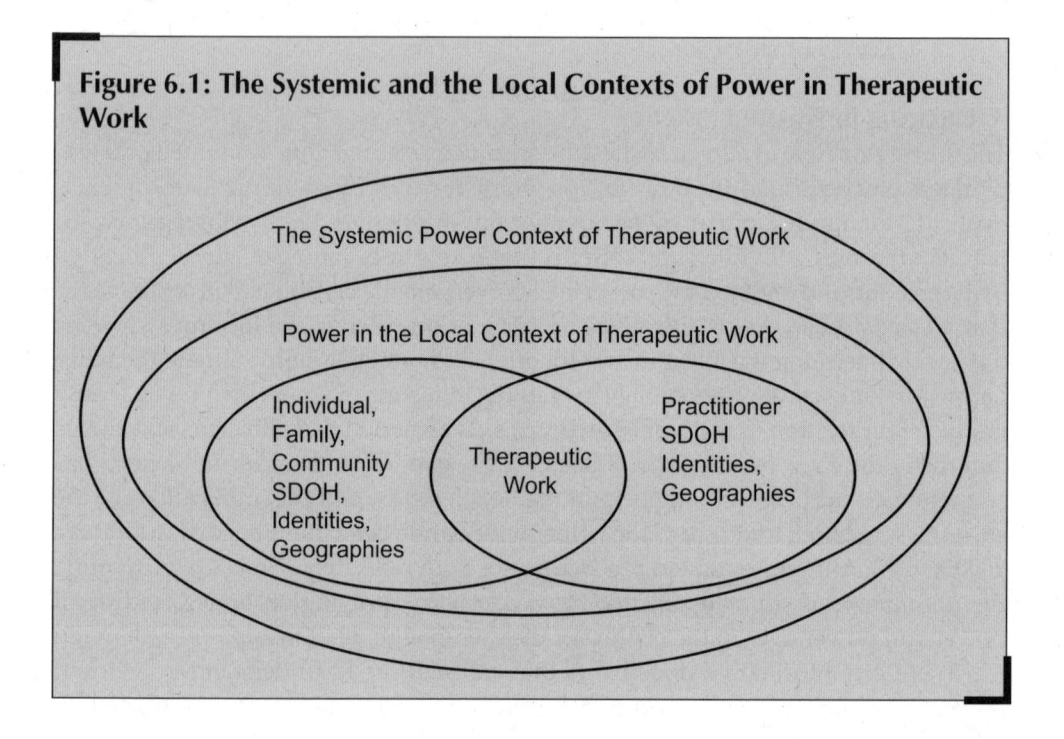

Figure 6.1: The Systemic and the Local Contexts of Power in Therapeutic Work

- The Systemic Power Context of Therapeutic Work
- Power in the Local Context of Therapeutic Work
  - Individual, Family, Community SDOH, Identities, Geographies
  - Therapeutic Work
  - Practitioner SDOH Identities, Geographies

When we consider the systemic contexts of power imbalances, we see that systemic power imbalances related to racism and other forms of oppression overlay all our therapeutic work. For example, when a mother arrives at the health centre for a prenatal visit, the clinician usually develops an ongoing relationship with the woman throughout her pregnancy. This is the one-to-one therapeutic work that underpins much of health care. There is an embedded power difference here, with the health care practitioner being in a power-over position by virtue of the historical nature of health care work in the Western world. This is the local, one-to-one context of power in therapeutic work. Local also refers to the family and community context. Also operating in the local context are the clinician's identities (e.g. gender, race). When the clinician has dominant identities (e.g. White, upper class), then this power difference is also embedded in the local, one-to-one therapeutic work, whether or not the clinician is aware of it. All of these aspects of power operate within the systemic power context described throughout this book.

In the example above regarding working with Indigenous peoples, the already existing and well-documented power imbalance created by virtue of the nature of the therapeutic relationship is further compounded by the power imbalance created by systemic oppression. If we have the attitude that Indigenous peoples are lazy, and were given everything by White people, then we bring a highly toxic and dangerous mix to our therapeutic work with Indigenous individuals, families, and communities. Thus, power and power over in clinical practice with individuals and families is a reflection of these same power structures in the larger societal context. If we are White, then a dedicated part of our ongoing practice incorporates the meanings of whiteness in terms of power in the local and systemic contexts of racism and oppression.

Practitioners are often reluctant to practise within the context of situated practice because situated practice involves another layer of meaning and responsibility in their everyday work. For example, consider a community health practitioner working with a diabetic pregnant woman who is a new immigrant from Guatemala. In situated practice, concerns would extend from usual and important intervention regarding diabetes in pregnancy, to acknowledgement of the dynamics of institutional power that health professions hold—power in the local, one-to-one context. By extension, the practitioner would think about the connections among power in the local context of therapeutic work, systemic power of police and legal institutions, and the woman's reluctance to disclose information due to her experiences of terror in a police state back home in Guatemala. Box 6.2 provides a clear and practical way for practitioners to think about power as it is situated in their practice.

5. Confronting the Myth of Neutrality

It is necessary to acknowledge the myth of neutrality—to think about why "the confused, middle, or neutral position is one of condoning racism and other forms of dominance" (Hagey & MacKay, 2000, p. 10). Neutrality, in the English language, usually brings to mind words such as impartial, uncommitted, objective, and free from opinion. The neutral observer listens and surveys the situation and retains neutrality. In the health professions, neutrality is often viewed as synonymous with objectivity. Practitioners often pride themselves in maintaining a neutral stance, and students and beginning practitioners often strive to treat everyone equally. When teachers and clinicians bring anti-racist ideas to faculty or staff meetings, into the classroom, or into clinical case conferences, they face the very real possibility of being accused of being biased. The status quo is somehow viewed as unbiased and objective. This is because we are immersed in the dominant view, and unless we see beyond this view, any information that challenges this view is immediately recognized as unusual, and therefore is considered to be introducing bias.

Over 10 years ago, one of us facilitated a large interdisciplinary, undergraduate workshop about sexuality. The students were from many different health-related

Box 6.2: Locating Yourself in Your Clinical Practice

Goal
This exercise is designed to help you think about your social location. In clinical practice in the health fields, we are educated to focus on the demographics and other identifying information of clients. Common sense tells us that our own gender and age, for example, make a difference in our everyday therapeutic work.

However, we are not usually accustomed to explicitly thinking about our own social location and how it forms the foundation of our interface with the world. The diagram below represents the multiple intersections of the various social locations: gender, race, age, ethnicity, to name a few. The diagram is based in Enid Lee's Power Flower (Arnold, Burke, James, Martin, & Thomas, 1991).

Instructions
1. Take a few moments to think about who you are in terms of these social locations and privately fill in the corresponding blanks. Notice that some of the social locations are changeable, such as social class and geography. Others, such as gender, are changeable as well. When you fill in the blanks, be sure to take note of your social locations of origin (at birth or in the early years), and your current social location. Note the circle with the question marks. This could be locations such as religion or spirituality (original or current).
2. After you have completed the diagram for your own social location, individually or in a group, fill in the blanks for the common stereotypes of the following client: An unkempt man with dark skin who enters your emergency department for assessment.
3. Beside your own identity, write in the identities that are dominant.
4. Discuss the questions in Box 6.3.

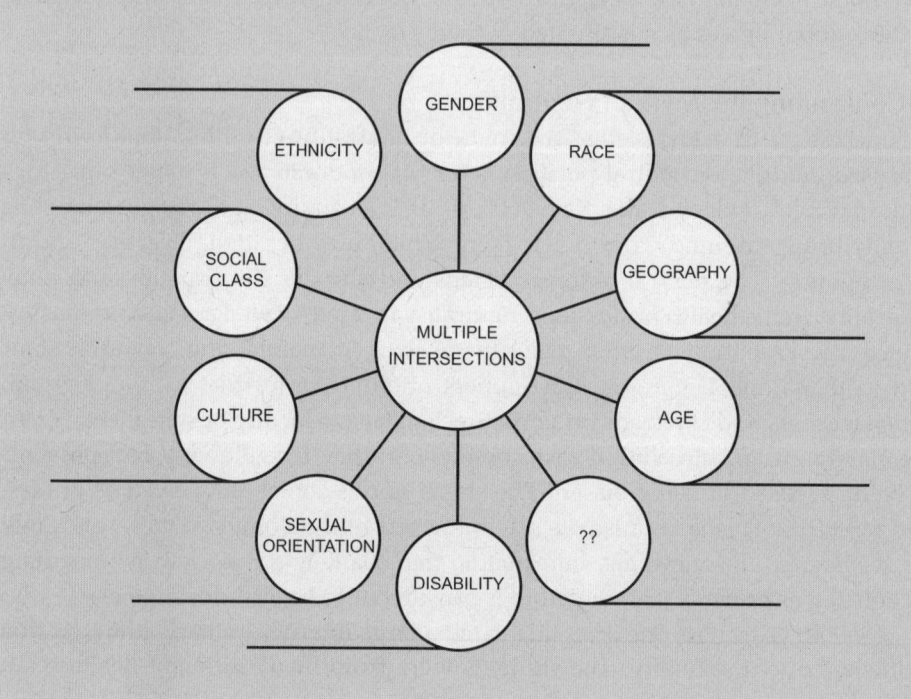

> **Box 6.3: Questions for Personal Reflection Group Discussion/Debate, and Action**
>
> 1. How are your own race, culture, and ethnicity related?
> 2. In your own life, what are some of the intersections of your social locations? (*Hint:* Gender and age, race and ethnicity, rural location, education, and so on.)
> 3. When we don't know a client's social location, do we tend to fill in the blanks with: (a) the dominant social location (i.e., heterosexual); and/or (b) the stereotypical social location (i.e., unkempt = lazy or poor)? Why?
> 4. In the diagram above, in Box 6.2 note the circle with the question marks. What other social locations would you add here?
> 5. Where do we get most of our messages/ideas about social location?
> 6. Is it possible to leave your social location at the door when you enter a therapeutic relationship?
> 7. Make a list of actions that clinicians can take to ensure that they are working in a context of situated practice. Make another list of actions that your institution can take. Write corresponding barriers to carrying out these actions, and possible solutions to overcome the barriers.

disciplines. One of the speakers, a Black man, talked about notions of sexuality in working with adolescents in his clinical practice. He introduced stories and reflections about the importance of being mindful of areas such as sexual orientation and racial and geographic origin when we engage in therapeutic work. He wove these stories together with his own personal experiences in one of the best presentations in the week-long workshop.

After each presentation, we formed small discussion groups. Most of the students in my group could not get past the notion that the speaker was biased and spent far too much time talking about race and sexual orientation: "We're tired of hearing about it; it's overkill." In fact, the speaker's mention of race and sexual orientation took up relatively little of his presentation time. The reason the students thought he did nothing but discuss race and sexual orientation was because they were so unaccustomed to hearing about these topics in an integrated way. These students were more comfortable with the usual presentation of race and sexual orientation in their curriculum: in discrete and one-time-only classes about "diversity" or "patient sexuality" — ideas safely constrained in a box, to be opened for exam study and then tossed back in. I could see that some of their peers were uncomfortable with their complaints; however, they were not willing or able to speak up at that particular time. For many of these students, the mention of race and sexual orientation was perceived as biased, as stepping beyond the necessary neutrality of clinical practice.

When one is immersed in the dominant culture — in this case White and heterosexual — any stepping into the world of the non-dominant groups is difficult to accomplish without careful reflection. This can be done in many interesting and inspiring ways:

- Ask yourself where you get your messages and your information about race, sexual orientation, and social class. Is it primarily from popular culture—TV, magazines, YouTube, and advertisements in all their electronic and material forms? If these are your main sources of information, then you do not have the opportunity to see the non-dominant side of the story. Making a specific and consistent effort to access this other side of the story is an important component of ethical practice.
- Make it a point to go to first-person presentations, where people talk about their experiences of being in the world as the Other—a member of one of the non-dominant groups—being gay, being Indigenous, being Black, being poor, being a Black woman, being an Inuit woman, being an adolescent with a learning disability, to name a few. If you do not hear first-person stories, how will you find any avenue into knowing about and beginning to understand the life experiences of people in non-dominant groups?
- Read, read, read to balance the relentless bombardment of stereotyped images from the media, from health education textbooks, and from the images on DVDs in the video store. If we are not reading alternative information and stories, it will be difficult to engage in everyday practice that is not discriminatory. Unless we create a window into the non-dominant world and keep it open, we will be stuck in the artificial position of neutrality.

6. Creating a New Meaning for Critical Thinking in the Health Fields

Encouraging critical thinking is becoming standard practice in health care settings, in educational settings, and in professional associations. In this context, critical thinking includes an attitude of inquiry involving the use of principles, abstractions, deductions, interpretations, and analysis of arguments (Green, 2000). Anti-racist practice includes all of these kinds of thinking. Green's emphasis on abstractions, deductions, and interpretations underscores the sometimes not-so-concrete nature of thinking about race, racism, and other forms of oppression. These are abstract terms that challenge our ability to bring anti-racist practice into our everyday worlds. Much of the emphasis in this book is to do just that.

Most discussions of critical thinking in the health fields also include notions of investigation, logical deduction, and scientific reasoning. These notions are particularly important if you are trying to understand problems such as the cause of an allergic reaction. However, they present barriers when one is attempting to understand racism in the health care system. There is no test or uniform set of logical indicators that can be applied in every situation or even in most situations. Biomedical protocols fall short of the critical thinking necessary to incorporate anti-racist principles into our practice. The influence of biomedical science is especially evident in the following critical thinking trait described as an "intellectual sense of justice" (Green, 2000):

> This trait implies that, as a critical thinker, you will assess all viewpoints similarly, without regard to vested interests or feelings of friends, communities, or nations. For

example, you may be discussing a new piece of equipment with a friend and several other colleagues. Your intellectual sense of justice will allow you to listen to everyone's viewpoints about the equipment and weigh them equally, without showing preference toward your friend's opinion (p. 6).

This quote exemplifies the persistence of believing the possibility of neutrality in clinical practice. One of the most interesting aspects of this thinking is that it is analogous to White people's claims that they are not racist, even when participating in racist stereotyping. The credibility of both of these claims, the neutrality of the listener in the above example, and the claim of non-racism rest squarely on the assumption that in order to violate fairness or to be racist, *we have to be able to identify when we are doing so*. This kind of logic tells us that if we walk away from the encounter *feeling and thinking* that we were not unfair or racist, then our *actions* must not have been unfair or racist. A newer version of critical thinking must encompass the ability to recognize and critique the illogical discrepancy in these claims. The point here is that opening up critical thinking to this kind of gaze frees us to stop attempting the impossible stance of neutrality, and to allow ourselves the space to question our own thinking.

A new meaning of critical thinking encompasses some of the core features of conventional definitions of critical thinking in the health fields; however, we expand on these conventional definitions to include the critical perspectives discussed in Chapter 4—critical theory, feminism, anti-racist, post-colonial, anti-colonial, human rights, and political economy perspectives. Here critical means an explicit analysis of societal power imbalances and how they are articulated to everyday practice and to health outcomes across the lifespan. As this discussion has indicated, conventional meanings of critical thinking may obscure and reinforce the power of dominant groups. Critical thinking, in addition to being about reflective reasoning, and the ability to make abstractions, deductions, and interpretations, must include an analysis of power and oppression in people's lives and in governing systems as an underlying feature. Box 6.4 introduces "The question lineup" as a group exercise that helps to critically analyze ideas and opinions about power.

The principles of anti-racist health care practice call for thinking and acting in new ways. The feeling of renewal that this change often brings is often accompanied by the experience of resistance from other people. The following sections discuss this resistance.

Working with Everyday Resistance to Anti-racism Practice

Resistance often flows along the same lines as resistance to anti-racism education, and the two are inseparable. The arguments in health practice tend to go something like this:

> **Box 6.4: The Question Lineup: Critical Thinking as Thinking about Power**
>
> *Goals*
> 1. To think about where we stand on important social issues.
> 2. To think about how our own stance relates to the stance of the other people in the lineup.
> 3. To explain our position and debate our differing perspectives with each other.
>
> *Instructions*
> Participants stand up and form a line along the side of the room, or whereever they can comfortably stand in a line. The facilitator asks one of the questions below, and everyone walks to the area along the line that best suits their personal opinion. Responses usually range all along the line, as illustrated below, from "strongly agree" to "strongly disagree." Sometimes there is also a cluster in the middle.
>
> | Strongly Agree | | Strongly Disagree | |
> |---|---|---|---|
> | X   X X   XX | XXXX   XX | XXXX | XX |
>
> *Suggested Lineup Questions*
> 1. If a person tries very hard, he or she can usually overcome obstacles to enroll in community college or university.
> 2. Lack of ambition is one of the main reasons why people don't succeed in life.
> 3. People can achieve a healthy lifestyle if they are really committed to changing their behaviour.
> 4. A woman can leave an abusive relationship if she really wants to.
> 5. People can stop smoking if they have sufficient willpower.
>
> *Questions for Reflection, Discussion and Debate, and Action*
> 1. What are barriers to achieving mental, spiritual, and physical wellness?
> 2. How do dominant societal power structures influence individual agency?
> 3. What are all the places and methods through which we get our ideas about how we might achieve wellness and illness?
> 4. What do our positions in the question lineup have to do with our world view?

1. Yes, some clinicians are racist, but I am not racist. This belief is often based in the belief that racism is an individual act. Many people struggle with and resist the concept of systemic racism and any claims that individual acts of racism are bound within societal racism. An individual focus obscures the need to acknowledge that racism is part of a complex system of oppressions. Also inherent in this thinking is the notion that in order to be racist, one has to be able to identify one's racist acts. In other words, if you cannot see racism in your own thinking and actions, then it does not exist. We are all immersed in a racist world. For example, images that perpetuate racism abound in popular culture, including stereotypical television programs; magazine advertisements that sexualize dark bodies in particular ways; and newspaper photos that portray Indigenous men as violent and unkempt. We internalize racism so that noticing racism is like a fish noticing water.

2. *She (a Black woman) could afford prenatal vitamins if she really wanted to. White people are poor too. In my town, White people are poorer than some of the Black immigrants.* This is the case-of-one argument, which is often used to discredit claims that people of colour consistently and increasingly experience higher rates of poverty than White people, regardless of geographies of place and space. Yes, sometimes people of colour earn more than White people. Volumes of evidence tell us that this is an unusual circumstance. The case-of-one argument is a common strategy for denying health issues that have a social, political, and economic foundation. It is called a case-of-one argument because it represents one unusual exception to a generally accepted and proven fact. One of the most popular case-of-one arguments goes like this: "My grandfather smoked every day of his life and lived to be 89." This is one of the most familiar arguments in denial of the relationship between cancer and tobacco smoking. No doubt there is the occasional truth to examples such as these. However, case-of-one arguments are sidetracking barriers that keep us from acting for change.

3. *Overall, with some exceptions, there is equality in health care. I strive to treat everyone equally.* Even in the face of overwhelming statistics regarding the existence of racism in health, this claim is often based on a lack of understanding of the meanings of equality and equity. In a related way, Razack (1998) refers to this as "rights thinking" (p. 17). "Rights thinking is based on the liberal notion that we are all individuals who contract with one another to live in a society where each of us would have the maximum in personal freedom. Starting from this premise, there are no marginalized communities of people and no historical relations of power ... we are all just human beings" (p. 17).

4. *My ability to be objective with patients helps to guard against the possibility of being racist in my practice.* This is an example of the difference between a biomedical approach and a critical social scientific approach to care. A biomedical framework is historically based on the possibility and desirability of objectivity in practice — personal bias contaminates scientific discovery and scientific practice. A critical social science approach acknowledges the impossibility of objectivity.

5. *Current theoretical models used in health care education, practice, and research already include racism. It's just not there explicitly.* There are literally thousands of theoretical models for explaining biophysical and mental health issues and phenomena. Given the well-documented dominance of biomedicine in health care, words such as racism, oppression, and discrimination do not exist in the majority of these models. Similarly absent are the words sexism, heterosexism, ageism, classism, and ableism. These ideas are not yet a meaningful part of mainstream health care language despite ongoing claims to the contrary. The addition of words or phrases such as inclusive or embracing diversity in the mission statement of a hospital or a professional school, in professional codes of ethics, or in curriculum guidelines does not ordinarily invoke a capacity to address oppression or to confront White privilege.

In our teaching and other academic work we have critiqued current models for a wide variety of health concepts and issues. These include prenatal health screening, heart health, ethical dilemmas in health care, occupational stress, traumatic stress, design of health services for street youth, and consumer involvement in health service delivery. A common response from the audience, or from readers, is to tell us that so-and-so's model actually does allow for racism. They then point out where, in the model being critiqued, that one might *imply* the insertion of such concepts.

An example is the use of the word environment, a common term in health care models. "Couldn't we just put racism under the area of 'environment'?" In a similar fashion, we have been asked why we cannot fit racism into the category of "support systems" in models of health service delivery for street youth. For us, these questions are akin to finding a needle in a haystack. Yes, theoretically the needle exists and can be found; however, without explicit guidance, this is very unlikely. More importantly, why do we want to keep it hidden?

6. *I can't incorporate anti-racism practice into my education of health professionals because there is already too much material to cover.* This is a common dilemma for many teachers. Despite the current health education talk of holistic care, this thinking assumes that the topics to be taught are mostly linear lists of various health and disease processes. For example, when teaching heart health, there are numerous important topics, such as the structure and electrical functioning of the heart, oxygen perfusion rates in damaged heart muscle, and interpretation of the nuances of electrocardiogram results. Adding yet another topic, such as heart health and African-Canadian women, simply will not fit into the schedule.

If one uses the list-of-topics approach to teaching heart health, this is certainly true. However, if an anti-racism, anti-oppression frame is used, then there are numerous places in any given lecture where the teacher may integrate knowledge about the relationship between racism and health. In the lecture on heart transplants, the teacher can list statistics about how much less likely people of colour are to be organ recipients. Similarly, in another lecture, the teacher can cite research about pathophysiology and Black women's heart health. In the lecture about pain, the teacher can cite research that people of colour are consistently offered less or no pain relief in the clinical setting. The ideas are incorporated just as many other ideas and examples are in any given lecture or learning situation. The crucial point is that the teacher makes a conscious choice to consistently incorporate examples that speak to oppression, along with her or his various other examples. Box 6.5 draws upon the principles in the field of brief therapy (Burgess, 1998) to promote working toward anti-racist education practices.

7. *The language of anti-racism practice is too harsh, too "in your face." You need to find a softer way to talk about racism.* Although we have noted a shift in this thinking over the past 15 years, the language of anti-racism practice still carries with it an element of extremism for many health clinicians. It is just not very nice to talk about. This is, in part, why terms such as "diversity" and "multicultural care" are so popular in the health fields. Resistance to using the language of anti-racism practice subverts and silences the brutal realities of racism and health care. There is no benign way to

> **Box 6.5: The Miracle Question: Imagining Anti-racist Education of Professionals in the Health Fields**
>
> Suppose one night there is a miracle while you are sleeping. When you wake up, anti-racist education is fully integrated into the education of professionals in the health fields. Because you were sleeping, you don't know that a miracle has happened.
>
> - The next morning, what do you suppose you will notice that may be different, indicating that there has been a miracle?
> - Who will be the first person to notice the next day that something is different after the miracle?
> - How will teachers and learners be different after the miracle?
> - Are there times now that some of this miracle happens, even just a little bit?
> - On a scale of 1 to 10 (1 is no anti-racist education, and 10 is fully integrated anti-racist education), where are you now in your educational institution?
> - If you are, say, at 3, what would it take to move to a 4? To eventually move to a 10?

actively resist racism. The continued lack of anti-racism language in the health fields is an effective mechanism to sustain racism.

8. *What are you talking about? My best friend is Black. I invite Black people to my home. I never see Black. I don't even see colour.* These claims are still very prevalent and it is important to explicitly address them. We encounter them often in our work, even though one of us is Black and one of us is White. Steeped in these statements are many concepts and ideas, particularly the assumed privilege of not having to see colour and race, and the colonial notion that if we (White people) let "them" into our houses and our circle of acquaintances, we must not be racist. Table 6.1 provides a detailed list of common points of resistance to anti-racist practice along with strategies for change.

Wijeyesinghe, Griffin, and Love (1997) explain that working for social justice happens along a continuum from actively practising racism to confronting oppression.

Working for Social Change: The Action Continuum

Action for social change happens on a continuum from supporting oppression to confronting oppression (Wijeyesinghe, Griffin & Love, 1997). The work of these authors sums up many of the ideas in this chapter, and indeed in this book. On one end of the continuum, we actively participate in oppression. On the supporting oppression end of the continuum, we work to maintain colonial dominance. It is crucial to note that we can support oppression *without actually noticing* that we are doing so. For example, this is frequently a conundrum for White people because the prevailing thinking is that we must actually be able to identify our White privilege

Table 6.1: Strategies for Overcoming Common Points of Resistance to Anti-racist Action

Point of Resistance in Practice	Strategy for Change
Some clinicians are racist, but I'm not racist.	Read Peggy MacIntosh's "White Privilege: Unpacking the Invisible Knapsack" (1990). Post it at school and at work. Include it in your course syllabus, and teach it in your classroom and in continuing education. Let go of the notion that we are not immersed in a racist culture. It is not about blame. It is about collective action for change.
I already strive to treat everyone equally.	Be clear about the difference between equality and equity. If we attempt to treat everyone equally, we erase their identities, which is surely not an ethical mode of practice.
My clinical objectivity guards against racism in my practice.	Embrace the impossibility of objectivity—you cannot leave yourself in a little box at the patient's door (your gender, your motherhood or fatherhood, your current and former social class, your race, your age, your sexuality, and so on). Ask yourself what will be left of you to engage in therapeutic practice. Learn about the therapeutic use of your identity in your practice, while still honouring therapeutic boundaries. Ask for education in professional schools and in the workplace about how to do this.
White people are poor too.	Yes, increasing numbers of White families are living in poverty in Canada. The point is that people of colour are even poorer, and this is a result of systemic racism. Numbers talk. Seek and use the volumes of statistical evidence about the relationships among educational opportunity, educational level, income, job security, economic status, and race. Post graphs and charts at school and at work. Even skeptics have a difficult time ignoring the mounting evidence that racism is a determinant of health. Practise recognizing and speaking up about the case-of-one argument.
The theoretical models I use for teaching, research, and publication already include notions such as racism.	Take up the challenge to insist on, and expect, the words of anti-racist practice in models, frameworks, and course syllabi. If the following words are not present, the models, frameworks, etc., are not anti-racist: "oppression," "power," "White privilege." Silencing these words is racism by omission.
I can't incorporate course materials about racism because I already have to cover too many topics in my course.	Relax. It is not that difficult. Start with one idea or statistic per lecture. Go on Google Scholar and type in: "First Nations and diabetes"; "immigrant and access to health care"; "Black women and cardiac assessment"; "geography, health, and racism"; "rural, remote, fly-in, and access to cancer care." It is more an issue of resistance to change than an issue of time.

	(*Note:* We suggest Google Scholar because it includes a wide array of important and current grey literature from local and national perspectives that are not necessarily included in academic databases.)
I think that the language of anti-racism is too harsh and unnecessarily argumentative.	Read about, talk about, and reflect on the historical context of oppression: the death, starvation, brutality, and attempted extinction of Indigenous peoples in Canada (the successful extinction in the case of the Beothuk people of Newfoundland); the existence of slavery in Canada and the brutal rape of women of colour as a strategy of colonization. Naming the words of racism helps to free us to move for action.
I'm not racist. My best friend is Black.	Try to dismantle the logic of this statement. We are all immersed in a racist culture. It is like saying there is no such thing as sexism because we all have a close friend or family member who is a woman.

before it can be said to exist. The same holds true for the other oppressions such as classism, heterosexism, or sexism. One of the most important starting points in working for social change is to embrace the fact that oppressions often flourish without the oppressors being willing or able to name oppression.

We support oppression when we actively participate in oppression; deny or ignore oppression; or recognize oppression, but take no action. Unfortunately, the latter describes many health care professionals. Noticing or witnessing oppression, and taking the moral stance that it is none of our business or that it is someone else's responsibility to speak up is the same as not doing anything in the face of need. A quote from Dante's *Inferno*, frequently cited by the late Martin Luther King Jr., has become a hallmark of social justice work around the world: "The hottest places in hell are reserved for those who remain neutral in times of great need." The people who sit silent in the case conference room when another clinician claims that Indigenous peoples were given everything by the Canadian government are actively perpetuating colonialism. In fact, this is one of the key covert reasons why colonial oppression continues so successfully in modern Canada. Silence is assent.

> *In Germany they first came for the Communists, and I didn't speak up because I wasn't a Communist. Then they came for the Jews, and I didn't speak up because I wasn't a Jew. Then they came for the trade unionists, and I didn't speak up because I wasn't a trade unionist. Then they came for the Catholics, and I didn't speak up because I was a Protestant. Then they came for me and by that time no one was left to speak up. (Rev. Martin Niemöller, 1946)*

Figure 6.2 is an adaptation of Wijeyesinghe, Griffin, and Love's (1997) action continuum. The following discussion describes each of the steps along the continuum:

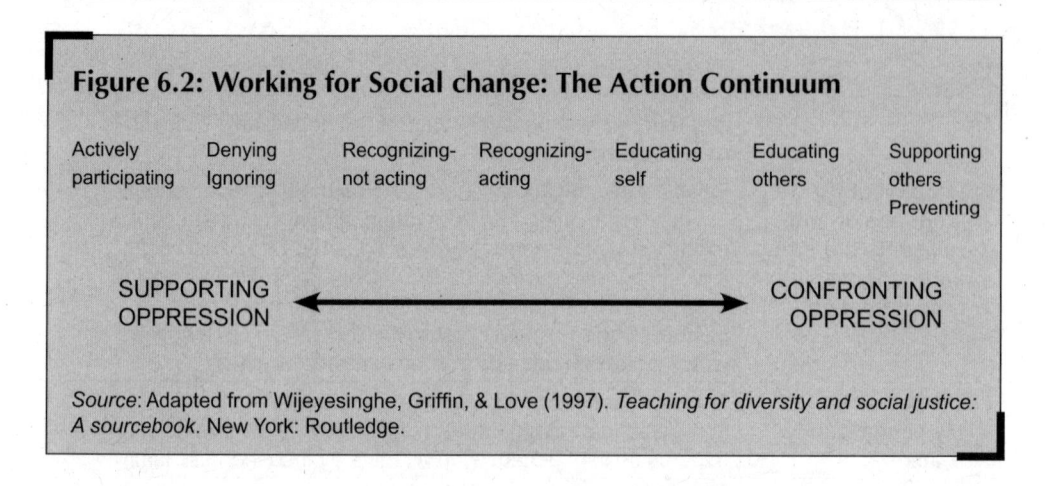

> **Figure 6.2: Working for Social change: The Action Continuum**
>
> | Actively participating | Denying Ignoring | Recognizing- not acting | Recognizing- acting | Educating self | Educating others | Supporting others Preventing |
>
> SUPPORTING OPPRESSION ←――――――――→ CONFRONTING OPPRESSION
>
> Source: Adapted from Wijeyesinghe, Griffin, & Love (1997). *Teaching for diversity and social justice: A sourcebook.* New York: Routledge.

Actively participating: Telling oppressive jokes; putting down, intentionally avoiding, or discriminating against marginalized or racialized peoples; or verbally or physically harassing people from marginalized or racialized groups. In the health fields this would include failing to conduct a thorough physical exam, or failure to refer for specialist treatment when indicated.

Denying or ignoring: Enabling oppression by denying that people from marginalized or racialized groups are oppressed. In this step, people do not actively oppress, but by denying that oppression exists, they collude with oppression. In the health fields, this might be refusing to believe that oppression at the hands of White colonial governments is directly related to current day mental health struggles of Indigenous peoples.

Recognizing, taking no action: Being aware of oppressive actions by self or others and their harmful effects, but taking no action to stop this behaviour. This inaction is often the result of fear, lack of information, or confusion about what to do. In this step, people experience discomfort at the contradiction between their awareness and lack of action. For example, during a case conference a clinician may recognize racism in the team's decision not to refer a Black adolescent for dental braces because the parents won't bother to follow through with their recommendation. If the clinician does not speak up, she or he is colluding in a racist act.

Recognizing, taking action: Being aware of oppression, recognizing oppressive actions of self and others, and taking action to stop it. This is when the clinician speaks up: "Yes we must still refer him for braces. We don't know much at all about his parents, and even if we did, we should still refer the young man for proper treatment."

Educating self: Taking action to learn more about oppression and the experiences and heritage of people from marginalized or racialized groups by reading; attending workshops, seminars, or cultural events; participating in discussions; joining organizations or groups that oppose oppression; and attending social action and social change events. An example of this step is when health professionals attend a cultural safety workshop in their institution.

Educating others: Moving beyond only educating self to questioning and engaging in dialogue with others as well. Rather than only stopping oppressive comments or behaviours, also engaging people in discussion to share why you object to a comment or action. In this step the health professionals are organizing the cultural safety workshop.

Supporting, encouraging: Supporting others who speak out against oppression or who are working to be more inclusive of people from marginalized or racialized groups by publicly backing up others who speak out, forming an allies group, or joining a coalition group. This includes encouraging a fellow clinician when she or he suggests that your institution seek funding to routinely administer sickle cell anemia screening for all Black newborns.

Initiating, preventing: Working to change individual and institutional action and policies that discriminate against people from marginalized or racialized groups, planning and implementing educational programs or other events, working for passage of legislation that protects people from marginalized or racialized groups from discrimination, being explicit about making sure that people from marginalized or racialized groups are full participants in organizations or groups (1997, p. 109). An example is when groups of health care practitioners collectively lobby their government for routine administration of sickle cell anemia screening for all Black newborns.

Box 6.6 is an example of the "initiating, preventing" end of the working for change action continuum. This example of increasing diversity in a professional program has been used as a template for other regional schools of nursing. The program's success rests on embracing of action for social change. Box 6.7 provides an exercise to stimulate thinking about examples of the action continuum in your own clinical practice. The exercise is also relevant for policy-makers and researchers interested in social change.

Conclusions

Engaging in anti-racist health care practice is often a messy business. It involves a great deal of thinking about our own locations and the tricky territory of acknowledging our privilege and our disadvantage. In many ways, anti-racist practice upends assumptions that we have held for a long time, yet this unease is at the heart of working for change. In Chapter 7 we bring this change to the policy realm, where racism is created and maintained. This realm is also a rich avenue for social change. Practitioners are generally not accustomed to thinking at this level on a day-to-day basis. Our hope with Chapter 7 is that it will expand the context of anti-racist practice as well as the possibilities for anti-racist action.

> **Box 6.6: Institutional Change at Dalhousie School of Nursing to Promote Diversity**
>
> The School of Nursing acknowledged that the limited enrolment of diverse populations from Nova Scotia was problematic, and equitable representation of Black members in nursing education was crucial. Increasing the number of Black nurses in the health care system became a priority because a diverse workforce can respond to a diverse population to improve the health of all citizens. A multiphase project for recruitment and retention of ANS (African Nova Scotians) was initiated with funding from external and internal sources for the first four years of the project.
>
> *Recruitment*
> - Community liaison person
> - Summer camp for four consecutive years
> - Targeted recruitment to junior high
> - Reserved number of seats in admissions
>
> *Retention Activities*
> - Listserv
> - Peer-support group sessions
> - Faculty advisers
> - Mentorship with Black registered nurses
>
> *Outcome of Activities to Date*
> - Black student nursing population increased exponentially
> - Summer camps successful based on evaluations, including parents' feedback
> - Increased demand for summer camps
> - Black students invited the broader student population to peer-support sessions
> - Some students have a registered Black nurse mentor
>
> *Reflexivity of Efforts*
> Recruitment and retention must be done concurrently; community partnerships are critical to the success of targeted initiatives; increased communication informing all stakeholders of activities promotes progress and enhances change; change is incremental and requires a concerted effort by students, faculty, post-secondary schools, community leaders, and family members; curriculum and program changes are necessary and ongoing to support diversity.
>
> *Sources:* Vukic, Adele. 1994. Master of Nursing Thesis Dalhousie University School of Nursing, Halifax.
> Etowa, J., Foster, S., Vukic, A. & Youden, S. (2005). Recruitment and retention of minority students: Diversity in nursing education. *International Journal of Nursing Education Scholarship, 2*(1), Article 13. Available at www.bepress.com/ijnes/vol2/1551/art13

Box 6.7: Thinking of Examples from Education and Clinical Practice

Goals
1. To relate the action continuum to everyday professional education and clinical practice
2. To develop strategies for change that are locally relevant to your work

Instructions
Individually or in groups, brainstorm examples of each of the actions along the continuum.

Questions for Reflection, Discussion and Debate, and Action
1. What are some of the specific consequences for not speaking up in the context of professional practice?
2. How is not speaking up in clinical practice different than not speaking up in general?
3. What are some of the barriers to speaking up in your education or clinical practice?
4. What supports would you suggest in your educational or practice area in terms of making it easier to speak up?

Action	Professional Education Example	Professional Practice Example
Actively participating		
Denying or ignoring		
Recognizing but not acting		
Recognizing and acting		
Educating self		
Educating others		
Supporting and encouraging		
Initiating and preventing		

CHAPTER 7

Racism, Public Policy, and Social Change

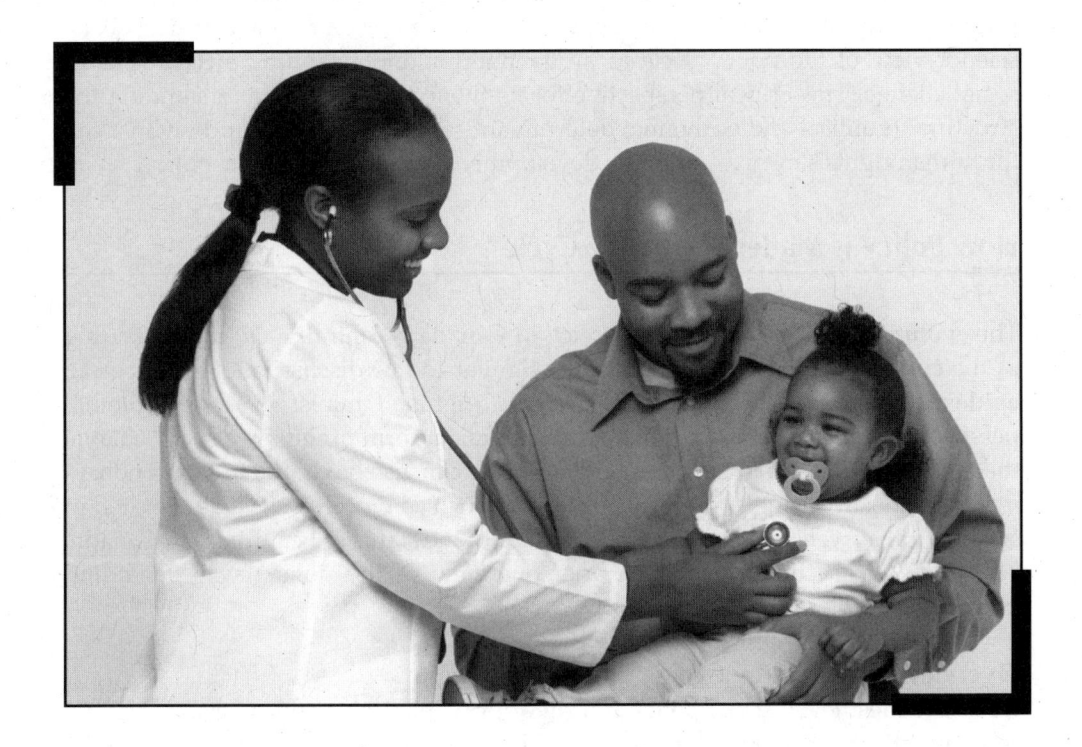

The myth that Canada is a land in which human rights have always been protected and respected is so deeply engrained in the minds of Canada. However, Canada's racist past is readily observable, requiring only an overview of legislation that has been implemented in the course of Canada's history that there is often a refusal to acknowledge that Canada has a racist history, which has been echoed in modern policies. (Roy, 2008, p. 1)

Introduction

This chapter brings the relentless perpetuation of racism to a health and social policy perspective. Although the discussion focuses primarily on Canadian policy, we emphasize that the methods of creating and recreating racism are global. We begin with a detailed description of the policy cycle and discuss the application of the policy cycle to everyday clinical practice. The role of policy-making in the promotion of inequity is described using Canadian examples of policy-created poverty, gender pay inequity, and democratic racism. Careful attention to context in policy formulation and implementation is stressed. We provide a critical social science view of the policy cycle as an avenue for understanding mechanisms of social change. This critical perspective forms the foundation of understanding the structural (political and economic) determinants of health. We conclude with a call for human rights stewardship in the development of anti-racist public policy.

How Policy Is Made: The Policy Cycle

The evolution of health and social policy in Canada is central to an understanding of the current context of health inequity. Similar to our discussion of sociological, epidemiological, political economy, human rights, feminist, and anti-colonial perspectives in Chapter 3, the policy context must inform progressive social change that addresses racism. In fact, these perspectives can also be central forces in policy-making. Not surprisingly, political economists such as Vincente Navarro are cited in sociological as well as policy-centred analyses of the status of health care in Canada. The following sections provide a brief overview of the policy cycle, including practical examples of each phase of the cycle.

Overview of the Policy Cycle

At its broadest level, social policy is a set of principles that guide decision-making regarding the human needs of citizens. In this sense, social policy may be said to be "synonymous with public policy and encompasses all the actions of governments in their continuing but not always consistent attempts to regulate social and economic structures and citizens' quality of life" (Wharf & McKenzie, 2004, p. 1). The most common way to understand policy-making is through the policy cycle. Although policy development is not a linear process, or even a strictly circular process, the policy cycle nonetheless provides a framework to understand, critique, and advocate for healthy public policy. There are numerous descriptions of the policy cycle and each variation has unique features. However, all policy cycles refer to common stages and processes that describe policy-making, whether it is in government or in non-governmental organizations.

It is only recently that the training of health professionals has included specific and comprehensive education regarding the policy cycle. Policy is often seen as something in procedure manuals or more in the realm of administration or government rather than an integral aspect of clinical practice. In our own experience as clinicians, the urgency of human need in everyday practice can be all-consuming, especially when we work in chronically underfunded areas such as mental health and addictions or in non-profit, street-level health services. In these circumstances, and in many other practice areas, thinking about policy can seem esoteric and not feasible.

As discussed in Chapter 4, biomedical dominance has also played its part in encouraging a more microscopic analysis of social problems, yet the policy realm is a central aspect of working for change. This is why an understanding of the policy cycle is an important tool for health and human service professionals who seek to promote anti-racist practice and policies. We have specifically adapted several versions of the policy cycle to incorporate multiple areas of possible policy intervention for anti-racist health care practice. These include policy in educational and health care institutions; non-profit social and health service agencies; and municipal, provincial, territorial, and federal governments. After describing the policy cycle, we offer examples of how the policy cycle can be successfully harnessed to promote anti-racist practice in each of these domains.

Stages of the Policy Cycle

Figure 7.1 illustrates the four stages of the policy cycle. The policy cycle begins with the identification of a social problem or issue. In Halifax, Nova Scotia, for example, the plight of homeless young people received national attention when a large, abandoned downtown building burned down one evening over a decade ago. It became evident that a group of homeless young people were living in the building in a city that barely acknowledged their existence. The combination of clear and graphic media attention to the problem, and non-profit agencies' already well-developed concerns about homelessness in Halifax, moved the problem of homelessness onto the municipal and provincial governments' policy agendas. This did not happen overnight. A complex and arduous advocacy process took place in which key people brought the case forward that there were, in fact, many homeless young people in their city, and that more services, including health services, were needed.

The second stage of the policy cycle involves moving from policy to action. In the homeless youth example, agencies such as the North End Community Health Centre and the Long-Term Services for Youth Association, already well-recognized agencies in the city, worked with policy-makers in municipal and provincial governments and in hospital administrations to formulate strategic policies to address youth homelessness. The iterative back-and-forth nature of the policy cycle was illustrated as these key people revisited the initial social problem of youth homelessness and negotiated issues such as the meaning of homelessness and jurisdictional boundaries regarding policy formulation: Whose problem was it? Communities and individuals, including homeless youth, were consulted regularly in the policy-formulation process.

The third stage of the policy cycle is where the policy is actually implemented. This is a difficult stage because abstract ideas must be translated into concrete

Figure 7.1: The Policy Cycle

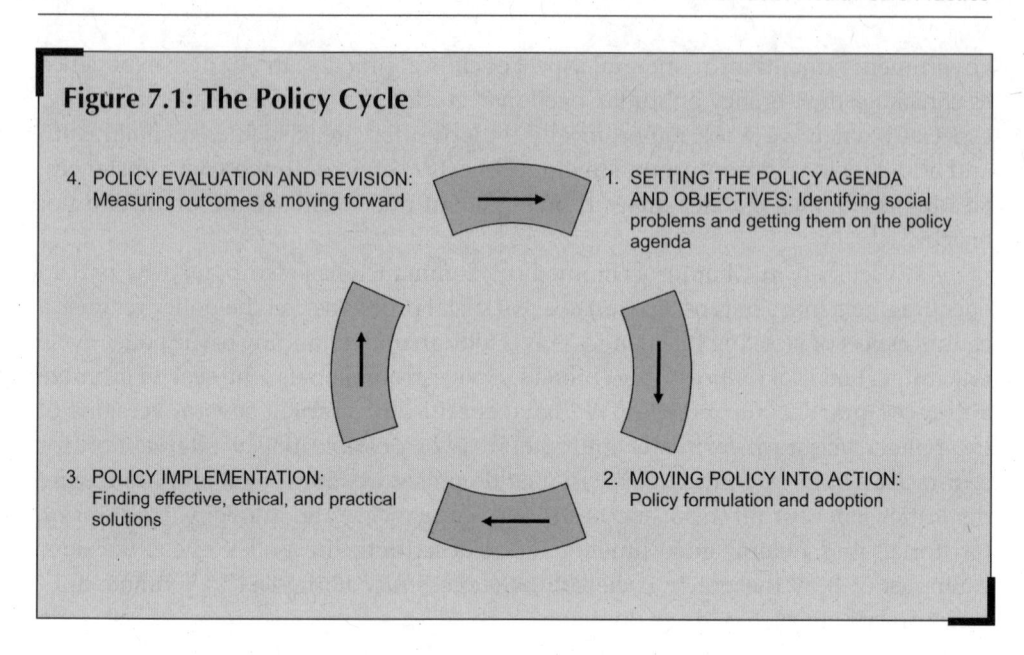

4. POLICY EVALUATION AND REVISION: Measuring outcomes & moving forward

1. SETTING THE POLICY AGENDA AND OBJECTIVES: Identifying social problems and getting them on the policy agenda

3. POLICY IMPLEMENTATION: Finding effective, ethical, and practical solutions

2. MOVING POLICY INTO ACTION: Policy formulation and adoption

activities and processes. Even though consensus may have been reached in the policy-formulation stage, debates continue about just how to make change happen to solve a problem. Youth homelessness in Halifax was addressed through the design and implementation of Phoenix Center for Youth where young people could go for counseling, health care, and referral services. In another example, an academic department may agree on the policy that social justice will be a core thread in the curriculum, but how will this policy translate into actual teaching-learning strategies and approaches? How will social justice be linked to related core areas such as human rights and anti-oppressive, anti-racist practice? What are reasonable timelines and who will be responsible for organizing the strategic planning that will be necessary to implement the policy? What are the indicators that will allow the department to track success of policy implementation and who will be responsible for progress reports? These questions point to the complexity of policy implementation and some of the common challenges and barriers. If the answers to questions such as these are not openly and collectively discussed and debated, it is unlikely that a policy can be meaningfully integrated into overall organizational planning. Box 7.1 describes an exercise that encourages the application of the policy cycle to everyday practice.

The fourth stage of the policy cycle, evaluation, is present in any successful solution to a social problem or issue. Formative evaluation involves integration of evaluation efforts throughout the policy cycle. Ideally, formative evaluation will involve qualitative and quantitative processes. Participatory evaluation involves individuals and communities who seek to benefit from the policy. Specifically, these people are involved in the evaluation process in much the same way as participants are involved in participatory action research—all the way from the design of the evaluation questions to the interpretation of results and the recommendations to

> **Box 7.1: Applying the Policy Cycle to Your Practice**
>
> *Goal*
> To identify the phases of the policy cycle and discuss how they apply in a practical example. The emphasis is on everyday examples that bring the policy cycle into plain view so that it may be harnessed for change.
>
> *Instructions*
> 1. Form groups of about three to five people. You can also do this exercise as a large group; however, smaller groups will help to uncover a rich variety of policy cycle examples.
> 2. Identify a policy in your area (public policy/government-based, institution-wide, or department-specific, etc.) that is related to or includes racism. Examples include: equity and discrimination guidelines; anti-racism policies, mission statements, etc.
> 3. Discuss the following questions:
>   (a) How did the policy get on the policy-making agenda (who, where, when, why)? If you don't know the exact answer to this question, discuss the steps you would have taken to get it on the agenda.
>   (b) What was the policy-formulation process (who, where, when, why)? In other words, how was the issue translated into actual policies?
>   (c) How was/is the policy implemented (who, where, when, why)?
>   (d) How is the policy evaluated (who, where, when, why)?
> 4. Now discuss a policy that you think is much needed in your practice area or in your institution. Walk through the policy cycle as described above and document your answers. Think about how you would actually initiate the policy cycle, especially the identification of key allies.
>
> *Questions for Personal Reflection, Discussion/Debate, and Action*
> 1. Why don't health care practitioners usually have specific education in the policy cycle? Think of local and systemic answers.
> 2. What are the institutional supports that need to be in place for you to go ahead with the much-needed policy you devised in step 4 above?
> 3. What are some of the barriers to implementing the policy? What might be some of the corresponding solutions? Note that at this point, some of you will feel a sense of futility, especially if your institution is in need of a lot of improvement in anti-racist, anti-oppressive practice. The key here is usually to find a few like-minded people and start small.

work for continued social change. As you may have noted, participatory evaluation is in its infancy when it comes to government policy implementation.

Quantitative evaluation can also be very useful in assessing a policy and either changing or adjusting the policy, or abandoning it altogether and starting anew. Quantitative measures need to be discussed in detail from the beginning of the policy cycle. For example, if we want to measure the nature of attendance to a new diabetic outreach program, we will need to set up a database before the program begins. A critical perspective will lead us to include the following questions in our evaluation database for the diabetic outreach program: What is the family income of program participants? Are gender, age, race, or disability, related to income among the program participants? Although we know that this is certainly the case on a population health level, the data will help to verify national data in a smaller geographic area, and specifically with people with diabetes. Since successful diabetes management is so closely related to food security, your evidence will provide a powerful argument to promote policy change for better service delivery. Table 7.1 summarizes key considerations in each stage of the policy cycle.

Table 7.1: Summary of Key Considerations in the Policy Cycle

Stage of Policy Cycle	Key Considerations
1. Setting the policy agenda and objectives: Identifying social problems and getting them on the policy agenda	- Gather evidence to make a solid case. - Identify allies to help bring your case forward. - Tailor message to your policy audience. Is it a government policy brief or a verbal presentation to a hospital or academic administration? - Consider timing: Where are the resistance points and how might you overcome them?
2. Moving policy to action: Policy formulation and adoption	- Policy analysis involves designing policy alternatives and considering intended and unintended consequences of the policy. - There are always battles and choices in formulating policy. - Find avenues to be a consultant and a watchdog when new policy is being implemented (e.g. community forums, report cards).
3. Policy implementation: Finding effective, ethical, and practical solutions	- How will the world be different if the issue is addressed? - Battles and choices continue in policy implementation (e.g. in interpretation of policy). - Formulated policies don't necessarily translate into implementation—they may need to be reformulated for the real world. - Consultation is central to implementation success: Find or insist on avenues to be part of the process. - Consider time frames, resource allocation, marketing, instruments used to implement policy (laws in government; brochures and manuals in institutions; programs in health care).
4. Policy evaluation, reassessment, and revision: Measuring outcomes and moving forward	- What does the formative evaluation say (e.g. the ongoing evaluation of the first three steps in the policy cycle)? - What are the overall success or failure indicators? What has been the impact of the policy? - Evaluation can be quantitative (how many clinicians attended a cultural competence training course?) and qualitative (what are patients' experiences with these same clinicians?). - Evaluations always point to ways to move forward.

Although a detailed description of the policy cycle is beyond the scope of this chapter, the above discussion and the accompanying exercise provide a background for working with policy change. This foundation will be important in any actions for systemic change to support anti-oppressive, anti-racist practice. The policy cycle provides clear entry points to interrupt racist practices in clinical practice, professional associations, educational institutions, and at all levels of government. The key is always to figure out a strategic way to get anti-racist ideas on the policy agenda. This process may involve a great deal of negotiation, even if the change you desire is relatively small. However, there are many examples of successful anti-racist programs and initiatives in Canada. The following section helps to translate policy principles into their impact on everyday life in Canada.

How Policy-making Promotes Inequity: Some Canadian Examples

Canadian examples such as government policy regarding wages and incomes further explain how policies play themselves out in the everyday lives of individuals and families. Since poverty is the best predictor of poor health status across the lifespan (Raphael, 2007), some of the policy-based origins of poverty in Canada are especially important to highlight. We then add a policy-based gender lens through a discussion of gender inequity in Canada's federal budgets. We conclude the section with a discussion of democratic racism, or entrenching racism in ostensibly democratic policies and laws in Canada.

Entrenching Poverty through Public Policy

Provincial, territorial, and federal government policies create poverty for citizens. In Canada, government policy makes it very difficult for many families to feed, clothe, and shelter themselves at a level that promotes health and well-being. In other words, in public policy realms such as setting the minimum wage, employment insurance, and pay equity, the policy cycle is sometimes designed to maintain chronic struggle. This view seems counterintuitive to conventional thinking about how the policy cycle operates. Public policy-making ostensibly works for the common good of all citizens, and aims to reduce poverty for Canadian families. This is how policies are presented in public documents about government policy, and during election campaigns: all political parties offer detailed policy platforms that generally claim to have the best interests of individuals and families as a policy goal.

So, if the Canadian government is developing policies to improve the lives of Canadians, why is the child poverty rate increasing for some children? As discussed in previous chapters, the number of children living in poverty for any nation is considered a clear and valid gauge of the health of a nation. Figure 7.2, from the Child Poverty League (United Nations International Children's Emergency Fund, 2005), illustrates the performance of several countries in the area of child poverty.

Figure 7.2: The Material Well-being of Children
Three components were selected to represent children's material well-being: relative income poverty, households without jobs and reported deprivation. The figure averages each country's score over three components, and is scaled to show each country's distance above or below the average (set at 100) for the countries featured.

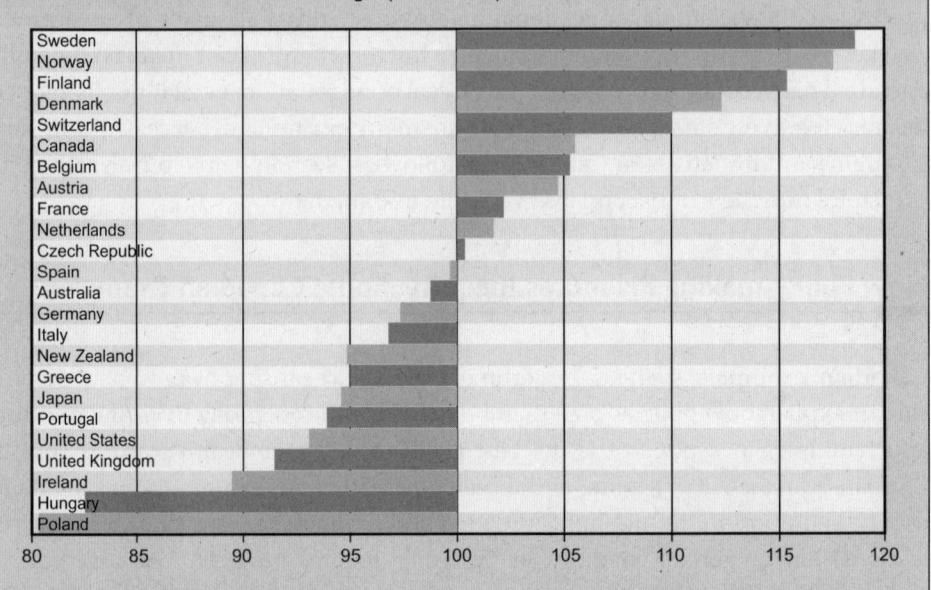

Country	Score
Sweden	~120
Norway	~119
Finland	~117
Denmark	~114
Switzerland	~112
Canada	~111
Belgium	~110
Austria	~108
France	~106
Netherlands	~105
Czech Republic	~100
Spain	~99
Australia	~98
Germany	~97
Italy	~95
New Zealand	~94
Greece	~93
Japan	~91
Portugal	~90
United States	~88
United Kingdom	~87
Ireland	~86
Hungary	~82
Poland	~81

Note: Material well-being as presented in this chart is made up of equally weighted components of (a) relative income poverty, (b) households without jobs, and (c) reported deprivation (as reported by children themselves). Each country has been placed on a scale determined by the average score for the group. The unit used is the standard deviation (the average deviation from the average). To ease interpretation, the results are presented on a scale with a mean of 100 and a standard deviation of 10.

Source: UNICEF, United Nations International Children's Emergency Fund (UNICEF, 2005). Child poverty in rich countries. Florence: UNICEF Innocenti Research Centre.

Linking poverty statistics with a nation's public policy helps to broaden the context of why people live in poverty. For example, a commonly held view is that poverty is caused by being lazy, not bothering with training to get a job, or wanting to be a freeloader living off public funds. When we actually link poverty statistics with public policy, we begin to view the broader political and economic context of poverty. This link is particularly evident in the areas of minimum-wage legislation, employment insurance, income assistance (social assistance or welfare), education and training supports, pay equity, and pensions. Lucille Harper (2007) traced statistics for the province of Nova Scotia and linked living in poverty with policy in each of these areas.

According to Statistics Canada, the low income cut-off point (LICO) is the amount of annual income below which a family is considered to be living in poverty. LICOs are commonly used to analyze the implications of poverty for individuals and families living in poverty. The following analysis is taken from Harper's (2007) document *Poverty Is Policy Created*. Although minimum wage has since been increased slightly in Nova Scotia, the evidence presented below remains painfully relevant for people living in poverty. While you read these statistics, actively link them to your practice. Ask yourself questions such as: How would I feed, clothe, and shelter my own family for $167 per week? What policies make 57 percent of unemployed people ineligible for employment insurance benefits? What does the phrase "the lived experience of poverty" mean to me? The following list of public policies is taken from Harper's (2007) document:

- *Minimum wage:* In Nova Scotia, government policy has set the minimum wage at $7.60 per hour as of May 1, 2007. The gross earnings of someone working 40 hours per week at minimum wage would be $15,808. The gross earnings of a single parent in Nova Scotia who is working full-time, full-year at minimum wage and raising one child would fall $2,000 to $6,468 below the 2005 poverty line. The gross earnings of two parents working full-time, full-year at minimum wage and raising two children in Halifax would fall $1,635 below the 2005 poverty line.
- *Employment Insurance benefits:* Employment insurance policy means that only 43 percent of unemployed people qualify for employment insurance benefits (National Anti-poverty Organization, 2005). Those who do qualify are faced with a two-week unpaid waiting period, which places the poorest and most vulnerable in real danger. After two weeks an eligible person will receive 55 percent of his or her earnings averaged over the last 26 weeks. This means a single mother earning minimum wage would have to support herself and her child(ren) on a weekly benefit of $167 for 14–45 weeks depending upon the region. This amounts to $2,341–$7,524 respectively. Annually, this is $10,028 below the LICO for a family of two living in a rural area and $19,935 below the 2005 LICO in Halifax.
- *Income assistance:* The Nova Scotia Employment Supports and Income Assistance (ESIA) Program is a last stop for people with little or no income. It is supposed to provide for basic expenses that include food, rent or mortgage, utilities like heat and electricity, clothing, and taxes. ESIA policy sets the monthly income of a single mother with one child living on income assistance in Nova Scotia at $1,076 ($12,917 annual income), including the child tax benefits (National Anti-poverty Organization, 2005). This income is $4,890 (rural) to $9,359 (Halifax) below the LICO. If these families had an extra $4,000 (rural) or $9,000 (Halifax) per year, they would still be living in poverty.
- *Education and training supports:* To move out of poverty, a single mother with one child needs to earn at least $11 an hour. Most jobs that pay this wage require post-secondary education. According to policy guidelines, single parents on income assistance are not allowed to retain their income-

assistance benefits while they attend university. A mother attending university cannot pay her tuition and support both herself and her children on a student loan.
- *Pay equity:* Women earn approximately 71 percent of what men earn for full-time, full-year work. In the world's 29 most developed countries, Canada has the 5th largest wage gap (Canadian Research Institute on the Advancement of Women, 2005).
- *Pensions:* Senior women who are single, widowed, or divorced and over the age of 65 have a 41.5 percent chance of living in poverty (Canadian Research Institute on the Advancement of Women, 2005). This is because many women throughout their lives earn low wages, work in insecure jobs, and carry the main responsibility for child rearing. Therefore, women are more likely than men to depend upon public pensions as their primary source of income. Pensions for senior women are 58 percent of those of senior men (Barnwell, 2006).

These statistics help us to look at public policy with an explicit anti-oppressive lens. This lens brings forward some of the ways in which the policy cycle results in inequity and poverty for large groups of citizens. The one-size-fits-all approach to policy-making is being sharpened to increasingly include questions from a critical, anti-oppressive perspective. In what ways do cutbacks in public spending on income assistance differentially affect racialized peoples, including women, children, seniors, and people with disabilities? How do cutbacks affect the health outcomes of these citizens from a longitudinal perspective? These questions help to politicize the policy cycle and direct attention to political decision making and the world views of the various political parties — the structural determinants of health. According to Raphael (2007), "poverty in Canada is a result of political decisions that shape the distribution of resources within the population" (p. 303). The above snapshot of policy and poverty in the province of Nova Scotia also holds true for Canada as a whole.

Grace-Edward Galabuzi detailed the statistical evidence of the racialization of poverty in Canada (Galabuzi, 2006, 2008). He described the economic plight of racialized peoples in Canada as Canada's economic apartheid. Apartheid is racial segregation. It can take the form of geographic segregation, such as the creation of reservations for Indigenous peoples in North America and it can also take the form of segregation in schools and in the workplace. Many subtle forms of segregation also operate in Canada and globally. These include exclusion of opportunity to enter professional schools through the many forms of racism in public schools. Ultimately, apartheid is a well-developed system of oppression that permeates all aspects of everyday life. Economic apartheid refers to the policies and processes that ensure ongoing high poverty rates and social exclusion — the use of policy-created economic hardship to maintain oppression.

Economic apartheid can be seen through inequities in access to employment for racialized groups, which produces increasingly high poverty rates. Unemployment rates for immigrants and racialized groups in 2001 were almost twice as high when compared with the total rates for the Canadian labour force (Statistics Canada, 2001). In the year 2000, the income gap between university-educated immigrants and university-educated Canadian-born citizens grew to 28.6 percent for men and 20.9 percent for women. For both immigrant and Canadian-born women, the gender inequality gaps persisted. Canadian-born women earned 38 percent less than men. After 10 years in Canada, immigrant women with a university degree earned 21 percent less than their Canadian-born counterparts, 32 percent less than immigrant men, and 51 percent less than Canadian-born men (Statistics Canada, 2001). Figure 7.3 compares average earnings of immigrants with average earnings of Canadian-born adults.

Figure 7.3: Average Earnings of Immigrants and Canadian-born with a University Degree (2000)

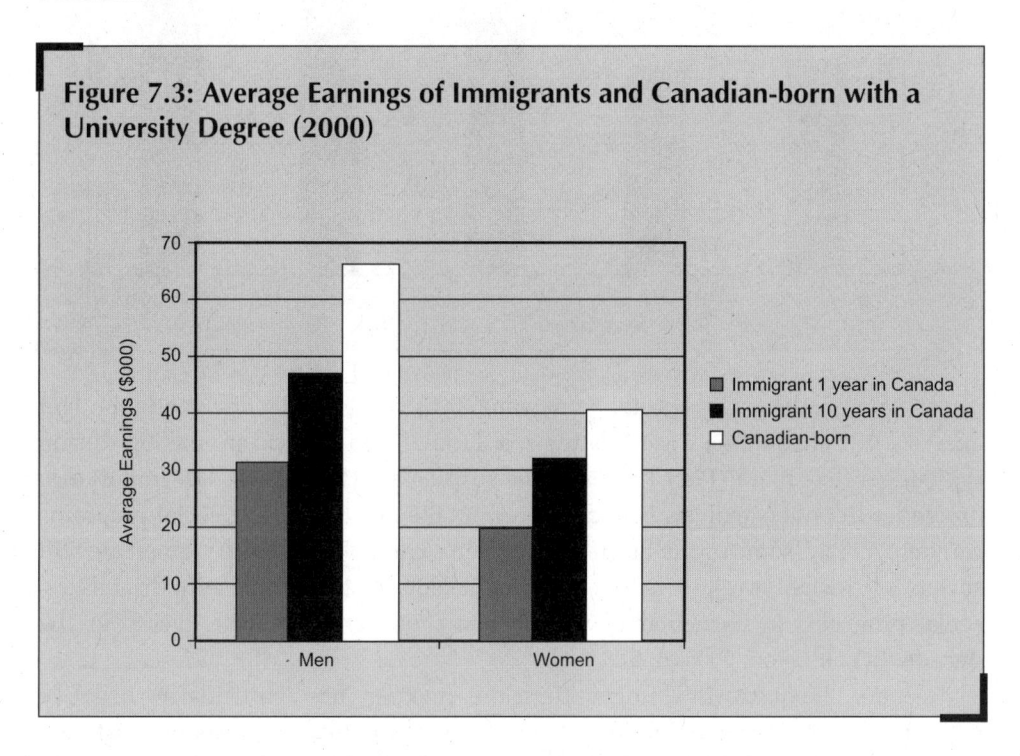

Figure 7.4 illustrates the unfair distribution of unemployment rates in Canada. This evidence is an excellent example of how a critical analysis of inequities in income can inform the policy-change agenda. In the case of average earnings of university-educated immigrants and Canadian-born citizens, we see an unfair distribution of individual and family economic instability. This unfair distribution is evident regardless of education level, which is so often used as the commonly held, or common-sense, reason for lower incomes. Women fare worse across all categories, demonstrating the economic impact of interlocking oppressions.

Gender Inequity and Federal Budgets

Canada's performance in the area of gender equity in federal budgets serves as another case example of how public policy, or lack of progressive public policy,

Figure 7.4: Unemployment Rates, Total Labour Force, Canadian-born, All Immigrants, Recent Immigrants, Racialized Groups. (%)

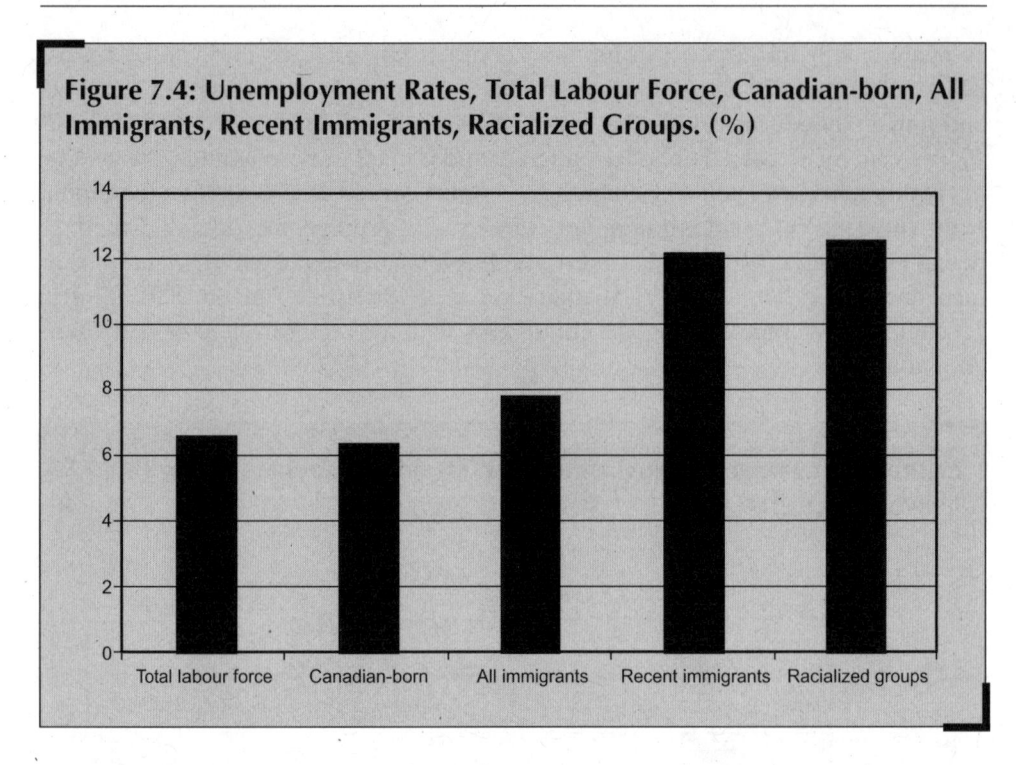

can sustain gender pay inequity. Yalnizyan (2005) prepared the first gender budget analysis in Canada. She traced patterns of federal policy decision making during the budget deficit era (1995-1997) and the surplus era (1998-2004). The importance of gender in policy analysis is underscored by the fact that strong social programs can help to ease some of the burden of women's caregiving. "Since women are still society's principal care-givers for children, the elderly, and people with disabilities, social programs in particular have played a central role in their lives over the decades" (Yalnizyan, 2005, p. 5).

Gender inequity in budget decision making has particularly negative consequences for women, and especially for women of colour. Gender must be a fundamental category of policy analysis because it explicates the gendering that results from public policy that advantages men and disadvantages women, even if not intentionally (Bensimon & Marshall, 2003). For example, income security and many other social programs were steadily eroded in Canada over the past decade. The deficit era between 1995 and 1997 affected women in a disproportionate way with billions of dollars in reduced funding for social programs (Yalnizyan, 2005). When the benefits of social programs such as income assistance, employment insurance, and pensions are reduced, women are disproportionately affected due to the burden of caregiving.

But even in the budget surplus era of 1998–2004, the way that the surplus was allocated did not alleviate the damage done in the deficit era. During this period, the federal government allocated $152 billion to tax cuts, mostly to higher-income earners and large corporations, and $61 billion to pay down the debt. Yet only $34 billion net of new resources were transferred to the provinces for health care and child care (Yalnizyan, 2005). These budget-related policy decisions about funding meant that large corporations received five times the funding that health and child care received during the same period. Although an in-depth discussion of gender equity is beyond the scope of this chapter, these numbers indicate the entrenchment of gender inequity in public policy decision making in federal budgets. As each of the chapters in this book has demonstrated, women of colour will be even further disadvantaged by inequitable federal budgets. Sexism and racism in public policy amplify oppression in Canada.

Health as a Human Right and Policies of Democratic Racism

The state has a pivotal role in the pursuit of a just society. Federal, provincial, and municipal governments carry a special responsibility to assert leadership in the eradication of racism through public policy (Henry, Tator, Mattis & Rees, 2000).

> *The fundamental rights and freedoms to which Canada adheres include the right of all residents to full and equal participation in the cultural, social, political, economic, and political life of the country. This right is based on the principle of fundamental equality of individuals. The rights of equality of access, equality of opportunity, and equality of outcomes for all communities are therefore implicit. (Henry, Tator, Mattis & Rees, 2000, p. 334)*

Although human rights are enshrined in many national and international policies and laws, the right to health is not realized for many people, particularly racialized groups. And, as we describe here, even if additional laws are put into place to ensure adherence to human rights legislation, democratic racism continues to prevent the enjoyment of basic human rights.

Health and Human Rights

The relationship between health and human rights has evolved through several national and international agreements. In 1976 the United Nations passed the International Covenant on Civil and Political Rights. In 1977, the Canadian Human Rights Act was passed, and in 1982, after almost 15 years of political and legal battles, the Canadian Charter of Rights and Freedoms became part of the Constitution of Canada. The Charter legalized citizens' fundamental freedoms, such as freedom of association and freedom of religion. The Charter listed, for the first time in Canadian law, the grounds upon which citizens could not be discriminated against before the law: race, national or ethnic origin, colour, religion, sex, age, or mental or physical disability.

The Charter also provided for affirmative-action programs in stating that this non-discrimination clause "does not preclude any law, program, or activity that has as its object the amelioration of conditions of disadvantaged individuals or groups, including those that are disadvantaged because of race, national or ethnic origin, color, religion, sex, age, or mental or physical disability" (Government of Canada, 1982). A separate section of the Charter, the "Rights of the Aboriginal Peoples of Canada," specified rights such as the recognition of existing Aboriginal and treaty rights. Since their inception, the persistent social justice and policy challenge has been to find mechanisms to require governments to honour these legal entitlements. Not surprisingly, the translation of basic human rights laws into ethical and legal everyday practices has proved elusive in many areas, including in institutional systems such as the health care system.

Addressing racial inequalities in health care is part of the unfinished civil rights agenda in the United States (Smith, 2005a). Racial inequalities in Canada create and sustain inequities in access to health care, and Canada, too, has an unfinished civil rights agenda regarding the health of people of colour. Racial discrimination and other forms of intolerance infringe on the human rights and dignity of those who experience this injustices. In addition, discrimination harms their health and reduces the lifespan of millions of people who suffer from it. Thus, inequities in health and health care cannot be reduced by medical and other health interventions alone. Instead, a human rights approach is necessary to recognize racism and other forms of discrimination as major factors impairing the health of millions of people. It is also crucial to acknowledge the link between the right be free of racism and the right to have an optimal standard of health.

The foundations have been clearly laid for the relatively recent global social movement to consider health as a human right. The United Nations (UN) implemented the first worldwide public health and human rights strategy in the 1980s through its global program on AIDS. Further, World Health Organization (WHO) initiatives in the 1990s, based on the UN Charter of Rights and Freedoms, brought health and human rights together in international law (Gruskin, Mills & Tarantala, 2007). Decades earlier, in the challenge of the Jim Crow laws that legalized the dehumanization of African Americans, leaders in the civil rights movement in the United States linked civil rights with the right to health care based on the lack of access to basic health care for African-American people.

The successful challenge of these laws led to the creation of a civil rights report card, which detailed the results of human rights violations in the United States health care system (Smith, 2005a). This direct link between human rights and health care remains one of the earliest strategies to address health inequities through legalization of equitable health care treatment. A human rights perspective on health care reframes healthy population outcomes as a legal entitlement rather than a desired, but not always achievable, goal. The movement toward defining health as a human right requires a social injustice-based analysis of the relationships among health and social policy decisions, health and social service expenditures, population health outcomes, and the social determinants of health.

The Canadian Charter of Rights and Freedoms (1982) and a number of international human rights instruments that Canada has ratified, provide a legal and social policy-based imperative for civil society pressure to remove barriers in access to health care. Relevant international documents include: The United Nations Universal Declaration of Human Rights (1948); the International Covenant on Economic, Cultural, and Social Rights (1966); the Convention on the Elimination of All Forms of Racial Discrimination (1969); and the Convention on the Elimination of All Forms of Discrimination against Women (1979). The last convention obligates the state to uphold the right of rural women to "have access to adequate health care facilities, including information, counseling and services in family planning ... to enjoy living conditions, particularly in relation to housing, sanitation, electricity and water supply, transport and communications" (1979). The Convention on the Rights of the Child (1989), Article 24, requires that states "recognize the right of the child to the enjoyment of the highest attainable standard of health and to facilities for the treatment of illness and rehabilitations of health ... and strive to ensure that no child is deprived of his or her right of access to such health care services" (1989). Canada's Charter of Rights and Freedoms, Section 15, states that inequitable access to health care is unconstitutional.

Canada's first nationwide action to bring social justice to health care policy began with Tommy Douglas. Douglas, known as the father of Canadian social medicine, successfully lobbied for a universally accessible health care system, which was nationally legislated in 1966. Douglas's vision for the health of Canadians focused squarely on designing and sustaining public policy to promote equity and dignity in the provision of health care. However, government commitment to Tommy Douglas's vision for health care has gradually shifted from concerns about universal and equitable access to the development of an increasingly market-driven health care system. Privatization of health care is underway in Canada, reinforced by the Canadian Medical Association's Medicare Plus recommendations: "If, and only if, the public system fails to provide timely care, Canadians should have access to private insurance that can cover the cost of obtaining care in the private sector" (Canadian Medical Association, 2007, p. 685). The Canadian Medical Association fails to acknowledge the complex, systemic implications of promoting a parallel private-pay system, despite such clear evidence of its pitfalls from our United States neighbours. The view that we can have two successful health care delivery systems, one private and one public, naively ignores the far-reaching dynamics of corporate profit. A two-tier health care system, with private-pay clients, will create differential access based on ability to pay—the very problem that prompted Douglas to fight for social medicine in the 1960s (McGibbon, 2008). Private payment for health services is an example of a public policy that reinforces racism because racialized families already experience inequities in income.

Inequitable access to health care, even in the publicly funded system, is not supported by Canadian law. Although the Canada Health Act (1984) legislated universality and accessibility in Canada's health care system, equitable access to health care is a human right that has not been realized for millions of Canadians. Violations of the basic human right to health will be integral to the growing social movement to hold the state accountable for its deplorable performance on the social determinants of health (SDOH) in Canada. Almost 30 percent of children of colour live in poverty in Nova Scotia (Ministerial Advisory Council on Rural Health, 2002). This fact alone is sufficient evidence for focussed attention on Canadian violations of rights such as the right to education and the right to non-discrimination on the basis of race and gender in the Canadian workplace. As discussed in detail in Chapter 2, the intersections of the SDOH, identity, and geography create powerful and very real barriers in access to health services. Although most evidence is based in the U.S., Canadian scholars such as Etowa, Thomas Bernard, and Loppie are already building a strong case that racism is at the core of barriers in access to physical and mental health care for people of colour in Canada.

Democratic Racism: When Rights Are Not Enough

As the evidence in this and in earlier chapters demonstrated, racism is clearly a determinant of health. In fact, there has been a deliberate shift among anti-racism scholars and practitioners from the phrase "race as a determinant of health'" to "racism as a determinant of health." This shift acknowledges the structural or policy-based causes of increasing ill health for racialized individuals, families, and communities. So why, in a democratic society such as Canada, does racism flourish to the point of creating such differences in the social determinants of health and in health outcomes? Nationally ratified United Nations covenants, the Canadian Charter of Rights and Freedoms, multiculturalism policy, employment-equity policy, and human rights codes and commissions are all designed to integrate the principles of democracy in policy-making so that Canada is a more just society. However, some of these legal and democratically formulated initiatives actually reinforce racism. "The liberal discourses of multiculturalism, rights, and equality are largely framed on a passive model of state intervention that ignores collective or group rights based on race" (Henry, Tator, Mattis & Rees, 2000, p. 343).

The case study in Box 7.4 about human rights codes and commissions illustrates a case study about democratic racism. Although these policies and laws were designed within the principles of democracy in a democratic country by democratically elected officials, they often reinforce racism and further perpetuate racist acts. As these authors argue, human rights codes and commissions place the burden of responsibility on the individual rather than on the state. It is very difficult to imagine what this burden might be like unless you have experienced it yourself, or have witnessed or helped another person to navigate a complaints process. The complainants, and in many cases their families, must have a considerable reserve of

Box 7.4: Case Study: Human Rights Codes and Commissions

Background

Ontario's Racial Discrimination Act of 1944 was the first provincial legislation to prohibit racial discrimination. In 1962, the Ontario Human Rights Code was the first such provincial legislation to be enacted. The code prohibited discrimination on the grounds of race, creed, colour, nationality, ancestry, or place of origin. Today, all the provinces, two of the three territories (at the time of writing, Nunavut had just been established), and the federal government have a human rights code and most have a human rights commission to administer their codes. Provincial human rights codes have quasi-constitutional status. The Canadian Human Rights Act is, of course, subject to the Canadian Charter of Rights and Freedoms, which in section 52 states that the Constitution is the supreme law of Canada.

Human rights laws are codes of conduct to which society is expected to adhere. Although the prohibited grounds of discrimination vary from province to province, several jurisdictions prohibit discrimination in accommodation, facilities, services contracts, and employment. All the codes prohibit discrimination on the basis of race, creed, colour, ethnicity, religion, gender and in Ontario, sexual orientation.

Canada's system of human rights is activated by the complaint mechanism. Under various human rights codes, claims must be handled by a human rights commission, which investigates claims and attempts to settle them by conciliation and mediation. If this is not possible, the commission either dismisses the claim or sends it to hearings conducted by a human rights board of inquiry. The board of inquiry is a quasi-juridical tribunal and an independent body. If a claim goes to a board of inquiry, lawyers acting for the commission present the case and argue for the "appropriate" remedy. Boards of inquiry make decisions to uphold or reject claims and can order redress, such as back pay and damages (Ontario Human Rights Code Review Task Force, 1992:17).

Discussion

The present model of human rights has been criticized (Day, 1990; Duclos, 1990; *Equality Now*, 1984) for being a reactive model that comes into play only when a complaint is launched. Critics argue that commissions do not have a sufficiently broad mandate to combat discrimination effectively. A principal criticism is that a complaint-motivated system cannot effectively address a problem that is so widespread in society.

The Canadian human rights commissioner reinforced the criticism of the complaint model: "I am convinced that one of the reasons our scheme of human rights laws has become prey to bureaucratic delays and judicial haggling is that it so predominantly a complaint-driven model," which requires several conditions to be met: a victim must come forward; that person must be able to relate particular actions to one or more of the forbidden types of discrimination; and the treatment must be demonstrably discriminatory, not just unfair or different. He proposed that the commissions complement the complaint system by creating a non-discriminatory environment that includes employment equity (Yalden, 1990:2).

In resolving human rights complaints, the present model allows for persuasion and conciliation where necessary and, alternatively, for punitive measures when such persuasion fails. Human rights commissions are therefore under tremendous pressure to settle complaints. In attempting to reach conciliation, staff are often unaware of the impact of their behavior on victims. In the hearings of a task force established to examine the procedures of the Ontario Human Rights Commission, delegations representing various community groups stated that the "process can be coercive and unfair. Claimants argued that sometimes they are specifically told that if they do not accept a settlement, which in their view is unjust, their case will be dismissed by the commission. Since they have

> no other choice, they feel forced to accept the settlement" (Ontario Human Rights Code Review Task Force, 1992:116). Often, settlements involve the payment of a certain sum of money. Several people believe that such settlements are offensive and unprincipled as it appears that human rights are being bought and that the underlying questions of discrimination are not been addressed.
>
> This complaint-driven approach is viewed as inadequate in addressing the complex, pervasive, and intractable forms of racism in Canadian society. A re-evaluation of the "effectiveness of a human rights system that is based on a model developed in the 1960's" (Mendes, 1997:2.v.) is clearly called for. Analyzing statistics for the various commissions, Mendes came to the conclusion that, due to a variety of factors, including the inability to deal with race complaints, there is a general tendency for "race complaints to be treated differently than other complaints ... they are dismissed more frequently than cases based on other grounds of discrimination." He concluded his analysis of human rights commissions by noting that the human rights system existing in most jurisdictions in Canada is not affording the victims of discrimination of the recourse necessary to enforce their rights. In particular, cases of racial discrimination are proving to be too much for the present system to handle (Mendes, 1997).
>
> Two other reviews of the structure of human rights commissions in Ontario and British Columbia have suggested a radical reorganization of the commissions and their operations (Ontario Human Rights Code Review Task Force, 1992; Black, 1994).
>
> *Source:* From HENRY. *The color of democracy: Racism in Canadian society.* Copyright 2006 Nelson Education Ltd. Reproduced by permission, www.cengage.com/permissions.

mental and physical energy to withstand the close and often damning scrutiny of counter-arguments. Inquiries or investigative processes can take months or years to come to a conclusion. The case study highlights many of these policy-based problems with human rights codes and commissions.

Although the efforts of individuals working for human rights commissions or institutional equity boards are to be solidly commended in many ways, the crux of the matter is that the state is still leaving the burden of proof on the shoulders of people experiencing racism. This is a policy-based situation of having your cake and eating it too. Governments can claim to be formulating and implementing solid policies to uphold human rights, all the while leaving the enforcement largely up to individuals who have the tenacity to take up the battle. The burden of responsibility for just outcomes must shift to its proper place in a democratic country—to the governing mechanisms and bodies that have been elected and mandated to do the work.

Context in Policy Formulation and Implementation

Policy-making always happens within the context of evolving social movements. The likelihood of policy adoption and implementation is based on many key areas, such as political will, the complexity of the issue, and public support. It is important to explore the political basis of public policy choices because it turns out that the thinking of reigning political parties is a central predictor of the health outcomes of citizens over time. This claim runs counterintuitive to much of the current health promotion-related thinking in the health fields. For example, the popular healthy lifestyles approach in health promotion demonstrates the importance of a political perspective when we consider the relationship between public policy and health outcomes.

The Importance of a Critical Social Science View in Policy Change

The examples of policy-created poverty, gender pay inequity, and democratic racism demonstrate the importance of context in the ways that public policy is formulated and implemented. Without a critical social scientific analysis, we may continue to locate social problems such as poverty within the realm of individual shortcomings rather than in their socio-political origins. Since racialized peoples continue to be overall the poorest in the country, there is a profoundly racist undertone to blaming families in poverty for their plight. These contextual aspects of analyzing social problems are foundational in working for change. In the health fields and in other practice-based fields as well, context is becoming increasingly recognized. However, it is not often brought to a sufficiently critical level to help understand problems and to advocate for change. There are few practitioners who could not list important contexts such as personal, environment, history, social, economic, genetic, political, and so on, but what do these words actually mean? Depending on your world view, the answer to this question will be significantly different.

For example, historical contexts are fully recognized as important determinants of present-day circumstances. Some people think that bad things happened to Indigenous peoples in Canada, but that is over now and it is time to move forward and think more positively about how we can all live together in this country. On the other hand, some believe that land was stolen, and Indigenous peoples were systematically brutalized and annihilated (the Beothuks of Newfoundland) at the hands of White people. The solution to this social problem will vary widely according to how the context is viewed. In the first instance, we might continue to treat everyone equally, and frown upon any extra attention given to Indigenous students, such as university tuition assistance. White students consistently bring this up in classroom settings, claiming reverse discrimination because they do not have these benefits. In the second instance, historical trauma transmission will be affirmed and policies and programs will reflect the deep and lasting nature of trauma, the effects of ongoing racism against Indigenous peoples, and the reconciliation that is imperative.

Another example is the use of the terms social inclusion rather than social exclusion in public policy. Although some versions of social inclusion emphasize attention to discrimination in society (Saloojee, 2002), overall, most definitions of social inclusion stress participation, integration, and co-operation. Social inclusion refers to "a social lens through which we can understand social wellbeing, equality and citizenship. Valued recognition is central to this understanding, as are notions of social and economic proximity and participation" (Gilbert, 2003, p. 3) These kinds of definitions, while acknowledging difference and sometimes stressing inequity and discrimination, fail to bring their analysis to the structural, systemic causes of inequity. Incorporating some of the language of social inclusion tends to add the veneer of social change to policy documents. However, social exclusion involves: (1) denial of participation in civil affairs through institutional sanctions, as is often experienced by status and non-status migrants; (2) denial of access to education, health care, and housing; (3) denial of opportunity to participate actively in society, such as the exclusion of people of colour from the professions (note that this is caused by endemic racism rather than overt policies in professional associations and in educational institutions); and (4) economic exclusion, as evidenced by the policy-created poverty statistics mentioned earlier in this chapter (Galabuzi, 2006; White, 1998). In order to tackle the systemic origins of oppression, we must direct our gaze to their structural, systemic origins in public policy.

Creation of fairness across the social determinants of health is an important public policy goal, but this goal will not be achieved until public policy includes explicit and action-oriented attention to *how* people become marginalized and racialized *through the public policies themselves*. Social inclusion descriptions, although acknowledging disadvantage, "still don't commit to the need for transformative action, choosing instead to focus on unequal outcomes" (Galabuzi, 2006, p. 175). Even when racism is mentioned in social inclusion documents, it is listed as a source of exclusion without making explicit links to public policy that creates and maintains racism (Laidlaw Foundation, 2003). Mentioning racism and oppression in health and public policy documents without attending to White privilege, and clearly identifying dominant social structures, may be described as appropriation of the language of social change without actually getting at the causes of the causes.

Social exclusion occurs because privilege and dominance always occur at the expense of others:

> *Historically in Canada, the dominance of Eurocentric culture has granted non-racialized populations privileged access to resources while first decentering Aboriginal culture, and then marginalizing other ethnic cultures. In key institutions like the labor market, school system, health care system, and criminal justice system, this devaluation of racialized experiences has become a key source of social exclusion. (Galabuzi, 2006, p. 176)*

Social exclusion is much deeper than lack of access, and lack of chances for participation. It originates in state-based hierarchical power structures. According to Galabuzi (2006), social exclusion is characterized by the following considerations:

- Social exclusion describes the structures and processes of inequality and unequal outcomes among groups in society.
- In industrialized societies, social exclusion arises from uneven access to the processes of production, wealth creation, and power.

- Social exclusion is a form of alienation and denial of full citizenship experienced by particular groups of individuals and communities.
- The characteristics of social exclusion occur in multiple dimensions and are often mutually reinforcing. (p. 177)

Table 7.2 shows what a critical social science approach to thinking about policy context might look like. The examples also provide a way to understand the difference between a critical perspective and other kinds of perspectives. This differentiation is becoming increasingly important because the language of social justice is sometimes applied without recognition or knowledge of the critical perspective that underpins it. Context has many layers, like an onion. If the commonly held or dominant view is the first layer of the onion, the critical social science view uncovers the deeper layers of the onion. Note that the examples interlock in many, if not all, cases.

The Structural Determinants of Health

It is important to direct our analysis squarely at political, policy-based determinants of health if we are to improve the health of racialized and marginalized peoples in Canada. These are the structural determinants of health. According to Navarro (2004), "we cannot study public policies without comprehending the political context which determines them" (p. 3). As discussed in Chapter 2, Navarro stresses the political economy of inequalities. A political economy approach to analyzing health inequities is relatively new in Canada and globally, and it brings discussions about public policy and health inequity into an uncomfortable realm for some people. If we decrease our emphasis on locating poorer health in individual shortcomings, then where must our gaze be directed? If we direct our gaze at the policies of political parties, then we bring health thinking to a much larger context, and, in particular, a public policy context. If we bring our gaze to a political context, then the gaze becomes personal because it perhaps points to our own political views and possible complicity in the problem. The ways in which we and our governments frame our thinking about the causes of ill health very much direct our level of policy commitment to solving social problems such as persistent child poverty.

There are several approaches to social policy in contemporary Canada: neo-liberal, neo-conservative, social democratic, feminist, and anti-oppressive. We discuss each of these ideologies in terms of their importance in understanding health and social policy in Canada. This understanding is central to strategic action for change. The addition of the prefix *neo-* (new) tells us that although liberal and conservative political thinking has existed in Canadian politics since Confederation, the newer versions of these areas of policy have changed since their original inception. Table 7.3 summarizes the relationship among political ideologies and social policy. Conservative, liberal, and social democratic ideologies are generally associated with the corresponding major formal political parties in Canada (the Conservative Party, the Liberal Party, and the New Democratic Party). However, it is important to note

Table 7.2: Policy Context: Comparing a Dominant View and a Critical View

Policy Context	Dominant View	Critical Social Science View
Historical	Although White people were responsible for wrongdoings toward Indigenous peoples, this was long ago. The government makes compensation now with policies such as tuition assistance.	Land was stolen. Indigenous peoples were systematically brutalized by White people. Policies and programs must reflect historical trauma, ongoing racism, and the imperative of reconciliation.
Geographic	Displacement of Indigenous peoples by means of reservations was unfair, but there are many policies in place now that give Indigenous peoples extra help so that they can live decent lives.	Placing Indigenous peoples on reservations was an integral part of public policies that aimed to destroy Indigenous cultures, languages, and spiritual connections to the land.
Personal	White clinicians in the health fields must be careful to be objective when they work with people of colour, and to not let any bias enter their practice. Policies ensure objectivity.	White privilege is a core aspect of therapeutic encounters. It operates whether or not the clinician is aware of it. Professional and institutional policy must reflect that neutrality is a myth.
Political and Economic	Some families will always be poor because they don't have the will, the education level, or other knowledge about how to escape poverty. People of colour are usually poor anyway.	Poverty is policy-created by elected governments. Canada's economic apartheid is what makes families of colour poor.
Social	Social inclusion is important because everyone needs social supports. Participation, integration, and cooperation are core principles of social inclusion.	Social exclusion refers to denial of participation, denial of opportunity, and policy-based exclusion that has been described as Canada's economic apartheid.
Genetic	Sickle cell anemia affects relatively few Canadians, so routine testing should not be a public health priority.	Legislated post-natal testing for sickle cell anemia should be a policy priority, since it affects a much larger percentage of African Canadians when compared to the general population.

Environmental	Detailed scientific, environmental, and social assessments are carried out by municipal and other government departments. Policy decisions about landfill location are based on this science.	Systemic racism is responsible for translating these scientific assessments into policy decisions that locate most landfills around the globe near communities of colour.
Psychological	Individual acts of racism are uncomfortable for Black and Indigenous adolescents, but adolescence is a stressful time for all children.	Everyday racism is relentless, and it creates chronic stress for Black and Indigenous adolescents that their White peers do not experience. Policies that direct therapeutic practice must reflect the fact of racism.

that the ideologies represent a particular approach to shaping policy. For example, Conservative governments can and do sometimes adopt neo-liberal policies. The main point in learning to think about policy, and in advocating for just policies, is to consider the underlying ideology of policies.

Social democratic, anti-racist, and anti-oppressive perspectives attend to the creation and maintenance of societal power imbalances. In other words, these perspectives focus on the causes of the causes. For example, poverty causes poorer health outcomes, but what is the cause of poverty? Feminist and anti-racist analyses of public policy have added important dimensions to our ability to critically analyze policy. Social democratic political parties were the first to explicitly acknowledge gender equity as a policy priority.

Many of us are accustomed to thinking about what left-wing and right-wing ideas are and where we are situated in terms of left or right thinking. If you have never really thought about these ideas, then the test in Box 7.5 will help to bring them forward for you. The political compass (Ray, 2002) includes right and left thinking, and also adds other dimensions regarding the ways that people think. We usually think of the word compass as describing a guiding geographic direction: north, south, east, and west. Each of us has a political compass as well—the guiding direction for our thinking and our decision-making about many issues, including social problems. Box 7.5 expands on the political compass concept, and guides the reader in analyzing their own political compass. Please note that we make no claims about the validity of the test. Our sole aim is to provide a forum for openly discussing political stance and world view.

Table 7.3: The Relationship between Ideologies and Public Policy

Ideology of Policy Orientation	Selected Proponents	Relationship to Public Policy
Neo-conservative	Stephen Harper George W. Bush Margaret Thatcher Ralph Klein	Individuals are ultimately responsible for their own well-being and state intervention weakens initiative. Market forces determine resource distribution. Provision of social programs is only a last resort.
Neo-liberal	Lester Pearson Pierre Trudeau	Public social programs are important in addressing general risks to well-being, but these are subservient to economic issues. Advocates minimizing government interventions.
Social Democratic	Rosemary Brown Alexa McDonough Ed Broadbent Tommy Douglas	The organizing principle is social rights—reduction of poverty, inequality, and unemployment. Advocates commitment to universal social programs and stipulates that social policy and economic policy must be considered inseparable.
Feminist	Nelly McClung Patricia Hill Collins Dorothy Smith	The goal is to critique and deconstruct conventional explanations and reveal the gender biases (as well as racial, sexual, and social class biases) inherent in commonly accepted practices. Involves analyzing policy with a critical awareness of how androcentrism is embedded in conventional policy-making.
Anti-racist Anti-oppressive	Marie Battiste George Sefa Dei Agnes Calliste	Focuses on historical colonial roots of inequality and the racialization of social inequality. Recognition of interlocking impacts of oppression is emphasized as central to ameliorating social problems (race, class, gender, sexual orientation, age, disability).

Source: Adapted from: Wharf, B. & McKenzie, B. (2004). *Connecting policy to practice in the human services* (p. 4). Toronto: Oxford University Press.

> **Box 7.5: What Is Your Political Compass?**
>
> This exercise is meant to be fun, as well as a starting point for reflection and discussion about your world view. The Political Compass was developed by Paul H. Ray (2002). The goal of the Political Compass is to help people take a closer look at their world view: the social and political lens that we use to make decisions, vote in elections, decide which governments and policies we like and don't like, and so on.
>
> Most of us are accustomed to thinking about what left-wing and right-wing ideas are and where we are situated in terms of left or right thinking. If you have never really thought about these ideas, then this test will help to bring them forward for you. The Political Compass includes right and left thinking, and also adds another dimension regarding the ways that people think. That's about all we should tell you before you take the test. Please note that we make no claims about the validity of the test. Our sole aim is to provide a forum for bringing political stance and world view forward for discussion in an open manner that is not otherwise available.
>
> *Instructions for Locating Yourself on the Political Compass*
> 1. Log on to http://www.politicalcompass.org
> 2. Start on the home page. *Before* you go beyond the home page, take the Political Compass Test. It is a set of multiple-choice questions. It will take about five minutes.
> 3. Follow the directions on the website regarding analyzing your own political compass.
>
> *Questions for Reflection, Discussion and Debate, and Action*
> 1. Were you surprised about your location on the compass? Why?
> 2. Have a look at some of the famous people whose political compass is said to be close to yours. What does this mean to you?
> 3. Does your location on the political compass match your voting patterns in municipal, provincial, and federal elections? In professional associations?
> 4. What does your own personal political compass have to do with your clinical practice?
> 5. What strategies can you develop and implement in your educational program or in your workplace to relate your world view to your therapeutic work?

Human Rights Stewardship for Anti-racist Public Policy

In order to create equity in health care, we must consider the ways in which inequity is created and maintained through policy decision-making across many organizations and institutions, including but not limited to municipal, provincial, territorial, and federal governments; professional associations; and educational and health care institutions. We require human rights stewardship across all these aspects of governance. Since policy-making is complex, it is difficult to locate starting points. One example is our call for making social justice a core accountability measure in more professional codes of ethics in Canada, described as in Chapter 5. Another example is the Canadian Nurses Association's (CNA) Social Justice Gauge (Canadian Nurses Association, 2006).

According to the CNA, "social justice should be considered at all stages of policy development and at all levels of work within an organization" (p. 18). The gauge describes a process for assessing whether policy proposals and their supporting documentation reflect the attributes of social justice. The attributes include equity, human rights, democracy and civil rights, capacity building, just institutions, poverty reduction, and ethical practice. The gauge brings together many of the ideas described in this book, especially the explicit attention to human rights, democracy, and poverty. The following list of strategies draws upon the main ideas in the book to call for human rights stewardship for racial justice in the Canadian health care system. We draw upon McGibbon's (2008) framework for human rights stewardship in Canadian health care:

- *Build on existing critical perspectives:* The critical perspectives discussed in Chapter 4 are relevant for finding points of resistance. Critical theory, critical race theory, anti-colonial, feminist, political economy, and human rights perspectives are all important as a foundation for change.
- *Make public engagement a policy priority:* Since Canada has a representative democracy, people vote to elect representatives in an electoral system to formulate and implement policy. Although there are some avenues for citizen participation in the policy-making process, policies are largely made by government employees. In terms of professional practice, the involvement of practitioners in policy-making has proven to be elusive with the exception of relatively small numbers of involved individuals. National collective action will be a powerful tool for policy change.
- *Identify and address policy created and sustained inequities in access to health care:* Much of this book has discussed inequities in access to the goods and services of society. We are now losing social medicine in Canada. This is an important area for immediate national collective action.
- *Design and implement a human rights health report card:* A method of accountability must be developed to ensure equity in public policy, including health policy. A human rights health report card (Smith, 2003; Etowa & McGibbon, 2008) would link national policy directions with human rights by measuring Canada's outcomes over time on indicators such as cardiovascular health, the amount of time babies spend in the neonatal intensive-care unit, and the incidence of depression. The report card would be designed with an intersectionality lens in order to illuminate the different forms of oppression and how they compound to create even more disadvantage for people of colour. A human rights health report card would operate in much the same way as any report card. There would be clear pass and fail marks accompanied by the qualitative and quantitative evidence to support the marks. The results of the report card over time would paint a

very clear picture to inform social change for ant-racist practice in our health care system and in our society as a whole.

Box 7.6 provides a clear example of how the complexity of public policies and public systems must be embraced rather than reduced to more basic models that cannot accommodate inequity. If we are to address human rights in health care, we will need to more fully appreciate and understand this complexity. McPherson's (2008) study focused on child health networks as a mechanism to address complex social problems such as child poverty. The example further reinforces the synergistic effects of sorting out the complexity of health inequities within the already very complex health and public service system.

Box 7.6: On Public System and Health Complexity

Complexity scientists tell us that a simple pattern of interaction can create a huge number of potential outcomes and that may have relevance for population and public health issues (Homer-Dixon, 2008). The integrated character of people, institutions, and nature is often ignored as theoretical perspectives based on different world views simplistically fracture disciplines and contextual scales (Homer-Dixon, p. 234).

Complexity science extends our view of systems readiness, contextual paradoxes, and the interactive effect of the macro-environment through the external political context. Placed under a complex adaptive systems lens, the dynamic, entangled, emergent, and robust qualities of the child health network are evidenced. The large-scale impact of seemingly inconsequential changes (such as relationship building) supported large-scale impacts (such as increased system responsiveness) across multiple child and youth service organizations. Further, as this case study has revealed, what may have appeared random in terms of Network development, evolution, and sustainability, in fact had an underlying orderliness to it. Simple rules of behaviour guided the Network as it produced complex changes (p. 235).

Finally, attention to complexity science, social science theory, and a deeper understanding of socio-cultural systems issues for students in health and human service professional programs is essential. This layer of theoretical understanding is germinal if we are going to develop a workforce that recognizes the importance and complexity of these micro- and macro-level factors in networked arrangements and more broadly within our health care system (p. 242).

Further analysis of the micro-, meso-, and macro-level dynamics at play within evolving public service networks is required, with more emphasis on the socio-cultural dynamics of these evolving organizational forms. Given the highly contextual, relational, and political nature of the child health networks, future research on similar organizations should use an explicit socio-political theoretical framework to guide the research. The absence of a socio-political frame in health network research would effectively divorce the organization and its actors from its very essence. Further, attention should be paid to the limitations of current public management theory, organizational theory, and coalition theory vis-à-vis interorganizational health networks (p. 242).

Source: McPherson, C. (2008). *Child health networks: A case study of network development, evolution, and sustainability.* Unpublished doctoral dissertation, McMaster University, Hamilton, ON.

Conclusions

There are many avenues to interrupt racism in public policy and in the policies of professional associations, and educational and health care institutions. As described throughout this book, a grounding in anti-racist principles provides clear paths to work for social change to stop racism. Although the policy cycle is complex, we must nonetheless learn how it operates and how to influence it if we wish to engage in anti-racist health care practice. Knowledge and understanding of critical perspectives have been stressed throughout this and the preceding chapters. Through a critical perspective, practitioners may become fully engaged in anti-racist practice. Critical perspectives instigate us to transgress commonly understood and accepted ways of thinking and behaving. This transgression is the key to the social change that is so urgently needed in Canada's health care system.

Further Reading

Chapter 1

Calliste, A. & Dei, G.S. (2000). *Anti-racist feminism: Critical race and gender studies.* Halifax: Fernwood Publishing.

This collection adds to our understanding and critical engagement of how gendered and racially minoritized bodies can and do negotiate their identities and politics across several historical domains and contemporary spheres. The contributors explore the relational aspects of difference and the implications for reconceptualizing anti-racism discourse and practice. The strength of this book lies in its centring of the experience of racial minority women (and other racialized bodies) in a variety of social sites, thereby inciting the reader to broaden the examination of social spaces through the lens of anti-racist feminist scholarship.

James, C. (2003). *Seeing ourselves: Exploring race, ethnicity, and culture.* Toronto: Thompson Educational Publishing.

This book uses a collection of personal comments and essays written by students from a wide variety of ethnic backgrounds to examine what it means to participate in the cultural and ethnic mosaic that comprises Canada today. The author creates a dialogue with students and readers that probes the meaning of ethnicity, race, and culture, both in terms of the meanings that individuals bring to these concepts, and how they are understood in Canadian society today.

Krieger, N. (2003). Does racism harm health? Did child abuse exist before 1962? On explicit questions, critical science, and current controversies: An ecosocial perspective. *American Journal of Public Health, 93*(2), 194–199.

Research on racism as a harmful determinant of population health is in its infancy. Explicitly naming a long-standing problem long recognized by those affected, this work has the potential to galvanize inquiry and action, much as the 1962 publication of the Kempe et al.'s scientific article on the "battered child syndrome" dramatically increased attention to—and prompted new research on—the myriad consequences of child abuse, a known yet neglected social phenomenon. To further work on connections between racism and health, the author addresses three interrelated issues: (1) links between racism, biology, and health; (2) methodological controversies over how to study the impact of racism on health; and (3) debates over whether racism or class underlies racial/ethnic disparities in health.

Paul, D.N. (2007). *We were not the savages: First Nations history – collision between European and Native American civilizations.* Halifax: Fernwood Publishing.

This fully updated 3rd edition of a vital text on the history of Indigenous peoples comes from the thorough research of a First Nations descendant. By turns revealing and deeply unsettling, the book details the brutal treatment and complete displacement of the Mi'kmaq civilization at the hands of European settlers. The author's ongoing research casts doubt on the recorded tales of Canadian colonization and reveals that the mistreatment of First Nations peoples is not confined to the past.

Smith, D.B. (2005). Racial and ethnic health disparities and the unfinished civil rights agenda. *Health Affairs, 24*(2), 317–325.

This article traces civil rights-era efforts to end disparities in health care in federally financed health programs in the U.S. These efforts faced three successively more difficult challenges: (1) ending Jim Crow practices; (2) eliminating more subtle forms of segregation; and (3) assuring non-discriminatory treatment in integrated settings. Federal efforts peaked with the implementation of the medicare program. Visible symbols of Jim Crow disappeared, and most crude disparities in access were eliminated. The unfinished parts of the civil rights-era agenda, the persistence of more subtle forms of segregation, and the failure to assure non-discriminatory treatment pose major challenges to current efforts to eliminate health care disparities.

Chapter 2

Canadian Research Institute for the Advancement of Women (2006). *Intersectional feminist frameworks: A primer*. Ottawa: Author. Retrieved on December 8, 2006 from: http://www.criaw-icref.ca/IFF/The%20IFFs-%20An%20Emerging%20Vision.pdf

This document provides an overview of intersectionality and its relevance for women's inequality. Although gender-based analysis has been important in looking at gender impacts of discrimination, incorporation of identities such as race and social class are necessary for achieving social justice for women. The Canadian Research Institute for the Advancement of Women (CRIAW) provides tools and research to organizations taking action to advance social justice and equality for all women. CRIAW recognizes women's diverse experiences and perspectives, creates spaces for developing women's knowledge, bridges regional isolation, and provides communications links among researchers and organizations actively working to promote social justice and women's equality.

Carter, S. (2003). *Aboriginal people and colonizers of Western Canada to 1900*. Toronto: University of Toronto Press.

The history of Canada's Aboriginal peoples after European contact is a hotly debated area of study. In this book, the author looks at the cultural, political, and economic issues of this contested history, focusing on the western interior, or what would later become Canada's Prairie provinces. This wide-ranging survey draws on the wealth of interdisciplinary scholarship of the last three decades. Topics include the impact of European diseases, changing interpretations of fur trade interaction, the Red River settlement as a cultural crossroad, missionaries, treaties, the disappearance of the buffalo, the myths about the Mounties, Canadian "Indian" policy, and the policies of Aboriginal peoples toward Canada.

Curry-Stevens, A. (2001). *When markets fail people: Exploring the widening gap between rich and poor in Canada*. Toronto: Canadian Social Justice Foundation for Research and Education.

This report asserts that growing inequality is fundamentally tied to our market system and that both in periods of recession and recovery, the inequality between rich and poor continues to grow. This is why income inequality is at its largest spread than at any point in the last generation. This study challenges commonly held beliefs about the relationship between poverty rates and the market system. It examines market performance during periods of recession and recovery in Canada over the past 25 years with startling results.

Raphael, D. (2008). *The social determinants of health*. Toronto: Canadian Scholars' Press Inc.

This book is the 2nd edition of Canada's main volume on the social determinants of health. The book brings a critical social science perspective to the political and economic origins of health and illness in Canada.

Smith, L.T. (2005). *Decolonizing methodologies: Research and Indigenous peoples*. London: Zed Books Ltd.

From the vantage point of the colonized, the term "research" is inextricably linked with European colonialism; the way that scientific research has been implicated in the worst excesses of imperialism remains a powerful remembered history for many of the world's colonized peoples. In this book, an Indigenous researcher issues a clarion call for the decolonization of research methods. This book is in its 8th printing.

Chapter 3

Anderson, J.M. (2006). Reflections on the social determinants of women's health. Exploring intersections: Does racialization matter? *Canadian Journal of Nursing Research 38*(1), 7–13.

This article addresses the important question of why culture is a determinant of health and identifies additional variables that should be considered as determinants of health. The book also provides an analysis to unmask the complex intersections of race, gender, class, and other social locations, and how they are played out to impact on the health of marginalized people.

Comeau, L.M. (2007). Towards White, anti-racist mothering practices: Confronting essentialist discourses of race and culture. *Journal of the Association of Research on Mothering 9*(2), 20–30.

This article proposes that essentialist discourses of race and culture discipline mothering practices in ways that reproduces racial hierarchies. It also presents an anti-racist mothering practice to disrupt the normal patterns of "White racial superiority." It also provides an analysis of the construction of Indigenous and Black women as racially degenerate and inferior mothers and their White counterparts as "paragons of moral virtue."

Morrow, M., Hankivsky, O. & Varcoe, C. (2007). *Women's health in Canada: Critical perspective on theory and policy*. Toronto: University of Toronto Press.

This book provides a critical analysis of the ways that social conditions and inequities shape health, especially for women with multiple forms of oppression. It explicates women's health in a manner that is not limited by gender, and contextualizes women in their diverse social and economic situations. It also acknowledges the inseparable interaction of gender and other forms of social difference such as race, ethnicity, culture, class, sexual orientation, gender identity, and ability.

Stewart, M., Reutter, L., Veenstra, G., Love, R. & Raphael, D. (2007). "Left out": Perspectives on social exclusion and social isolation in low-income populations. *Canadian Journal of Nursing Research 39*(3), 209–212.

This article presents the findings of a study that examined the impact of socio-economic status on exclusion/inclusion and isolation/belonging, and their impact on the health and quality of life. It also identified strategies for enhancing inclusion and belonging for people living in poverty. The article makes a contribution to knowledge in the area of psychosocial and economic, as well political, factors that facilitate or hinder participation in activities of daily life.

Srivastava, R.H. (2007). *The health care professional's guide to clinical cultural competence.* Toronto: Mosby-Elsevier.

This book is an introduction to cultural competence as an important aspect of working effectively across cultural contexts. It uses a unique framework to examine the variety of theoretical perspectives of cultural diversity and the ways in which they inform cultural competence care in Canada. It starts with the fundamentals of clinical cultural competence and how the Canadian health care contexts have shaped the understanding of cultural competence. The book explicates the complexity and opportunities created by cultural diversity. It also identifies the cultural knowledge required to work effectively across populations and with specific subpopulations.

Chapter 4

Armstrong, P., Armstrong, H. & Coburn, D. (2001). *Unhealthy times: The political economy of health and care in Canada.* Toronto: Oxford University Press.

This unique work assembles, in a readily accessible format, an enormous amount of research in the areas of health and health care within a broadly defined political economy framework. Divided into three sections, it covers home care, globalization, and the comparisons between the Canadian system and the British National Health Service; research in health services, women, and the pharmaceutical industry; and environmental contamination and poverty.

Battiste, M. (2000). *Reclaiming Indigenous voice and vision.* Vancouver: UBC Press.

This book clarifies post-colonial Indigenous thought at the beginning of the new millennium. It represents the voices of the first generation of global Indigenous scholars, and converges those voices, their analyses, and their dreams of a decolonized world. In moving and inspiring ways, *Reclaiming Indigenous Voice and Vision* elaborates a new inclusive vision of a global and national order, and articulates new approaches for protecting, healing, and restoring long-oppressed peoples, and for respecting their cultures and languages.

Gruskin, S., Mills, E.J. & Tarantala, D. (2007). Health and human rights I: History, principles, and practice of health and human rights. *Lancet, 370,* 449–455.

Individuals and populations suffer violations of their rights that affect health and well-being. Health professionals have a part to play in reducing and preventing these violations and ensuring that health-related policies and practices promote rights. This needs efforts in terms of advocacy, application of legal standards, and public-health programming. The changing views of human rights are discussed in the context of the HIV/AIDS epidemic and the authors propose further development of the right to health by increased practice, evidence, and action.

Henry, F., Tator, C., Mattis, W. & Rees, T. (2000). *The color of democracy: Racism in Canadian society.* Toronto: Harcourt Canada.

This book examines institutional racism from a uniquely anti-racist perspective. Linking theory with practice, the personal with the political, and the community with the state, its authors focus on the central ideological struggle for Canadians—the existence and persistence of racism within a seemingly democratic and equitable society.

Navarro, V. (2004). The political and social contexts of health. New York: Baywood Publishing Company.

Our lives are largely determined by health, and our health is largely determined by the social and political contexts in which we live. This book explains and documents how and why using a cross-cultural perspective. Edited by the world's expert in the political economy of public health, this volume is a major contribution both to scholarly research and to policy debates in the field. It should be mandatory reading for students of social policy and planning, as well as for all concerned citizens facing the consequences of the health crisis around the world.

Chapter 5

Bishop, A. (2002). *Becoming an ally: Breaking the cycle of oppression in people.* London: Zed Books.

Anne Bishop is an anti-racism trainer and popular educator who felt inspired to write this book out of concern for "how many people deeply engaged in the liberation of their own group seem not to be able to see their role in oppressing others, and how that comes full circle in perpetuating their own oppression." This is a guidebook for would-be allies, underscoring the complementary process of becoming aware of one's own oppression, and one's possible role in the oppression of others.

Cole, L. & Foster, S. (2000). *From the ground up: Environmental racism and the rise of the environmental justice movement.* New York: New York University Press.

This is a book on an important issue—the environmental justice movement—that is timely and relevant. The phenomenon of environmental racism—the disproportionate impact of environmental hazards, particularly toxic-waste dumps and polluting factories, on people of colour and low-income communities—has gained unprecedented recognition. The authors effectively use social, economic, and legal analysis to illustrate the historical and contemporary causes for environmental racism. Environmental justice struggles, they demonstrate, transform individuals, communities, institutions, and even the nation as a whole.

Galabuzi, G.-E. (2006). *Canada's economic apartheid: The social exclusion of racialized groups in the new century.* Toronto: Canadian Scholars' Press Inc.

Canada's economic apartheid calls attention to the growing racialization of the gap between the rich and poor. Despite the dire implications for Canadian society, the rift is increasing with minimal public and policy attention. The myths about the economic performance of Canada's racialized communities that are used to deflect public concern and to mask the growing social crisis are challenged in this relevant work. Galabuzi points to the role of historical patterns of systemic racial discrimination as essential in understanding the persistent overrepresentation of racialized groups in low-paying occupations. While Canada embraces globalization and romanticizes cultural diversity, there are persistent expressions of xenophobia and racial marginalization that suggest a continuing political and cultural attachment to the concept of a White, settled society.

Hagey, R. & McKay, R. W. (2000). Qualitative research to identify racialist discourse: Towards equity in nursing curricula. *International Journal of Nursing Studies, 37*(1), 45–56.

Professional curriculum planning is beginning to address issues of equity. The authors report on findings from a research initiative to integrate anti-racism into an undergraduate curriculum. Theory and methods of Essed, Fanon, Frankenberg, Hall, van Dijk, and Woodward are synthesized for interpreting racialist discourse. The findings support the principle of normalizing accountability for discourse practices that construct whiteness and "Otherness" in their representations. Essentialist discourse practices are implicated in the perpetuation of racism, ableism, heterosexism, ageism, etc. Hence, the ideal of equity is expanded to include the enactment of non-essentialist discourse. The logic is revealed as either/or: either equity or dominance through normalized perpetuation of essential categories assigning negative value to others constructing difference, marginalization, problematization, exclusion, and containment. The confused, middle, or neutral position is one of condoning racism and other forms of dominance.

MacIntosh, P. (1990). White privilege: Unpacking the invisible knapsack. *Independent School*, Winter, 31–36. Available online at: http://www.case.edu/president/aaction/UnpackingTheKnapsack.pdf

This is a classic article on recognizing the meaning of White privilege and its relevance for anti-racism work. Written almost two decades ago, it is one of the most-cited works about White people's unrecognized role in creating and maintaining racist disadvantage.

Chapter 6

Calliste, A. (2000). Nurses and porters: Racism, sexism, and resistance in segmented labor markets. In A. Calliste & G. Sefa Dei (Eds.), *Anti-racist feminism: Critical race and gender studies* (pp. 143–163). Halifax: Fernwood Publishing.

This chapter is based on a study that traced similarities between African-Canadian women's resistance to professional exclusion and marginality in nursing from the 1970s to the 1990s, and sleeping car porters' anti-racist struggles against the submerged split labour market on Canadian railways in the 1950s and 1960s. Calliste described how Black nurses, like porters, tend to be streamed into the least desirable and least skilled areas of practice, regardless of their qualifications or experience. The chapter is an excellent overview of marginality and exclusion in the profession of nursing.

Canadian Mental Health Association. (2007, June 7). *Discussion paper: Power, paternalism, and partnerships*. Available online at: http://www.cmha.ca/data/1/rec_docs/1336_Power%20Paternalism%20and%20Partnerships.pdf

The purpose of this discussion paper is to invite discussion within the Canadian Mental Health Association about power in therapeutic and other partnerships, in order for the association to develop a more consistent understanding of its importance to consumers. The paper also serves as an excellent core reading about the meaning of power in therapeutic relationships.

hooks, b. (2004). *Teaching to transgress*. New York: Routledge.

This classic book combines practical knowledge of the classroom with a deeply felt connection to the world of emotions and feelings. This is a book about teachers and students that dares to raise critical questions about rage, grief, and the future of teaching itself: "To educate as the practice of freedom is a way of teaching that anyone can learn."

Pate, K. & Neve, L. (2005). Challenging the criminalization of women who resist. In Julia Sudbury (Ed.), *Global lockdown: Gender, race, and the rise of the prison industrial complex around the world* (pp. 19–34). New York: Routledge.

Poor, young, and racialized girls are among the fastest-growing prison populations in Canada and worldwide. Through the lens of Lisa Neve, this chapter explores factors contributing to the increasing criminalization and incarceration of women and girls in Canada. The authors explore the stereotypes about young women and violence that inform the treatment of poor, racialized, and disabled women.

Senate Canada. (2004). *Mental health, mental illness, and addiction: Overview of policies and programs in Canada*. Ottawa: Author. Available online at: http://www.parl.gc.ca/38/1/parlbus/commbus/senate/com-e/soci-e/rep-e/report1/repintnov04vol1table-e.htm#PDF%20FORMAT (See Chapter 3: "Stigma and Discrimination.")

This document describes mental health policies and programs in Canada. The document also provides numerous first-person stories of Canadians experiencing mental health struggles. Chapter 3 provides an overview of stigma and discrimination.

Chapter 7

Canadian Council on Social Development. (2000). *Urban poverty in Canada: A statistical profile.* Ottawa: Author.

This document details the rate and nature of poverty in Canadian cities. Published in April 2000 by the Canadian Council on Social Development, this study used the most recent statistics available to compare poverty rates among Canadian cities and provides a profile of Canada's urban poor. Special attention is given to poverty rates among visible minorities, immigrants, and Aboriginal peoples living in urban areas.

Gilson, L., Doherty, J., Loewenson, R. & Francis, V. (2007). *Challenging inequity through health systems: Final report, knowledge network on health systems.* Geneva: The World Health Organization Commission on the Social Determinants of Health.

This report presents the arguments for health systems as a social determinant of health in the context of inequities and civil society engagement. The paper concludes with the urgent need for initiating and sustaining health system transformation.

Illich, I. (1999). *Limits to medicine: Medical nemesis, the expropriation of health.* London: Marion Boyars Publishing Ltd.

This book is a reprint of Illich's 1974 germinal text regarding the medicalization of human experience and the limited utility of applying biomedical solutions to social problems.

Morrow, M., Hankivsky, O. & Varcoe, C. (2007). *Women's health in Canada: Critical perspectives on theory and policy.* Toronto: University of Toronto Press.

Gender is one of the most powerful determinants of health and health care access. This book includes critical analyses of women's health in a Canadian historical and current context. Topics include gender-based policy analysis and the social determinants of women's health.

Raphael, D. (2006). *Staying alive: Critical perspectives on health and health care in Canada.* Toronto: Canadian Scholars' Press Inc.

Staying Alive provides a fresh perspective on the issues regarding health, health care, and illness. In addition to the traditional approaches of health sciences and the sociology of health, this book unpacks the impact that human rights issues and political economy have on health. This provocative volume takes up these issues as they occur in Canada and the United States, while placing these analyses in an international context. No book to date has taken such an in-depth look at the construction of health care and illness internationally. With its emphasis on political economy and power distribution, and its global perspective, *Staying Alive* will become an essential text for those teaching the sociology of health in North America.

Related Websites

Chapter 1

Centre for Social Justice
http://www.socialjustice.org/
 The Centre for Social Justice conducts research, education, and advocacy in a bid to narrow the gap in income, wealth, and power, and enhance peace and human security. The centre brings together people from universities and unions, faith groups, and community organizations in the pursuit of greater equality and democracy. As such, the centre is committed to working for social change in partnership with various social movements. Although the centre is based in Ontario, their work increasingly takes them across Canada and into the international sphere.

Harvard Center for Society and Health (HCSH)
http://www.hsph.harvard.edu/centers-institutes/society-and-health/
 The HCSH's work is focused on researching the ways in which social and economic inequalities affect the public's health and well-being; formulating public- and private-sector policies that strive to improve people's health and quality of life; and communicating new findings on the social determinants of health to the general public.

International Society for Equity in Health (ISEqH)
http://www.iseqh.org/journal_en.htm
 The purpose of ISEqH is to promote equity in health and health services internationally through education, research, publication, communication, and charitable support. Goals include promoting equity and exposing inequity in health and in health care services internationally, and facilitating scientific interchange and research regarding equity in health and health care services.

National Anti-racism Council of Canada (NARCC)
http://www.narcc.ca
 This organization has a vision of a Canada that is fully equitable and inclusive, that truly respects human dignity and reflects ethnoracial equality, and that honours these foundational principles across all spheres of community and society. NARCC is committed to being a national, community-based, member-driven network that provides a strong, recognized, effective, and influential national voice against racism, racialization, and all other forms of related discrimination in Canada. They strive to effectively address racism, racialization, and all other forms of related discrimination by sharing and developing information and resources; by building, supporting, and helping to coordinate local, regional, national, as well as international initiatives, strategies, and relationships; and by responding to issues and events in a timely and effective manner.

Worldmapper
http://www.worldmapper.org/
Worldmapper is a collection of world maps, where territories are resized on each map according to the subject of interest. An index of nearly 600 maps provides a pictorial representation of global inequities in a wide variety of areas such as child poverty distribution, education of women, toxic environmental emissions, and water consumption. Many of the maps are also available as PDF posters. This is an outstanding method to help understand global health inequities.

Chapter 2

First Nations and Inuit Regional Longitudinal Health Survey
http://rhs-ers.ca/english/search/search.cgi?zoom_and=1&zoom_cat=-1&zoom_page=5&zoom_per_page=10&zoom_query=nations&zoom_sort=0
　　The site not only provides detailed health information, it also describes the participatory research process that is used to conduct this ongoing survey — background and governance, cultural framework, and survey results. In 1996 the Assembly of First Nations Chiefs Committee on Health mandated that a First Nations health survey be implemented every four years across Canada. This resulted in the creation of the First Nations and Inuit Regional Longitudinal Health Survey. This is a First Nations and Inuit-controlled project that documents the health of First Nations and Inuit peoples across Canada over time. The project also originated the ownership, control, and access principles for research with Aboriginal peoples. The project reports provide the detailed self-reported health of First Nations and Inuit physical and mental health.

Harvard Center for Society and Health (HCSH)
http://www.hsph.harvard.edu/centers-institutes/society-and-health/
　　The HCSH's work is focused on researching the ways in which social and economic inequalities affect the public's health and well-being; formulating public- and private-sector policies that strive to improve people's health and quality of life; and communicating new findings on the social determinants of health to the general public.

The International Society for Equity in Health (ISEqH)
http://www.iseqh.org/journal_en.htm
　　The purpose of ISEqH is to promote equity in health and health services internationally through education, research, publication, communication, and charitable support. Goals include promoting equity and exposing inequity in health and in health care services internationally; and facilitating scientific interchange and research regarding equity in health and health care services.

Pan American Health Organization Equidad Listserv Archive Website
http://listserv.paho.org/archives/equidad.html
　　This global archive includes up-to-date resources, articles, and tool kits regarding equity and health, health economics, health legislation, gender, bioethics, ethnicity, human rights, health disparities, information technology, virtual libraries, and research and science concerns around the globe.

World Health Organization Commission on Social Determinants of Health (CSDH)
http://www.who.int/social_determinants/en/
　　The CSDH supports countries and global health partners to address the social factors leading to ill health and inequities. It draws the attention of society to the social determinants of health that are known to be among the worst causes of poor health and inequalities among and within countries. The determinants include unemployment, unsafe workplaces, urban slums, globalization, and lack of access to health systems.

Chapter 3

The Antiracist Alliance
http://www.antiracistalliance.com/

The Antiracist Alliance is a movement to undo structural racism. It is an organizing collective of human service practitioners and educators whose vision is to bring a clear and deliberate anti-racist structural power analysis to social service education and practice. Its members work to undo structural racism from a common understanding and move beyond a focus on the symptoms of racism to an understanding of what racism is, where it comes from, how it functions, why it persists, and how it can be undone. The organization works with people from diverse backgrounds.

The Canadian Race Relations Foundation
http://www.crr.ca/eraceit/

The Canadian Race Relations Foundation is Canada's leading agency dedicated to the elimination of racism in the country. The foundation is committed to building a national framework for the fight against racism in Canadian society. It sheds light on the causes and manifestations of racism; provides independent, outspoken national leadership; and acts as a resource and facilitator in the pursuit of equity, fairness, and social justice. Its goal is to help bring about a more harmonious Canada that acknowledges its racist past, recognizes the pervasiveness of racism, and is committed to creating a future in which all Canadians are treated equitably and fairly.

Diversity Rx
http://www.diversityrx.org/HTML/ESWEL.htm#map

Diversity Rx is a clearinghouse of information on how to meet the language and cultural needs of minorities, immigrants, refugees, and other diverse populations seeking health care. It provides information, resources, and technical assistance to design and implement linguistically and culturally appropriate health care programs and policies. Information on this website is organized into different sections to make it easier for people to find their way around.

The National Multicultural Institute (NMCI)
http://www.nmci.org/

The NMCI is one of the first organizations to have recognized the need for new services, knowledge, and skills in the growing field of multiculturalism and diversity. It is a private, non-profit organization funded through fees for service, contracts, foundation grants, and corporate and individual contributions. It works with individuals, organizations, and communities to facilitate personal and systemic change in order to build an inclusive society that is strengthened and empowered by its diversity. Through the development of strategic initiatives, partnerships, and programs that promote an inclusive and just society, NMCI addresses critical and emerging issues in the diversity field.

Chapter 4

Canadian Civil Liberties Association
http://www.ccla.org/

On this site, you will find information about CCLA's efforts to protect Canadians' rights and freedoms, as well as information on how to join and get involved. The CCLA is a non-profit, non-governmental, law-reform organization dealing with issues of fundamental civil liberties and human rights that affect those who live in Canada. The CCLA was established in 1964, and now has more than 6,000 paid individual supporters, seven affiliated chapters, and more than 50 associated group members who represent several additional thousands of people. The membership includes people from all walks of life: lawyers, homemakers, writers, academics, artists, retirees, broadcasters, trade unionists, clergy, educators, and representatives of most racial, ethnic, and religious constituencies. Policy is guided by a volunteer board.

Canadian Council on Social Development (CCSD)
http://www.ccsd.ca/home.htm

The CCSD is a non-governmental, not-for-profit social research organization that was founded in 1920. Their mission is to develop and promote progressive social policies inspired by social justice, equality, and the empowerment of individuals and communities. This is accomplished through research, consultation, public education, and advocacy. The CCSD's main product is information. Sources of funding include research contracts, the sale of publications and memberships, and donations.

C. Wright Mills' Home Page
http://www.faculty.rsu.edu/~felwell/Theorists/Mills/index.htm

This website provides a comprehensive overview of sociologist C. Wright Mills, including his major works, a bibliography, and links to detailed explanations of his life and works. This website also contains overviews of great social theorists such as Karl Marx and W.E.B. DuBois, and a glossary of social science from "absolute poverty" to "xenophobia." The website is maintained by Frank W. Elwell, of Rogers State University in Oklahoma.

Innocenti Research Centre
http://www.unicef-irc.org/aboutIRC/

The UNICEF Innocenti Research Centre (IRC) in Florence, Italy, was established in 1988 to strengthen the capacity of UNICEF and its co-operating institutions to respond to the evolving needs of children and to develop a new global ethic for children. It promotes the effective implementation of the Convention on the Rights of the Child, in both developing and industrialized countries, thereby reaffirming the universality of children's rights and of UNICEF's mandate.

International Union for Health Promotion and Education (IUHPE)
http://www.iuhpe.org/

The mission of IUHPE is to promote global health and to contribute to the achievement of equity in health between and within countries of the world.

Chapter 5

Canadian Association of Elizabeth Fry Societies (CAEFS)
http://www.elizabethfry.ca

The CAEFS is an association of self-governing Elizabeth Fry Societies that work with and for women in the criminal justice system. Together the Elizabeth Fry Societies develop and advocate the beliefs, principles, and positions that guide CAEFS. The association exists to ensure substantive equality in the delivery and development of services and programs through public education, research, legislative and administrative reform, regionally, nationally, and internationally.

Canadian Broadcasting Corporation Digital News: Expropriating Nova Scotia's Blacks
http://archives.cbc.ca/society/racism/topics/96/

This website contains a live description of the history of Africville, including stories from some of Africville's residents: When dump trucks roared in to move Africville residents out, it seemed like a good idea. By the 1960s, years of neglect and racism had made Halifax's oldest and largest black neighbourhood one of the worst slums in the country. But the relocation of Africville also meant the end of a vibrant community. As one former resident put it, they lost more than a roof over their heads, they lost their happiness. The broadcast date was July 27, 1973, so the website also offers a glimpse into the social construction of the experiences of the Africville residents.

Canadian Social Research Links
http://www.canadiansocialresearch.net/

This website is a virtual resource centre for Canadian social program information and contains a wealth of information in the form of links such as: successive federal budget decision making, the status of the Canada Health Act, social costs of gambling, homelessness and housing, human rights, anti-poverty strategies and campaigns, and asset-based social policies. The site is maintained by Gilles Seguin, who established Canadian social research links on his own time and, he says, on "my own dime, so that I could share my collection of web links with my colleagues in the social research community, whether in government, the non-governmental sector, or academia."

Dennis Raphael's Website
www.atkinson.yorku.ca/draphael

This site contains numerous papers and presentations related to poverty and health. These papers and presentations can be found in the website section entitled "Library." Raphael is a leading social and health policy expert in Canada. His work is grounded in a critical social science perspective.

Metropolis Canada Website
http://canada.metropolis.net/index_e.html

Metropolis is an international network for comparative research and public policy development on migration, diversity, and immigrant integration in cities in Canada and around the world. The international arm of the project involves partnerships with policy-makers and researchers from over 20 countries, including the United States, most of western Europe, Israel, and Argentina, and the Asia-Pacific region. Includes a page "Equity and Social Inequality in Canada."

Chapter 6

Canadian National Political Parties

These websites contain detailed explanations of the policies of some of the political parties in Canada. They serve as an overview of the various perspectives of the parties on the issues of social justice. Practitioners who have not had the opportunity to link their practice with policy and politics will find these websites an invaluable resource, especially during elections.

Conservative Party of Canada
www.conservative.ca
The website for the Conservative Party of Canada.
Green Party of Canada
www.greenparty.ca
The website for the Green Party of Canada.
Liberal Party of Canada
www.liberal.ca
The website for the Liberal Party of Canada.

New Democratic Part of Canada
www.ndp.ca
The website for the NDP of Canada.

National Anti-poverty Organization (NAPO)
http://english.napoonap.ca/Page.asp?IdPage=6605&WebAddress=NAPO2007
 This website will be of interest to practitioners who wish to broaden their understanding of the economic and political context of their clients' lives. NAPO's mission is to eradicate poverty in Canada by promoting income and social security for all Canadians, and by promoting poverty eradication as a human rights obligation. NAPO believes that poverty is a violation of the human right to security of the person and, with reference to the Canadian Charter of Rights and Freedoms and the International Covenant on Economic, Social, and Cultural Rights, the legal right to security of the person. NAPO further believes that poverty is an affront to the values of fairness, justice, and the inclusion of all people in Canadian society and, as such, poverty must be eradicated.

Research Principles and Protocols — Mi'kmaw Ethics Watch
http://mrc.uccb.ns.ca/prinpro.html
 This website contains a detailed overview of the principles and protocols inherent in research with Mi'kmaw peoples. It serves as an excellent example of the principles of ownership, control, and access, which have been developed to decolonize research with Indigenous peoples. The goal of the Principles and Protocols is to "protect the integrity and cultural knowledge of the Mi'kmaw people. These principles and protocols are intended to guide research and studies in a manner that will guarantee that the right of ownership rests with the various Mi'kmaw communities. These Principles and Protocols will guarantee only the highest standards of research." The site is maintained by the Mi'kmaw College Institute, Cape Breton University, Nova Scotia.

Social Justice: A Means to an End and an End in Itself (Canadian Nurses Association)
http://cna-aiic.ca/CNA/documents/pdf/publications/Social_Justice_e.pdf
 This website contains the full document: *Social Justice: A Means to an End and an End in Itself* by the Canadian Nurses Association. It is a clear overview of the concept of social justice and its application to everyday practice as well as policy.

University of Toronto's Quality of Life Website
http://www.utoronto.ca/qol/
 This website will be of interest to practitioners who wish to enrich their core knowledge about quality of life concerns from a social science perspective. The Quality of Life Research Unit has been developing conceptual models and instruments for research, evaluation, and assessment since 1991. In partnership with the Department of Occupational Therapy and the Centre for Health Promotion at the University of Toronto, the unit carries out quality of life research that relates to communities, families, and individuals from a variety of population groups. Instruments, reports, manuals, and other publications developed through their research are made available on a cost-recovery basis.

Chapter 7

Campaign 2000
http://www.campaign2000.ca/
 On November 24, 1989, the House of Commons unanimously passed a resolution to seek to achieve the goal of eliminating poverty among Canadian children by the year 2000. Two

years later, Campaign 2000 "committed to promoting and securing the full implementation of the House of Commons Resolution of November 24, 1989." Campaign 2000 urges all federal parties to set minimum targets of a 25 percent reduction in child poverty rate over the next five years, and a 50 percent reduction over 10 years. This website provides a comprehensive collection of timely, action-oriented information related to child poverty in Canada.

Canadian Centre for Policy Alternatives (CCPA)
http://www.policyalternatives.ca/

The CCPA is an independent, non-partisan research institute concerned with issues of social and economic justice. Founded in 1980, the CCPA is one of Canada's leading progressive voices in policy debates. By combining solid research with extensive outreach, the centre enriches democratic dialogue and ensures that Canadians know there are workable solutions to the issues we face. The CCPA offers analysis and policy ideas to the media, general public, social justice and labour organizations, academia, and the government. The website has links to CCPA publications (reports and studies, editorials, news releases) that are all freely accessible. Topics include federal budget analyses, poverty and social exclusion, and Canada's productivity under various governments.

Canadian Social Research Links: Political Parties and Elections in Canada
http://www.canadiansocialresearch.net/politics.htm

Policy positions of all major political parties in Canada and related social research website links.

Government of Canada Status of Women Policy Research Publications
http://www.swc-cfc.gc.ca/pubs/pubspr/index_e.html

Numerous policy analyses of how policies impact marginalized and racialized individuals and groups. Includes a distinct section entitled "Factoring Diversity into Policy Analysis and Development: New Tools, Frameworks, Methods, and Applications."

Human Rights Watch, Global Issues
http://hrw.org/advocacy/index.htm

This website provides in-depth information on certain issues of concern to Human Rights Watch that cut across national boundaries. It has been designed to encourage advocacy efforts regarding these issues.

Glossary

Chapter 1

Bias: A way of thinking based on a stereotype or fixed image of a group of people. A common stereotype is that people who receive social assistance are lazy. When we begin to think that people on social assistance should be denied coverage for medications because they are lazy and don't deserve assistance, we are demonstrating biased thinking.

Culture: Refers to a group's shared set of beliefs, norms, and values. It is the totality of what people develop to enable them adapt to their world, which includes language, gestures, tools, customs, and traditions that define their values and organize social interactions.

Discrimination: Refers to denying members of a particular social group access to goods, resources, and services. Discrimination is an *action* that typically results from prejudice. *Inaction* in the face of need is also considered discrimination. Discrimination can occur at the individual, organizational, or societal level.

Ethnicity: Refers to belonging to a group that shares the same characteristics such as country of origin, language, ancestry, and culture. Ethnicity is drawn from the recognition that an individual's thoughts, perceptions, feelings, and behaviours in a given situation are often congruent with those of other members of the same ethnic group. People of the same race can be of different ethnicities. For example, Asians can be Japanese, Korean, Thai, or many other ethnicities.

Eurocentric: Eurocentric means being centred on belief systems, languages, cultures, and ways of thinking that have their historical origins in Europe.

-isms: The use of social power to systematically deny people access to resources, rights, respect, and representation on the basis of gender, race, age, income, or membership in any other group; *-isms* are based on the false belief that one group is superior to another group.

Nationality: Refers to the country of citizenship and is defined here because the concept of nationality is sometimes used to mean ethnicity, even though the two are technically different. People of one ethnic group do not necessarily live in one geographic location (such as a Chinese person residing in China and a Chinese Canadian living in Canada). Because of this, ethnicity and nationality are not always the same.

Oppression: Refers to discrimination that occurs and is supported through the power of public systems or services, such as health care systems, educational systems, legal systems, and/or other public systems or services; discrimination backed up by systemic power. Denying people access to culturally competent care is a form of oppression. See also "*-isms.*"

Prejudice: Refers to a negative way of thinking and attitude toward a socially defined group and toward any person perceived to be a member of the group. Like biases, prejudice is a belief and is based on a stereotype.

Race: Refers to a group of people who share the same physical characteristics such as skin tone, hair texture, and facial features. The transmission of human genes from one generation to another is a complex process that is examined in the field of genetics and is beyond this book. However, because people can be grouped by any number of physical differences (height, foot size, resistance to certain diseases), race is an artificial way to categorize people and what makes it salient is its use in signifying and symbolizing sociopolitical conflicts and interests in reference to different types of human bodies. Race is an important concept because people use racial differences as the basis for discrimination.

Religion: Is a system of faith and worship, such as Islam, Catholicism, Hinduism, and Protestantism. It is the formalization of a collection of faith-based principles. Religion is sometimes confused with ethnicity, and both have been used as a reason to brutalize individuals, families, and entire peoples. Powerful modern examples include the Holocaust perpetrated against Jewish people, and the recent conflation of Islam with political parties in Iraq.

Stereotype: A fixed image. Refers to an exaggerated belief, image, or distorted truth about a person or group; a generalization that allows for little or no individual differences or social variation.

White privilege: White privilege is a set of unearned advantages, opportunities, and authorities that are based solely on having white skin, and that confer lifelong increased access to the goods and services of society. White privilege is fundamental to the perpetuation of injustice based on race. An understanding of the ways in which White privilege operates in an everyday way is central to undertaking anti-racist practice.

Chapter 2

Assimilation: Refers to the process of denying, and erasing (where possible) the language, culture, ethnicity, beliefs, customs, and material possessions of a group of people, and forcing them to adopt the systems of the dominant group. Since assimilation involves erasing culture, it is sometimes referred to as acculturation.

Canada Health Act: The Act sets out the primary objective of Canadian health care policy, which is to protect, promote, and restore the physical and mental well-being of residents of Canada and to facilitate reasonable access to health services without financial or other barriers (Health Canada, 2008). The aim of the CHA is to ensure that all eligible residents of Canada have reasonable access to insured health services on a prepaid basis without direct charges at the point of service for such services. The following list provides a definition of the five criteria set out under the Canada Health Act (Health Canada, 2008):
    1. *Public administration:* Provincial and territorial health care insurance plans are administered and operated on a non-profit basis by a public authority, which

is accountable to the provincial or territorial government for decision making on benefit levels and services, and whose records and accounts are publicly audited.
2. *Comprehensiveness:* The health care insurance plan of a province or territory must cover all insured health services provided by hospitals, physicians, or dentists (i.e., surgical dental services which require a hospital setting) and, where the law of the province so permits, similar or additional services rendered by other health care practitioners.
3. *Universality:* All insured residents of a province or territory must be entitled to the insured health services provided by the provincial or territorial health care insurance plan on uniform terms and conditions. Newcomers to Canada, such as landed immigrants or Canadians returning from other countries to live in Canada, may be subject to a waiting period by a province or territory, not to exceed three months, before they are entitled to receive insured health services.
4. *Portability:* Residents moving from one province or territory to another must continue to be covered for insured health services by the home jurisdiction during any waiting period imposed by the new province or territory of residence.
5. *Accessibility:* Insured persons in a province or territory have reasonable access to insured hospital, medical, and surgical-dental services on uniform terms and conditions, unprecluded or unimpeded, either directly or indirectly, by charges (user charges or extra-billing) or other means (e.g., discrimination on the basis of age, health status, or financial circumstances). In addition, the health care insurance plans of the province or territory must provide.

Colonialism: Colonizers are groups of people or countries that come to a new place or country and steal the land from the inhabitants, steal natural resources such as copper, force the inhabitants to help them develop industries such as mining and farming for cash crops (usually with brutal and inhumane methods), and develop a set of laws and public processes that are designed to violate the human rights of the inhabitants, and, in some cases, to completely annihilate Indigenous inhabitants.

Indigenous peoples: Are the very first inhabitants of a geographic area. Examples of Indigenous peoples around the globe are the Maori in New Zealand, the Zulus in Africa, the Mayans in South America, the Mi'kmaq in eastern Canada, and the Cree in western Canada. All of these peoples have a long and disturbingly destructive history at the hands of White colonial oppressors.

Legalized racism: Legalized racism refers to racist practices that are enshrined in the laws and policies of a country. As such, racist acts are made legally defensible and enforceable by the police and other authorities across the region. For example, South Asian Canadians were excluded from the right to vote; denied entry into professional occupations; restricted in property rights; and discriminated against in housing practices.

Chapter 3

Cultural awareness: The ability of health care providers to appreciate and understand their clients' values, beliefs, practices, and problem-solving strategies; an in-depth self-examination of one's own culture, prejudices, and biases toward other cultures.

Cultural competence: A process in which the health care professional continuously strives to achieve the ability and availability to effectively work within the cultural context of a client. It is a journey, not a destination.

Cultural desire: The motivation of a health care professional to engage in caring for another regardless of conflict. It is characterized by compassion, authenticity, humility, openness, availability, and flexibility.

Cultural difference: A relationship between two or more perspectives. In the health care context, identifying difference requires contrasting two orientations: that of the client and that of the health professional.

Cultural diversity: The cultural differences that exist among people, such as language, dress, and traditions, and the way societies organize themselves, their conception of morality and religion, and the way they interact with the environment.

Cultural encounters: The ability of health care providers to competently work directly with clients of culturally diverse backgrounds. This is evident in the health care professional's verbal and non-verbal messages.

Cultural humility: A lifelong process of self-reflection and self-critique. It does not begin with an examination of the client's beliefs; instead, it starts with a thorough examination of the health care professional's assumptions and beliefs embedded in his or her own understanding, and the goals of the provider-client relationship.

Cultural knowledge: The ability of health care providers to have an educated knowledge base about various cultures to better understand their clients. It also requires health care providers to be knowledgeable about biological, psychosocial, and physiological variations among cultural groups.

Cultural safety: The provision of quality care for people of ethnicities different than the mainstream. Health care professionals provide such care within the cultural values and norms of the client.

Cultural skill: The ability of health care providers to conduct an accurate and culturally competent history and physical examination.

Culture: Patterns of human activity and the symbolic structures that make these activities salient. Culture has multiple definitions. It can be described as systems of symbols and meanings that lack fixed boundaries and that are constantly changing, and that interact and compete with one another. See Chapter 2 for more on culture.

Diversity: Most commonly refers to differences among cultural groups.

Health care inequity: The practice of intentionally treating people differently and unfairly because of their race, sex, national origin, disability, or other protected class.

Health inequity: Is the presence of systematic disparities in health (or in the major social determinants of health) among groups with different social advantage/disadvantage (e.g., wealth, power, and prestige).

Multicultural health care: Health care that recognizes the cross-cultural absolutes that all human beings share. It acknowledges racial and cultural diversity yet maintains a coordinated approach to overall health planning and service delivery.

Multiculturalism: The practice of acknowledging and respecting the various cultures, religions, races, ethnicities, attitudes, and opinions within a place.

Chapter 4

Anti-colonialism: Like anti-racism, anti-colonialism examines systemic power structures that create and maintain racism, and corresponding mechanisms to counteract racism. The historic racism of colonialism and the modern-day equivalent of colonialism are continuously examined with the goal of social justice for colonized peoples.

Anti-racism: Anti-racism examines systemic power structures that create and maintain racism. It explores and implements corresponding mechanisms to counteract racism. Understanding the White privilege that sustains racism is central to anti-racism work and achieving social justice for racialized peoples.

Conflict theory: Conflict theory emerged as a challenge to structural functionalism and the tendency for sociologists in general to seek theories that provided blanket explanations for all human behaviour. This theory stressed the limits of empiricism, the importance of examining power, and the need to study social problems within their historical institutional structures. Conflict theory laid much of the foundation for critical social scientific thought in the latter half of the 20th century.

Critical theory: Critical theorists critiqued common notions of the meaning of democracy and argued that democracy was no longer about having a voice in collective decision making and self-determination. Rather, democracy became a means of distribution of power among relatively few citizens. According to Habermas, a prominent critical theorist, democratic freedom was no longer tied to political equality in the sense of equal distribution of political power and the chances of exercising the power. Critical theory calls for liberation from oppressive societal power structures.

Feminism: The term "feminism," in its historical and current meanings, is by no means cohesive or static. Feminism is most widely known as women's political activism on behalf of women for the continued advancement of women's rights. The centrality of patriarchal dominance is emphasized as a core area for social change. Although feminism is popularly viewed as some sort of homogeneous set of ideas, there are many feminisms, such as Black feminism, which focuses on interrogating not only patriarchy, but White privilege. The "first wave" of feminism involved the fight for the right to vote and to be considered a person under the law.

Symbolic interactionism: Symbolic interactionists insisted that social theory be based or grounded in everyday activities and behaviours, hence the term "grounded theory." In this way, symbolic interaction became known as a micro-perspective due to its detailed attention to the nuances of human interaction. Symbolic interactionists, such as Goffman, also examined power relationships in institutions such as mental institutions and in professions such as psychiatry.

Systems theory: Systems theory, or structural functionalism, analyzes social systems in a way that is analogous to biological and engineering models (Kelly & Field, 2006). Systems have parts, which function together to ensure the stability of the overall system. Component parts have their own function and are functionally articulated to the larger system.

Chapter 5

Cultural racism: Refers to the culturally embedded network of beliefs and values that encourage and justify discriminatory practices, including the belief that the cultural practices and beliefs of one's own racial group are superior (Henry, Tator, Mattis & Reese, 2000). Cultural racism has its basis in ethnocentrism, which is "a tendency to view all peoples and cultures in terms of one's own cultural standards and values" (p. 57).

Environmental racism: Refers to the deliberate location of environmental toxins near the homes and communities of people of colour.

Individual racism: Takes the form of face-to-face stereotyping, prejudice, and discrimination. It involves discriminatory attitudes and resulting behaviours. More specifically, individual racism involves thinking and acting based on the belief that one's own racial group has superior values, customs, and norms. In a related way, individual racism is based on the belief that other racial groups are inferior (Henry, Tator, Mattis & Reese, 2000).

Internalized racism: Happens when people of colour adopt or internalize negative racist stereotypes about themselves as if they were true. All of us are profoundly influenced by the way people treat us in our everyday lives, and by the images we see of ourselves in the media and all around us. These influences become part of how we feel about ourselves to varying degrees. The relentless experiences of everyday racism, and the thousands of racist messages associated with these experiences, eventually start to influence the ways in which people of colour view themselves and their personal worth. Oppressive social structures reinforce racist messages in numerous ways.

Systemic racism: Is racism backed up by systemic power. At the core of racism is an unequal distribution of power. According to Sefa Dei (1996), institutional structures have the power to provide a space for individuals in society to discriminate against one another.

Chapter 6

Critical social science thinking: Involves bringing a critical perspective to bear on any form of analysis. A critical perspective includes examining societal power structures and how they are central in the creation and maintenance of social problems, including most population health problems in modern societies. Although critical social science thinking can encompass aspects of traditional thinking, the overarching emphasis is on the critical examination of the processes that maintain societal power hierarchies.

Critical thinking: Involves an attitude of inquiry involving the use of principles, abstractions, deductions, interpretations, and analysis of arguments. Most discussions of critical thinking in the health fields also include notions of investigation, logical deduction, and scientific reasoning.

Textual mediation and textually mediated racism: Refers to the process of using textual representations to mediate or reinforce ideas and ways of thinking. For example, when we examine social relations of power, the way that textual materials reinforce dominant power structures is very important to consider. The case example above shows how health-promotion pamphlets can reinforce the dominance of whiteness and the inferiority of people of colour. This is textually mediated racism. Textual mediation is a necessary and important part of maintaining power hierarchies in contemporary societies.

Chapter 7

Apartheid: Apartheid is racial segregation. It can take the form of geographic segregation, such as the creation of reservations for Indigenous peoples in North America, and it can also take the form of segregation in schools and in the workplace. Numerous and more subtle forms of segregation also operate in Canada and globally. These include exclusion of opportunity to enter professional schools through the many forms of racism in public schools. Ultimately, apartheid is a well-developed system of oppression that permeates all aspects of everyday life.

Economic apartheid: Refers to the policies and processes that ensure ongoing high poverty rates and social exclusion—the use of policy-created economic hardship to maintain oppression. Also see "Apartheid."

Low Income Cut-off (LICO): According to Statistics Canada, the low income cut-off point (LICO) is the amount of annual income below which a family is considered to be living in poverty. LICOs are commonly used to analyze the implications of poverty for individuals and families living in poverty.

Policy cycle: The most common way to understand policy-making is through the policy cycle. Although policy development is not a linear process, or even a strictly circular process, the policy cycle nonetheless provides a framework to understand, critique, and advocate for policy-making. There are numerous descriptions of the policy cycle and each of these descriptions has unique features. However, all policy cycles refer to common stages and processes that describe policy-making, whether it is in government or in non-governmental organizations: getting a social problem or issue on the policy agenda; translating the issue into policy formulation; implementing the policy; and evaluating the policy against its intended outcome.

References

Chapter 1

Anderson, K.N., Anderson, L. E., & Glanxe, W. D. (Ed.). (1994). *Mosby's medical, nursing, & allied health dictionary* (4th ed.).St. Louis: Mosby-Year book, Inc.

Bauer, Y. (2001). *A history of the Holocaust*. Danbury, CT: Franklin Watts.

Begley, S. (1996). Three is not enough: Surprising new lessons from the controversial science of race. *Newsweek, 13*, 67-69.

Benton, W. M. (1997). *The Evolution of African consciousness: The effects of R.A.C.I.S.M. on Afrikans in the Diaspora*. Unpublished Master of Social work thesis. Dalhousie University, Halifax, NS.

BLAC (Black Learners Advisory Committee) (1994). *Black report on education: Redressing inequity, Empowering Black learners*. Halifax, NS: Council on African Canadian Education.

Boyd, J. (1998). *Racism, whose problem: Strategies for understanding and dealing with racism in our communities*. Halifax: Fernwood Publishing.

Calliste, A. & Dei, G. S. (2000). *Anti-racist feminism: Critical race and gender studies*. Halifax: Fernwood publishing.

Canadian Islamic Congress (2008). *Islam and Canadian Muslims: A very short introduction*. Retrieved on September 4, 2008 from: http://www.canadianislamiccongress.com/about_islam.php

Dei, G. S. (2005). *Spiritual knowing and transformative learning*. Working Paper # 59: New Approaches to Life Long Learning. Retrieved on February 14, 2005 from: http://www.google.ca/search?hl=en&q=NALL&btnG=Google+Search&meta=

Dei, G, S. (2000). *Anti-racism education: Theory and practice*. Halifax: Fernwood Publishing.

Enang, J. (1999). *The childbirth experiences of African Nova Scotian women*. An Unpublished Master of Nursing Thesis. Dalhousie University. Halifax, Nova Scotia, Canada.

Erikson, E. (1959). *Identity and the life cycle*. New York: International Universities Press.

Etowa, J., Bernard, W. T., Clow, B. & Oyinsan, B. (2007) Participatory Action Research (PAR): Improving Black Women's Health in Rural and Remote Communities. *International Journal of Transcultural Nursing, 18*:349-359.

Freeman, E. M. (1990). The black family's life cycle: Operationalizing a strengths Perspective. In Logan, S. M. L., Freeman, E. M. & McRoy, R. G. (eds). *Social work practice with black families: A culturally specific perspective*. pp. 55-72. NY: Longman.

Galabuzi, G-E (2008). The economic exclusion of racialized communities- A statistical profile. In Barrington Walker (Ed.). *The history of immigration and racism in Canada: Essential readings*. Toronto: Canadian Scholar's Press.

Galabuzi, G-E (2006). *Canada's economic apartheid: The social exclusion of racialized groups in the new century*. Toronto: Canadian Scholar's Press Inc.

Henry, F., Tator, C., Mattis, W., & Rees. T. (2000). *The color of democracy: Racism in Canadian society*. Toronto: Harcourt Canada.

Houston, M. & Wood, J. T. (1996). Difficult dialogues, expanded horizons: Communicating across race and class. In J. T. Wood (ed.) *Gendered Relationships*. pp. 39-56. Mountain view. CA, Mayfield Publishing Co.

hooks, b. (1994). *Teaching to transgress*. New York: Routledge.

hooks, b. (2003). *Teaching community: A pedagogy of hope*. London: Routledge.

James, C. (2003). *Seeing ourselves: Exploring race, ethnicity, and culture*. Toronto: Thompson Educational Publishing Inc.

James, C. (1996). *Perspectives on racism and the human services sector*. Toronto: University of Toronto Press.

Logan, S. M. L. (1990). Black families: Race, ethnicity, culture, social class, and gender issues. In Logan, S. M. L., Freeman, E. M. & McRoy, R. G. (Eds) *Social work practice with black families: A culturally specific perspective*. pp. 18-37. NY: Longman.

MacIntosh, P. (1990). White privilege: Unpacking the invisible knapsack. *Independent School*, Winter, 1990, 31-36.

McAdoo, H. P. (1993). *Family ethnicity: Strength in diversity*. Thousand Oaks, CA: Sage Publications.

McGibbon, E., Etowa, J., & McPherson, C. (2008). Health care access as a social determinant of health. *Canadian Nurse*, 104(7), 22-27.

Miller, M. A. (1995). Culture, spirituality, and women's health. *Journal of Obstetric, Gynecologic and Neonatal Nurses (JOGNN)*, 24, 3, 257-263.

Ministerial Advisory Council on Rural Health (2002). *Rural health in rural hands: Strategic directions for rural, remote, northern and Aboriginal communities*. Ottawa: Health Canada.

Paul, D. (2007). *We were not the savages*. Halifax: Fernwood Publishing Company Limited.

Raphael, D., Bryant, T. & Curry-Stevens, A. (2004). Toronto Charter outlines future health policy directions for Canada and elsewhere. *Health Promotion International (19)* 2, 269-273.

Rodriguez-Wargo, T. (1993). Preparing for Cultural diversity through education. *Journal of Pediatric Nursing*, 8, 4, 272-273.

Schott, J. & Henley, A. (1996). *Culture, religion and childbearing in a multiracial society: A Handbook for health professionals*, London: Clays Ltd.

Spence, C. M. (2000). *The skin I'm in: Racism, sports, and education*. Halifax: Fernwood Publishing:

Smye, V. & Mussell, B. (2001). *Aboriginal health: What works best*. Vancouver: University of British Columbia Mental Health Evaluation and Community Consultation Unit.

Virtual Museum Canada (2008). *Open hearts, closed doors: Canadian immigration overview*. Gatineau, Quebec. Retrieved on August 23, 2008 from: http://www.virtualmuseum.ca/English/About/index.html

Welshing, F. (1991). Black children and the process of inferiorization (June 1974). Chapter in *The ISSIS Papers*. Chicago: Third World Press.

Wijeyesinghe, C., Griffin, P. & Love, B. (1997). Racism curriculum design. In M. Adams, L. A. Bell & Griffin, P. (Eds.). Teaching for diversity and social change (pp. 82-109). New York: Routledge

Witzig, R. (1996). The medicalization of race: scientific legitimization of a flawed social construct. *Annals of Internal Medicine*, 125, 8, 675-679.

World Health Organization (2003). *The social determinants of health: The solid facts*. Geneva, Switzerland: Author. Retrieved September 10, 2007 from: http://www.who.dk/document/e59555.pdf

Chapter 2

Aday, L.A. (1993). *At risk in America: The health and health care needs of vulnerable populations in the United States*. San Francisco: Jossey-Bass.

References

American Cancer Society. (2004). *Facts and Figures*. Atlanta: American Cancer Society.

American Heart Association. (2001). Heart and Stroke Statistical Update. Retrieved on March 20, 2001 from: www.americanheart.org/statistics/stroke.html

Ashing-Giwa, K. T., Padilla, G., Tejero, J., Kraemer, J., Wright, K., Coscarelli, A., Clayton, S. Williams, I., & Hills, D. (2004). Understanding the breast cancer experience of women: A qualitative study of African American, Asian American, Latina and Caucasian cancer survivors. *Psychooncology, 13*(6): 408-428.

Assembly of First Nations (2007). *First Nations Regional Longitudinal Health Survey*. Ottawa: Author.

Bach, P. B., Pham, H. H., Schrag, D., Tate, R. C., & Hargraves, J. L. (2005). Primary care physicians who treat blacks and whites. *The New England Journal of Medicine, 35*(6), 575-584.

Bach, P. B., Cramer, L. D., Warren, J. L. & Begg, C. (1999). Racial differences in the treatment of early-stage lung cancer. *New England Journal of Medicine, 341*, 1198-205.

Backlund, E, Sorlie, P.D., & Johnson, N.J. (1996). The shape of the relationship between income and mortality in the United States: Evidence from the national longitudinal mortality study. *Annals of Epidemiology, 6,*12-20.

Bernabei, R, Gambassi, G., Lapane, K., Landi, F., Gatsonis, C., Dunlop, R., Lipsitz, L., Steel, K., & Mor, V. (1998). Management of Pain in Elderly Patient with Cancer. *The Journal of the American Medical Association, 279*(23), 1877-1882.

Bernard, B. (2008). PM Stephen Harper apologizes to all Canadian Aboriginals. Circler of *Chance Monthly Newsletter, Mi'kmaw Legal Support Network*, August, 2008, p. 7.

Bernard, W.T. (2001). *Including Black Women in Health and Social Policy Development: Winning Over Addictions, Empowering Black Mothers With Addictions to Overcome Triple Jeopardy*. Halifax, NS: Maritime Centre of Excellence for Women's Health.

Blake, W. M. & Darling, C. A. (2000). Quality of life: Perceptions of African Americans. *Journal of Black Studies, 30* (3), 411-427.

Bolaria, B. S. & Bolaria, R., (Eds.) (1994). *Racial minorities, medicine, and health*. Halifax, NS: Fernwood Publishing.

Boyd, J. (1998). *Racism, whose problem: Strategies for understanding and dealing with racism in our communities*. Halifax: Fernwood Publishing.

Bradley, R., Schwartz, A.C., & Kaslow, N. J. (2005). Posttraumatic Stress Disorder Symptoms Among Low-Income, African American Women With a History of Intimate Partner Violence and Suicidal Behaviors: Self-Esteem, Social Support, and Religious Coping. *Journal of Traumatic Stress, 18*(6), 685-696.

Brancati, F.L., Kao, L., Folsom, A.R., Watson, R.L., & Szklo, M. (2000). Incident Type 2 Diabetes Mellitus in African American and White Adults: The Atherosclerosis Risk in Community Study. *Journal of the American Medical Association, 283*, 17.

Breen, N., Wesley, M., Merril, R., & Johnson, K. (1999). The relationship of socioeconomic status and access to minimum expected therapy among female breast cancer patients in the Black-White Cancer Survival Study. *Ethnicity and Disease, 9*, 111-125.

Brown, C., Shear, M. K., Schulberg, H.C., & Madonia, M. J. (1999). Anxiety Disorders Among African-American and White Primary Medical Care Patients. *Psychiatric Services, 50*, 407-409.

Bryant T. (2002). *The Current State of Housing in Canada as a Social Determinant of Health*. Paper given at The Social Determinants of Health Across the Life-Span Conference, Toronto, November 2002.

Bryant, T., Chisholm, C. & Crowe, C. (2002). Housing as a determinant of health. Paper presented at the Social Determinants of Health Across the Lifespan Conference, Toronto, ON, November, 2002.

Canadian Council on Social Development (2000). *Urban poverty in Canada*. Ottawa, ON: Author.

Canadian Institute for Health Information (2006). *How healthy are rural Canadians? An assessment of their health status and health determinants.* Ottawa: Author.

Canadian Research Institute for the Advancement of Women (2006). *Intersectional feminist frameworks: A Primer.* Ottawa: Author.

Carter, V. & Carter, L. (1993). *The Black Canadians: Their history and contributions.* Edmonton, AB: Reidmore Books, Inc.

Chronic Disease Prevention Alliance (CDPA) (2008). *Poverty and chronic disease: Recommendations for action.* Ottawa: CDPA.

Cloutterbuck, J., & Feeney Mahoney, D. (2003). African American Dementia Caregivers: The Duality of Respect. *Dementia,* 2, 221.

Cole, L. & Foster, S. (2000). *From the ground up: Environmental racism and therRise of the environmental justice movement.* New York: New York University Press.

Collins, P. H. (1990). *Black feminist thought: Knowledge, consciousness, and the politics of empowerment.* Boston: Unwin Hyman.

Cooper, R., Cutler, J., Desvigne-Nickens, P., Fortmann, S.P., Friedman, L., Havlik, R., et al (2000) Trends and Disparities in Coronary Heart Disease, Stroke, and Other Cardiovascular Diseases in the United States. *Circulation,* 102, 3137-3147

Coyte, P. & McKeever, P. (2001). Home care in Canada: Passing the buck. *Canadian Journal of Nursing Research,* 33(2), 11-25.

Curry-Stevens, A. (2001). *When markets fail people: Exploring the widening gap between rich and poor in Canada.* Toronto, ON: Canadian Social Justice Foundation for Research and Education.

Dana, R. H. (2002). Mental Health Services for African Americans: A Cultural/Racial Perspective. *Cultural Diversity and Ethnic Minority Psychology,* 8, 3-18.

DelBello, M.P., Lopez-Larson, M.P., Soutullo, C.A., & Strakowski, C.A. (2001). Effects of race on psychiatric diagnosis of hospitalized adolescents: a retrospective chart review. *Journal of child and adolescent psychopharmacology,* 11(1), 95-103.

Dixon, L., Green-Paden, L., Delahanty, J., Lucksted, A., Postrado, L., & Hall, J. (2001). Variables Associated With Disparities in Treatment of Patients With Schizophrenia and Comorbid Mood and Anxiety Disorders. *Psychiatric Services,* 52, 1216-1222.

Elliott, B. A., & Larson, J. T. (2004). Adolescents in mid-sized and rural communities: Foregone care, perceived barriers, and risk factors. *Journal of Adolescent Health,* 35, 303-309.

Enang, J. E. (2002). Black women's health: Health research relevant to Black Nova Scotians. In C. Amaratunga (Ed.). *Race, ethnicity and women's health.* Halifax, Nova Scotia: Halcraft Printers Inc. (pp. 43-82).

Enang, J. (1999). *The childbirth experiences of African Nova Scotian women.* An Unpublished Master of Nursing Thesis. Dalhousie University. Halifax, Nova Scotia, Canada.

Etowa, J., Weins, J., Bernard. W. T., & Clow, B. (2007). Determinants of Black women's health in rural and remote communities. *Canadian Journal of Nursing Research,* 39(3), 56-76.

Essed, P. (1991). *Understanding everyday racism: An interdisciplinary theory.* Newbury Park, CA: Sage Publications.

Ford, E., R. Cooper., A. Castaner, B., & Simmons, M. (1989). Coronary arteriography and coronary bypass survey among whites and other racial groups relative to hospital-based incidence rates for coronary artery disease: findings from NHDS. *American Journal of Public Health,* 79, (April): 437-40.

Galabuzi, G. E. (2005). *Canada's economic apartheid: The social exclusion of racialized groups in the new century.* Toronto: Canadian Scholar's Press Inc.

Gary, F.A. (2005). Stigma: Barrier to Mental Health Care among Ethnic Minorities. *Issues in Mental Health Nursing,* 26, 979–999.

Goldstein, R. B., Olfson, M., Wickramaratne, P. J., & Wolk, S. I. (2006). Use of outpatient mental health services by depressed and anxious children as they grow up. *Psychiatric Services,* 57, 966-975.

Green, C.R., Anderson, K. O., Baker, T. A., Campbell, L. C., Decker, S., Fillingim, R., Kaloukalani, D., Lasch, K., Myers, C., Tait, R., Todd, K. & Vallerand, A. (2003). The unequal burden of pain: Confronting racial and ethnic disparities in pain. *Pain Medicine*, 4(3), 277-294.

Harry, R. (2008). The British Columbia Restorative Health Project. Victoria: British Columbia Aboriginal Network on Disability Society. Retrieved on April, 2008 from: http://www.bcands.bc.ca/G.%20Kiesman/BC%20Aboriginal%20Restorative%20Health%20Project%20Summary.pdf

Hay, D. I. (1994). Social status and health status: Does money buy health? In B. Singh Bolaria & Rosemary Bolaria (Eds.), *Racial minorities, medicine and health* (pp. 9-52). Halifax, NS: Fernwood Publishing.

Health Canada (2008). *Canada's health care system*. Retrieved on January 23, 2008 from: http://www.hc-sc.gc.ca/hcs-sss/medi-assur/cha-lcs/index-eng.php

Health Canada (2003). Diabetes in Canada. Ottawa: Author.

Health Council of Canada. (2005). *The Health Status of Canada's First Nations, Métis and Inuit Peoples – A background paper to accompany Health Care Renewal in Canada: Accelerating Change*. Ottawa: Health Council of Canada.

Henry, F., Tator, C., Mattis, W & Rees. T. (2000). *The color of democracy: Racism in Canadian society*. Toronto: Harcourt Canada.

Jackson, L. (2002). *HIV prevention programmes and female prostitutes: The Canadian context In Striking to the heart of the matter: Selected readings on gender and HIV*. In Women's health in Atlantic Canada, C. Amaratunga & Gahagan, J. (Eds.). Atlantic Center of Excellence for Women's Health: Halifax, Nova Scotia.(87-104.)

Kafele, K. (2004). *Racial discrimination and Mental Health: Racialized and Aboriginal Communities*. Ottawa: Ontario Human Rights Commission.

Kim, J., Ashing-Giwa, K.T., Singer, M. K. & Tejero, J. S. (2006). Breast cancer among Asian Americans: Is acculturation related to health-related quality of life? *Oncology Nursing Forum*, November 2006. Retrieved on December 20, 2006 from: http://findarticles.com/p/articles/mi_6854/is_6_33/ai_n28391052/pg_1?tag=artBody;col1

Kirmayer, L., Brass, G., & Tait, C. (2000). The mental health of Aboriginal peoples: Transformations of identity and community. *Canadian Journal of Psychiatry*, 45,607-616.

Krieger, N. (2003). Does racism harm health? Did child abuse exist before 1962? On explicit questions, critical science, and current controversies: An ecosocial perspective. *American Journal of Public Health*, 93(2), 194-199.

Krieger, N., Rowley, D. L., Herman, A. A., Avery, B., & Phillips, MT. (1993). Racism, sexism, and social class: implications for studies of health, disease, and well-being. *American Journal of Preventive Medicine* 9(6), 82-122.

Krieger, N. (1987). Shades of difference: Theoretical underpinnings of the medical controversy on Black-White differences, 1830-1870. *International Journal of Health Service*, 17, 258-279.

Kuran, H. J. (2002). The Barriers to Healthy Living and Movement for Frail Aboriginal Elders. National Inuit & Community Health Representatives Organization (NICHRO). Retrieved on April 2, 2007 from: http://www.nichro.com/cfc_3.html.

Lasser, K. E., Himmelstein, D.U., Woolhandler, S. (2006). Access to Care, Health Status and Health Disparities in the US and Canada. Results of a Cross-National based Survey. *The American Journal of Public Health*, 96(7), 1300-1307.

Ross, L., Kohler, C., Grimley, D., Green, L., & Anderson-Lewis, C. (2007).Toward a model of prostate cancer information seeking:Identifying salient behavioral and normative beliefs among African American men. *Health Education & Behavior*, 34(3), 422-440.

Lynch, J.W. (1996). Social Position and Health. *Annals of Epidemiology*, 6, 21-23.

Lynch, J.W., Kaplan, G.A., & Shema, S.J. (1997). Cumulative impact of sustained economic hardship on physical, cognitive, psychological, and social functioning. *The New England Journal of Medicine*, 337, 1889-1995.

MacMillan, H. L., MacMillan, D. R., Offord, D. R., & Dingle, J. L. (1996). Aboriginal health. *Canadian Medical Association Journal*, 155(11), 1569-1578.

Mainous, A. G., King, D. E., Garr, D. R., & Pearson, W. S. (2004). Race, Rural Residence, and Control of Diabetes and Hypertension. *Annals of Family Medicine* 2, 563-568.

Maliski, S. L., Connor, S., Fink, A., & Litwin, M. S. (2006). Information desired and acquired by men with prostate cancer: Data from ethnic focus groups. *Health Education & Behavior,* 33(3), 393-409.

Marisa, N., Ugarte, C., Fuller, I., Haas, G. & Portenoy, R. K. (2005). Access to Care for Chronic Pain: Racial and Ethnic Differences. *The Journal of Pain,* Volume 6, Issue 5, Pages 301-314.

McDaniel, S. A., & Chappell, N. L. (1999). Health care in regression: Contradictions, tensions, and implications for Canadian seniors. *Canadian Public Policy,* 35(1), 1223-132.

McGibbon, E. (2008). Health and health care: A human rights perspective. In D. Raphael (Ed.). *Social determinants of health: A Canadian perspective.* Toronto: Canadian Scholar's Press.

McGibbon, E. Calliste, A., Arbuthnot, E, Bassett, R. Cameron, C., Graham, H., & MacDonald, D. (2005). *Barriers in Access to health Services for Rural Aboriginal and African Canadians: A Scoping workshop Report.* St. Francis Xavier University, Antigonish, Nova Scotia, June, 2005.

McGibbon, E., McPherson, C., & Etowa, J. (2007). Social determinants of health: Bringing advocacy to a health and public policy level. *Nursing in Focus, 8*(2), 17-19.

McIntyre, L. (2004). Food Insecurity. In D. Raphael (Ed.). *The social determinants of health: Canadian perspectives* (pp. 173-185). Toronto: Canadian Scholar's Press.

McPherson, C., Popp, J., & Lindstrom, R. (2006). Reexamining the paradox of structure: A child health network perspective. *Healthcare Papers, 7*(2), 46-52.

Meadows, L. M., Thurston, W. E., & Melton, C. (2001). Immigrant women's health. *Social Science & Medicine,* 52, 1451-1458.

Merkin, S. S., Stevenson, S., & Powe, N. (2002). Geographic socioeconomic status, race, and advanced-stage breast cancer in New York City. *American Journal of Public Health,* 92(1): 64–70.

Miller, B.A., Kolonel, L. N., & Bernstein, L. (1996). *Racial/ethnic patterns of cancer in the United States 1988-1992.* (NIH Pub. No. 96-4104). Bethesda, Md.: National Cancer Institute.

Ministerial Advisory Council on Rural Health (2002). *Rural health in rural hands: Strategic directions for rural, remote, northern and Aboriginal communities.* Ottawa: Health Canada.

Marisa, N., Ugarte, C., Fuller, I., Haas, G., & Portenoy, R. (2005). Access to care for chronic pain: Racial and ethnic differences. *The Journal of Pain,* 6(5), 301-314.

Mukamel, D.B., Murthy, A., & Weimer, D. (2000). Racial differences in access to high quality cardiac surgeons. *American Journal of Public Health* 90, 1774-1777.

Murray, S., Rudd, R. Kirsch, I., Yamamoto, K., & Grenier, S. (2007). *Health literacy in Canada: Initial results from the International Adult Literacy Skills Survey.* Ottawa: Canadian Council on Learning.

Navarro, V. (2004). *The political and social contexts of health.* New York: Baywood Publishing Company.

Oakley-Girvan, I., Kolonel, L., Gallagher, R., Wu, A. Felberg, A., & Whittemore, A.(2003). Stage at diagnosis and survival in a multiethnic cohort of prostate cancer patients. *American Journal of Public Health,* 93(10), 1753–1759.

Pappas, G., Queen, S., Hadden, W., & Fisher, G. (1993). The increasing disparity in mortality between socioeconomic groups in the United States, 1960 and 1986. *New England Journal of Medicine, 329,* 103-109.

Poland, B., Coburn, D., Robertson, A., & Eakin, J. (1998). Wealth, equity and health care: A critique of "population health" Perspectives on the determinants of health. *Social Science and Medicine, 46,* 785-98.

Portenoy, R., Ugarte, C., Fuller, I., & Haas, G. (2004). Population-based survey of pain in the United States: Differences among white, African American, and Hispanic Subjects. *The Journal of Pain,* 5(6), 317-328.

Quan, H., Fong, A., De Coster, C., Wang, J., Musto, R., Noseworthy, T. W, & Ghali, W. A. (2006). Variation in health services utilization among ethnic populations. *Canadian Medical Association Journal*, 174(6): 787–791.

Raphael, D. (2004). Strengthening the social determinants of health: The Toronto Charter for a healthy Canada. In Dennis Raphael (Ed.). *The social determinants of health: Canadian perspectives* (361-365).

Raphael, D. (2009). *The social determinants of health*. (2nd Edition). Toronto: Canadian Scholars' Press.

Raphael, D., Bryant, T. & Curry-Stevens, A. (2004). Toronto Charter outlines future health policy directions for Canada and elsewhere. *Health Promotion International (19)* 2, 269-273.

Razack, S. (1998). *Looking white people in the eye: Gender, race, and culture in courtrooms and classrooms*. Toronto: University of Toronto Press.

Richard, H., Harlan, L., Klabunde, C., Gilliland, F., Stephenson, R., Hunt, W., & Potosky, A. (2003). Racial differences in initial treatment for clinically localized prostate cancer. Results from the Prostate Cancer Outcomes Study. *Journal of General Internal Medicine*, 18(10): 845–853.

Rotimi, C. N., Cooper R. & Ward R. (1997). Hypertension in seven populations of African Origins. *American Journal of Public Health* 87 (2), 160-168

Rothenberg, B., Pearson, T., Zwanziger, J., & Mukamel, D. (2004). Explaining disparities in access to high-quality cardiac surgeons. *The Annals of Thoracic Surgery*, 78(1), 18-24.

Roy, J. (2008). Legalized racism. Toronto: Canadian Race Relations Foundation. Retrieved on April 20, 2008 from: http://www.crr.ca/content/view/224/377/lang,english/

Schrag, D., Cramer, L., Bach, P. & Begg, C. (2001). Age and adjuvant chemotherapy use after surgery for Stage III colon cancer. *Journal of the National Cancer Institute*, 93, 850-857.

Schraufnagel, T.J., Wagner, A.W., Miranda, J., & Roy-Byrne, P.P. (2006). Treating minority patients with depression and anxiety: what does the evidence tell us? *General Hospital Psychiatry*, 28(1), 27-36.

Schwartz, A. C., Bradley, R. L., Sexton, M., Sherry, A., & Ressler, K. J. (2005). Posttraumatic stress disorder among African Americans in an inner city mental health clinic. *Psychiatric Services*, 56, 212-215.

Seligman, H. K., Bindman, A. W., Vittinghoff, E., Kanaya, A. M. & Kushel, M. B. (2007). Food insecurity is associated with diabetes mellitus: Results from the National Health Examination and Nutrition Examination Survey (NHANES) 1999-2002 *Journal of General Medicine*, 22(7), 1018-1023.

Seng, J.S., Kohn-Wood, L.P., & Odera, L.A. (2005). Exploring racial disparity in posttraumatic stress disorder diagnosis: implications for care of African American women. *Journal of Obstetric, Gynecology and Neonatal Nursing*, 34(4), 521-30.

Shamian, J. (2007). *Home care: The unfinished policy*. Ottawa: Victorian Order of Nurses.

Shapcott, M. (2004). Housing. In D. Raphael (Ed.). *The social determinants of health: Canadian perspectives*. Toronto: Canadian Scholar's Press (pp. 201-216).

Sheppard, M. (2002). Mental health and social justice: Gender, race, and psychological consequences of unfairness. *British Journal of Social Work*, 32, 779-797.

Smith, D. B. (2005). Racial and ethnic health disparities and the unfinished civil rights agenda. *Health Affairs*, 24(2), 317-325.

Spezziani, G., Arrieta, C., Chirinos, J., Mallon, S., & Jimenez, J. (2006). 280 From symptoms of depression to diagnosis of depression: The gap among African American females with heart failure (ISHLT). *The Journal of Heart and Lung Transplantation*, 25(2), suppl.1, 141.

Statistics Canada (2008). *Ethnic origin, visible minorities, place of work and mode of transportation*. The Daily, Wednesday, April 2, 2008. Retrieved on August 9, 2008 from: http://www.statcan.gc.ca/daily-quotidien/080402/dq080402a-eng.htm

Statistics Canada (2007). *University tuition*. Statistics Canada: Ottawa, ON. Retrieved on September 4, 2007 from: http://www.statcan.ca/Daily/English/040902/d040902a.htm.

Statistics Canada (2005). *Women in Canada: A gender-based statistical report.* Statistics Canada, Ottawa, ON: Author.

Statistics Canada (2003). The Daily, Statistics Canada, Low income rates among immigrants. Thursday June 19th 2003. Retrieved on October 10, 2003 from: http://www.statcan.ca/Daily/English/030619/d030619a.htm)

Statistics Canada. (2002). The Daily, Statistics Canada, Health of the off-reserve Aboriginal population, 2000-2001. Retrieved November 7, 2006 from: http://www.statcan.ca/Daily/English/020827/d020827.pdf

Strothers, HS., Rust, G., Minor, P., Fresh, E., Druss, B. & Satcher, D. (2004). Disparities in antidepressant treatment in Medicaid elderly diagnosed with depression. *Journal of the American Geriatrics Society, 53*(3), 456-61.

Sullivan, K., Johnson, L., Cloyer, C., Beale, J., Willis, J., Harrison, J., & Welsh, K. (2003). *National indigenous palliative care needs study.* Canberra: Commonwealth of Australia.

Tarlow, B. J., & Mahoney, D. F. (2005). Creating parity in health education: Designing culturally relevant Alzheimer's disease information. *Health Informatics Journal,* 11, 211.

Trumper, R. (2004). *Health status and needs of Aboriginal children and youth: Literature review.* Calgary: Southern Alberta Child and Youth Health Network

United Nations International Children's Emergency Fund (UNICEF, 2005). *Child poverty in rich countries.* Florence: UNICEF Innocenti Research Center.

Utsey, S.O., Ponterotto, J.G., Reynolds, A.L., & Cancelli, A.A. (2000). Racial Discrimination, Coping, Life Satisfaction, and Self-Esteem Among African Americans. *Journal of Counseling and Development,* 78 (1), 72-80.

Viola, V., Rathore, S., Wenger, N., & Frederick, P. (2005). Sex and racial differences in the management of acute myocardial infarction, 1994 through 2002. *The New England Journal of Medicine,* 353(7), 671-683.

Vindigni, D., Griffen, D., Perkins, J., & DaCosta, C. (2004). Prevalence of musculoskeletal conditions, associated pain and disability and the barriers to managing these conditions in a rural, Australian Aboriginal community. *Rural and remote health* 3(4), p. 230.

Walks, R. A. & Bourne, L. S. (2006). Ghettos in Canada's cities? Racial segregation, ethnic enclaves and poverty concentration in Canadian urban areas. *The Canadian Geographer,* 50(3), 273-297.

Wells, K., Klay, R., Koike, A., & Sherbourne, C. (2001). Ethnic disparities in unment need for alcoholism, drug abuse, and mental health care. *The American Journal of Psychiatry,* 158(12), 2027-2032.

Wilkins, C.H., Wilkins, K.L., Meisel, M., Depke, M., Williams, J., & Edwards, D. F. (2007). Dementia undiagnosed in poor older adults with functional impairment. *Journal of the American Geriatrics Society,* 55(11), 1771-6.

Wilkinson, R. & Pickett, K. (2005). Income inequality and population health: A review and explanation of the evidence. *Social Science and Medicine,* 16, 1768-84.

Williams, D.R. (1999). Race, socioeconomic status, and health: The added effects of racism and discrimination. *Annals of the New York Academy of Sciences,* 896, 173-188.

Williams, R. F. G. & Collins, P. H. (2001). Racial residential segregation: A fundamental cause of racial disparities in health. *Public Health Reports,* 116, 404-416.

Williams, D.R., Gonzales, H.M., Neighbors, H., Nesse, R., Abelson, J.M., Sweetman, J., & Jackson, J.S. (2007). Prevalence and distribution of major depressive disorder in African Americans, Caribbean blacks, and non-Hispanic whites: results from the National Survey of American Life. *Archives of general psychiatry,* 64(3), 305-15.

World Health Organization (2003). *The social determinants of health: The solid facts.* Geneva, Switzerland: Author.

Wu, P., Hoven, C. W., Cohen, P., Liu, X., Moore, R. E., Tiet, Q., Okezie, N., Wicks, J., & Bird, H. R. (2001). Factors associated with use of mental health services for depression by children and adolescents. *Psychiatric Services,* 52, 189-195.

Chapter 3

Alleyne, J., Papadopoulos, I. & Tilki, M. (1994). Anti-racism within transcultural nurse education. *British Journal of Nursing, 3*(15), 1118-1121.

Anderson, L.M., Scrimshaw, S.C., Fullilove, M.T., Fielding, J.E., & Norman, J. (2003). Culturally Competent health care systems: A systematic review. *American Journal of Preventive Medicine, 24* (35), 68-79.

Betancourt, J.R., Green, A.R., Carrillo, J.E., & Park, E.R. (2005). Cultural competence and health care disparities: Key Perspectives and trends. *Health Affairs, 24* (2), 499-505.

Betancourt, J.R., Green, A.R., Carrillo, J.E., & Ananeh-Firempong, O. (2003). Defining Cultural competence: A practical framework for addressing racial/ethnic disparities in health and health care. *Public Health Reports, 118* (4), 293-30.

Boyd, J. (1998). *Racism: Whose problem? Strategies for understanding and dealing with racism in our communities.* Halifax: Fernwood Publishing.

Boyle D.P. & Springer, A. (2001). Towards a cultural competence measure for social work with specific population. *Journal of Ethnic and Cultural Diversity in Social Work, 9*(3-4), 53-71.

Brach, C. & Fraser, I. (2000). Can Cultural competence reduce racial and ethnic health disparities? A review and conceptual model. *Medical Care Research and Review* 57, (suppl.1), 181-217.

Campinha-Bacote, J. A. (2008). Cultural competence: An integral part of holistic nursing practice. Paper presented at American Holistic Nurses Association 25th Annual conference. Accessed on Sept. 8, 2008 at: http://www.medscape.com

Campinha-Bacote, J. A. (2002). The process of cultural competence in the delivery of health care services: A model of care. *Journal of Transcultural Nursing, 13* (3), 181-184.

Canadian Council for Refugees (2000). *Report on Systemic Racism and Discrimination In Canadian Refugee and Immigration Policies- In Preparation for the UN World Conference Against Racism, Racial Discrimination, Xenophobia, and Related Intolerance.* November 1, 2000. Retrieved on November 20, 2008 from: http://www.ccrweb.ca/arreport.PDF.

Canadian Heritage (2008). Canadian multiculturalism: An inclusive citizenship. Retrieved on September 10, 2008 from: http://www.pch.gc.ca/progs/multi/inclusive_e.cfm

Carpenter-Song, E. A. Schwaille, M.N., & Longhofer, J. (2007) Cultural competence reexamined: Critique and directions for the future. *Psychiatric Services* 58 (100) 1362-1365.

Culley, L. (2006). Transcending transculturalism? Race, ethnicity and health care. *Nursing Inquiry, 13* (2), 144-153.

Culley, L. (1996). A critique of multiculturalism in health care: the challenge for nurse education. Journal of Advanced Nursing, 23(3), 564-570.

Drevdahl, D.J., Canales, M.K., &, Dorcy, K.S. (2008) Of Goldfish tanks and moonlight tricks: Can cultural competence ameliorate health disparities? *Advances in Nursing Science 51* (1), 15-27.

Dugas, B. W. & Knor, E. R. (1995). Health and ethnicity. In *Nursing Foundations: A Canadian Perspective.* (pp 278-304). Scarborough, Ontario: Appleton and Lange.

Enang, J. (1999). *The childbirth experiences of African Nova Scotian women.* An Unpublished Master of Nursing Thesis. Dalhousie University. Halifax, Nova Scotia, Canada.

Etowa, J. & Adongo, L. (2007) Cultural Competence: Beyond Culturally Sensitive Care for Childbearing Black Women. *Journal of the Association for Research on Mothering, 9* (2), 73-85.

Foley, R. & Wurmser, T. A. (2004). Culture diversity: A mobile workforce command creative leadership, a new partnership, and innovative approaches to integration. *Nursing Administration Quarterly 28* (2), 122-128.

Giddings, L.S. (2005). A theoretical model of social consciousness. *Advances in Nursing Science, 28* (3), 224-239.

Giger, J. N. & Davidhizar, R. E. (2002). The Giger and Davidhizar's transcultural assessment model. *Journal of Transcultural Nursing, 13*(3), 185-188.

Henry, F. (2002). Canada's contribution to the 'management' of ethno-cultural diversity. *Canadian Journal of Communication, 27*(2), 231-242.

Henry, F., Tator, C., Mattis, W & Rees. T. (2000). *The color of democracy: Racism in Canadian society.* Toronto: Harcourt Canada.

Higham, M. (1988). *The training needs of health workers in a multiracial society. Training in health and race.* Cambridge: National Extension College.

Hunt, L.M. (2001) Beyond Cultural competence: Applying humility to clinical settings. *The Park Ridge Center for Health, Faith and Ethics, Bulletin, Issue 24.* Accessed on September 09, 2008 at: http://www.parkridgecenter.org

Jackson, J. S. (1991). *Life in Black America.* Newbury Park: Sage.

Keusch, G.T. Wilentz, J. & Kleinman, A. (2006). Stigma and global health: developing a research agenda. *Lancet* 367, 525-527.

Kim-Godwin, Y. S., Clarke, P. N., & Barton, L. (2001). A model for the delivery of culturally competent community care. *Journal of Advanced Nursing, 35*(6), 918-925.

Kleinman, A. & Benson, P. (2006). Anthropology in the clinic: The problem of cultural competency and how to fix it. *PLoS Medicine, 3*(10), 1673-1676.

Kumas-Tan, Z., Beagan, B. Loppie, C. MacLeod, A. & Frank, B. (2007). Measures of cultural competence: Examining hidden assumptions. *Academic Medicine 82*(6) 548-557.

Lee, S., Lee, M. Chiu, M, & Kleinman, A. (2005). Experience of social stigma by people with schizophrenia in Hong Kong. *British Journal of Psychiatry, 186,* 153-157

Leininger M. & McFarland, M.R. (2002). *Transcultural nursing: Concepts, theories, research and practice.* (3rd Ed). New York: McGraw-Hill, Medical Publishing Division.

Leininger, M. (1991). *Culture Care diversity and universality: A theory of nursing.* New York: National League for Nursing Press.

Masi, R., Mensah, L., & Macleod, K.A. (1993) *Health and cultures: Exploring the relationships, policies, professional practice and education.* New York: Mosaic Press.

Meleis, A. I. (1996). Culturally Competent Scholarship: Substance and Rigor. *Advances in Nursing Science. 19*(2), 1-16

Miranda, J., Duan, N., Sherbourne, C., Schoenbaum, M., Lagomasino, I., Jackson-Triche, M. & Wells, K. B. (2003). Improving care for minorities: Can quality improvement interventions improve care and outcomes for depressed minorities? Results of a randomized, controlled trial. *Health Services Research, 38*(2), 613-630.

Naidoo, J. C. & Edwards, R. G. (1991). Combating racism involving visible Minorities: A review of relevant research and policy development. *Canadian Social Work Review, 8*(2), 211-235.

Purnell, L. (2005). The Purnell model for cultural competence. Journal of Transcultural Nursing, Summer, 2005. Retrieved on December 6, 2005 from: http://findarticles.com/p/articles/mi_qa3919/is_200507?tag=untagged

Rounds, K. A., Weil, M. & Bishop, K. K. (1994). Practice with culturally diverse families of young children with disabilities. *Families in society: The Journal of Contemporary Human Services,* 74, 1, 3-15.

Santiago-Irizarry, V. (1996). Culture as cure. *Cultural Anthropology* 11, 3-24.

Schlickau J. & Wilson, M. (2005). Development and testing of prenatal breastfeeding education intervention for Hispanic women. *Journal of Perinatal Education,* 14 (4), 24-35.

Schott, J. & Henley, A. (1996). *Culture, religion and childbearing in a multiracial society: A handbook for health professionals,* London: Clays Ltd.

Spector, R. E. (1996). *Cultural diversity in health and illness.* Norwalk, CT: Appleton & Lange.

Smith, L. T. (1999). *Decolonizing methodologies: Research and indigenous people.* London: Zed Books.

Wailoo, K. (2001). *Dying in the city of the blues: Sickle cell anemia and the politics of race and health.* Chapel Hill (North Carolina) University Press.

Chapter 4

American Psychiatric Association (2000). *Diagnostic and Statistical Manual of Mental Disorders, Text Revision (DSM-IV-TR)*. Arlington, VA:American Psychiatric Publishing.

Bailey, G. & Gayle, N. (2003). *Social Theory: Essential Readings*. Don Mills, ON: Oxford University Press.

Bannerji, H. (2006). Building from Marx: Reflections on class and race. *Social Justice, 32*(4), 144-160.

Barbee, E. L. (1994) A Black feminist approach to nursing research. *Western Journal of Nursing Research, 16,* 495-506.

Battiste, M. (2000). *Reclaiming indigenous voice and vision*. Vancouver: UBC Press.

Becker, H. (1963). *The outsiders: Studies in the sociology of deviance*. New York: The Free Press.

Bourgeault, I. L. (2006). Sociological perspectives on health and health care. In D. Raphael, T. Bryant, & M. Rioux (Eds.). *Staying alive: Critical perspectives on health, illness, and health care* (pp. 35-57). Toronto: Canadian Scholar's Press International.

Breggin, P. (1991). *Toxic psychiatry: Why therapy, empathy and love must replace the drugs, electroshock, and biochemical theories of the "New psychiatry"*. New York: St. Martin's Press.

Bryant, T., Raphael, D., & Rioux, M. (2006). Toward the future: Current themes in health research and practice in Canada. In D. Raphael, T. Bryant, & M. Rioux (Eds.), *Critical perspectives on health, illness, and health care* (pp. 373-391). Toronto: Canadian Scholar's Press International.

Calliste, A. (2000). Nurses and porters: Racism, sexism, and resistance in segmented labor markets. In A. Calliste and G. Sefa Dei (Eds.). *Anti-racist feminism: Critical race and gender studies* (pp. 143-163). Halifax: Fernwood Publishing.

Calliste, A. & Dei, G. (2000). *Anti-racist feminism: Critical race and gender studies*. Halifax: Fernwood Publishing.

Campbell, M. (1990). Identifying the barriers to nursing power in hospitals. *Canadian Operating Room Nursing Journal, 8*(4), 9-12.

Campbell, M. (1988). The structure of stress in nurses' work. In B. S. Bolaria & H. Dickinson (Eds.), *Sociology of health care in Canada* (pp. 393-405). Toronto: Harcourt Brace Jovanovich.

Campbell, M. & Gregor, F. (2002). *Mapping social relations: A primer in doing institutional ethnography*. Aurora, ON: Garamond Press.

Canadian Nurses Association (2004). *Social determinants of health and nursing: A summary of the issues*. Ottawa: Author.

Cassin, M. (1990). *The routine production of inequality: A study in the social organization of knowledge*. Unpublished Doctoral Dissertation. University of Toronto.

Coburn, D. (2001). Health, health care and neo-liberalism. In D. Coburn (Ed.). *Unhealthy times: The political economy of health and care in Canada.* (pp. 45-65). Toronto: Oxford University Press.

Collins, P. H. (1990). *Black feminist thought: Knowledge, consciousness, and the politics of empowerment*. Boston: Unwin Hyman.

Collins, P. H. (2002). The politics of Black feminist thought. In C. R. McCann & Kim, S. (Eds.). *Feminist theory reader: Local and global perspectives* (pp. 318-333). London: Routledge.

Dei, G. S. (2005). *Spiritual knowing and transformative learning*. Working Paper # 59: New Approaches to Life Long Learning. Retrieved on February 14, 2005 from: http://www.google.ca/search?hl=en&q=NALL&btnG=Google+Search&meta=

Dei, G, S. (2000). *Anti-racism education: Theory and practice*. Halifax: Fernwood Publishing.

Dei, G. S. (1996). *Anti-racism education: Theory and practice*. Halifax: Fernwood Publishing.

Ehrenreich, B. (1971) *The American health empire: Power, profits, and politics*. New York: Random House.

Etowa, J., Weins, F., Thomas Bernard, W., & Clow, B. (2007). Determinants of Black women's health in rural and remote communities. *Canadian Journal of Nursing Research., 30*(3), 56-76.

Fletcher, R. H. & Fletcher, S.W. (2005). *Epidemiology: The essentials.* Baltimore: Lippincott, Williams and Wilkins, 4th Ed.

Galabuzi, G. E. (2006). *Canada's economic apartheid: The social exclusion of racialized groups in the new century.* Toronto: Canadian Scholar's Press Inc.

Garner, R. (2000). *Social theory, continuity and confrontation: A reader.* New York: Broadview Press, Ltd.

Gilligan, C. (1993). *In a different voice: Psychological theory and women's development.* Cambridge: Harvard University Press.

Goffman, E. (1961). *Asylums: Essays on the social situation of mental patients and other inmates.* New York: Doubleday & Company Incorporated.

Gruskin, S., Mills, E. J., & Tarantala, D. (2007). Health and human rights I: History, principles, and practice of health and human rights. *Lancet, 370,* 449-55.

Habermas, J. (1973). *Legitimation crisis.* Boston: Beacon Press

Hale, S. M. (1990). *Controversies in sociology: A Canadian introduction.* Toronto: Copp Clarke Pitman Limited.

Hall, S. & duGay, P. (1996). *Questions of cultural identity.* London: Sage Publications Inc.

Henry, F., Tator, C., Mattis, W & Rees. T. (2000). *The color of democracy: Racism in Canadian society.* Toronto: Harcourt Canada.

Herman, J. (1972).*Trauma and recovery: The aftermath of violence – from domestic abuse to political terror.* New York: BasicBooks.

hooks, b. (1994). *Teaching to transgress.* New York: Routledge.

Illich, I. (1976). *Limits to medicine, medical nemesis: The expropriation of health.* Middlesex, England: Penguin Books.

James, C. (2003). *Seeing ourselves: Exploring race, ethnicity, and culture.* Toronto: Thompson Educational Publishing.

Keddy, B. (1996). A feminist critique of psychiatric nursing discourse. *Issues in Mental Health Nursing, 17*(4), 381-391.

Kelly, M. P. & Field, D. (1998). Conceptualizing chronic illness. In *Sociological perspectives on health, illness, and health care.* (pp. 3-19). D. Field & S. Taylor (Eds.). Oxford: Blackwell Publishing.

Kitts, R. L. (2005). Gay adolescents and suicide: Understanding the association. *Adolescence, 40*(159), 621.

Krieger, N. (2001). Theories for social epidemiology in the 21st century: An ecosocial perspective. *International Journal of Epidemiology, 30,* 668-677.

Labonte, R. (2004). Understanding 'globalization' as a determinant of health determinants: A critical perspective. *International Journal of Occupational and Environmental Health, 10*(4), 360-367.

Labonte, R., Schrecker, T, & Gupta, A. S. (2005). *Health for some: Death, disease and disparity in a globalizing era.* Toronto: Center for Social Justice.

Laing, R. D. (1967). *The politics of experience.* New York: Random House.

Marmot, M. & Wilkinson, R. (1999). *The social determinants of health.* New York: Oxford University Press.

Marshall, A. (2007). *Keynote address.* Public Health Agency of Canada Summer KSTE Institute. Baddeck, NS, August, 2007.

Marx, K. (1991). *Capital: Volume 3.* London: Penguin Books.

McCann, C. R. & Kim, S. (2003). Introduction. In C. R. McCann & Kim, S. (Eds.). *Feminist theory reader: Local and global perspectives* (pp. 1-9). London: Routledge.

McGibbon, E. (2008). Health and health care: A human rights perspective. In D. Raphael (Ed.) *The social determinants of health: Canadian Perspectives.* Toronto: Canadian Scholar's Press International.

McGibbon, E., Etowa, J., & McPherson, C. (2008). Health care access as a social determinant of health. *Canadian Nurse, 104*(7), 22-27.

McGibbon, E. (2004). *An institutional ethnography of nurses' work in pediatric intensive care.* Unpublished Doctoral Dissertation: University of Toronto.

McGibbon, E. & Etowa, J. (2007). *Health Inequities and the social determinants of health: Spatial contexts of oppression.* Invited Keynote Presentation, Nova Scotia Health Research Foundation Health Geomatics Conference, Halifax, NS, October, 2007.

McPherson, C. (2008). *Child health networks: A case study of network development, evolution, and sustainability.* Unpublished doctoral dissertation. McMaster University, Hamilton, ON.

Mills, C. W. (1959). *The sociological imagination.* New York: Oxford University Press.

Muntaner C., Lynch, J.W., Hillemeier, M., Lee, J.H., David, R., & Benach J. (2002). Economic inequality, working-class power, social capital, and cause-specific mortality in wealthy countries. International Journal of Health Services, *32*(4): 629-656.

Navarro, V. (2002). A historical review (1965-1997) of studies on class, health, and quality of life: A personal account. In V. Navaro (Ed.) *The political economy of social inequalities: Consequences for health and quality of life* (pp. 13-30). New York: Baywood Publishing Company.

Navarro, V. (2004). *The political and social contexts of health.* New York: Baywood Publishing Company.

Parsons, T. (1961). An outline of the social system. Reprinted with permission of The Free Press from *Theories of Society* by Talcott Parsons, Edward Shils, Kaspar Naegle, & Pitts, J.

Perleth, M., Jakubowski, E., & Busse, R. (2001). What is 'best practice' in health care? State of the art and perspectives in improving the effectiveness and efficiency of the European health care systems. *Health Policy, 56*(3), 235-250.

Raphael, D. (2006). *Poverty and policy in Canada.* Toronto: Canadian Scholar's Press

Raphael, D. (2004). *Social determinants of health: Canadian perspectives.* Toronto: Canadian Scholar's Press International.

Raphael, D. (2006). Social determinants of health: Present status, unanswered questions, and future directions. *International Journal of Health Services, 36*(4), 651-677.

Raphael, D. (2008). Getting serious about the social determinants of health: New directions for public health workers. *Promotion and Education, 15*(3), 15-20.

Rawls, J. (1971). *A theory of justice.* Cambridge, Mass.: Belknap Press of Harvard University Press.

Razack, S. (1998). *Looking white people in the eye: Gender, race, and culture in courtrooms and classrooms.* Toronto: University of Toronto Press.

Rich, A. (1980). Compulsory heterosexuality and lesbian existence. *Signs: Journal of Women, Culture, and Society, 5*(4), 1-32.

Rich, A. (1976). *Of woman born: Motherhood as experience and institution.* New York: W. W. Norton and Company.

Shamian, J. (2007). *Home care: The unfinished policy.* Ottawa: Victorian Order of Nurses.

Sharif, N. R., Dar, A. A., & Amaratunga, C. (2002). Ethnicity, income and access to health care: In C. Amaratunga (Ed.) *Race, ethnicity, and women's health* (pp. 121-151). Halifax: Atlantic Center of Excellence for Women's Health.

Shaw, M., Dorling, D., Gordon, D. & Smith, G. D. (1999). *The widening gap: Health inequalities and policy in Britain.* Bristol: The Policy Press.

Smith, D. B. (2005). Racial and ethnic health disparities and the unfinished civil rights agenda. *Health Affairs, 24*(2), 317-325.

Smith, D. (1987). *The everyday world as problematic: A feminist sociology.* Toronto: University of Toronto Press.

Smith, D. (1990a). *The conceptual practices of power.* Boston: Northeastern University Press.

Smith, D. (1990b). *Texts, facts, and femininity: Exploring the relations of ruling.* London: Routledge.

Smith, D. (1999). *Writing the social: Critique, theory and investigations*. Toronto: University of Toronto Press.

Smith, G. (1995). Accessing treatments: Managing the AIDS epidemic in Ontario. In M. Campbell & A. Manicom (Eds.), *Knowledge, experience and ruling relations: Studies in the social organization of knowledge* (pp. 18-34). Toronto: University of Toronto Press.

Stevens, P. E. (1992). Applying critical theories to nursing in communities. *Public Health Nursing, 9*(1), 2-9.

Szasz, T. (1961). *The myth of mental illness*. New York: Delta Books.

Thomas Bernard, W. (2002). Including Black women in health and social policy development: Winning over addictions. In C. Amaratunga (Ed.) *Race, ethnicity, and women's health* (pp. 153-182). Halifax: Atlantic Center of Excellence for Women's Health.

Wesley-Esquimaux, C. C. & Smolewski, M. (2004). *Historic trauma and Aboriginal healing*. Ottawa: Aboriginal Healing Foundation.

Wilkinson, R. (2000). The need for an interdisciplinary perspective on the social determinants of health. *Health Economics, 9*(7), 581-583.

Wilkinson, R. & Marmot (2003). *The social determinants of health: The solid facts*. Geneva: World Health Organization.

World Health Organization (2007). *International Classification of Diseases*. 10th Revision. Geneva: Author.

Yankauer, A. (1950). The relationship of fetal and infant mortality to residential segregation: an inquiry into social epidemiology. *American Sociological Review, 15*, 644-648.

Zola, I. (1972). Medicine as an institution of social control. *Sociological Review, 4*, 487-504.

Chapter 5

American Psychiatric Association (2000). *Diagnostic and Statistical Manual of Mental Disorders*, Text Revision (DSM-IV-TR). City: American Psychiatric Publishing.

Bach, P. B., Pham, H. H., Schrag, D., Tate, R. C., & Hargraves, J. L. (2005). Primary care physicians who treat blacks and whites. *The New England Journal of Medicine, 35*(6), 575-584.

Barbee, E. L. (1994) A Black feminist approach to nursing research. *Western Journal of Nursing Research, 16*, 495-506.

Bernabei, R., Gambassi, G., Lapane, K., Landi, F., Gatsonis, C., Dunlop, R., Lipsitz, L., Steel, K., & Mor, V. (1998). Management of Pain in Elderly Patient with Cancer. *The Journal of the American Medical Association, 279*(23), 1877-1882.

Bishop, A. (2002). *Becoming an ally: Breaking the cycle of oppression in people*. Halifax: Fernwood Publishing.

Boyd, J. (1998). *Racism, whose problem: Strategies for understanding and dealing with racism in our communities*. Halifax: Fernwood Publishing.

Breen, N., Wesley, M., Merril, R., & Johnson, K. (1999). The relationship of socioeconomic status and access to minimum expected therapy among female breast cancer patients in the Black-White Cancer Survival Study. *Ethnicity and Disease, 9*, 111-125.

Bryant, T., Raphael, D., & Rioux, M. (2006). Toward the future: Current themes in health research and practice in Canada. In D. Raphael, T. Bryant, & M. Rioux (Eds.), *Critical perspectives on health, illness, and health care* (pp. 373-391). Toronto: Canadian Scholar's Press International.

Bullard, R. D. (2007). *The Black metropolis in the 21st century: Race, power, and politics of place*. Lanham, MD: Roman & Infield Publishers Inc.

Calliste, A. (2000). Nurses and porters: Racism, sexism, and resistance in segmented labor markets. In A. Calliste and G. Sefa Dei (Eds.). *Anti-racist feminism: Critical race and gender studies* (pp. 143-163). Halifax: Fernwood Publishing.

Canadian Association of Elizabeth Fry Societies (2008). *Mission statement*. Ottawa: Author. Retrieved on May 14, 2008 from: http://www.elizabethfry.ca/caefs_e.htm

Canadian Association of Social Workers (2005).*Code of Ethics*. Ottawa: Author.

Canadian Criminal Justice Association (CCJA) (2000). Aboriginal Peoples and the criminal Justice system. *Bulletin of the CCJA*, Ottawa, May 15, 2000. Retrieved on August 3, 2000 from: http://www.ccja-acjp.ca/en/abori1.html

Canadian Institute for Health Information (2006). *How healthy are rural Canadians? An assessment of their health status and health determinants*. Ottawa: Author.

Canadian Medical Association (2007). Responding to the Globe. *Canadian Medical Association Journal, 177*(6), 685.

Canadian Nurses Association (2006). *Social Justice: A means to an end and an end in itself.* Canadian Nurses Association: Author. Retrieved November 10, 2006 from http://cna-aiic.ca/CNA/documents/pdf/publications/Social_Justice_e.pdf

Canadian Psychological Association (2000). *Canadian code of ethics for psychologists*. Ottawa: Author.

Coburn, D. (2006). Health and health care: A political economy perspective. In D. Raphael, T. Bryant, & M. Rioux (Eds.), *Critical perspectives on health, illness, and health care* (pp. 59-110). Toronto: Canadian Scholar's Press International.

Cole, L. & Foster, S. (2000). *From the ground up: Environmental racism and the rise of the environmental justice movement*. New York: New York University Press.

Dei, G. S. (1996). *Anti-racism education: Theory and Practice*. Halifax: Fernwood Publishing.

Etowa, J. (2006). Fostering healthy work environments for minority nurses in Nova Scotia. Nursing in Focus, Fall, 2006, pp. 15-17. College of Registered Nurses of Nova Scotia.

Etowa, J. (2005). *Surviving on the margins of a profession: Experiences of Black nurses*. Unpublished Doctoral Dissertation, University of Calgary, Calgary, AB.

Etowa, J. & McGibbon , E .(2003). *Oppression and racial discrimination: Everyday inequalities in health care* Paper Presented at the Canadian Association of Schools of Nursing (CASN) Conference, Halifax, NS., April, 2003.

Fine, M. (2004). Witnessing whiteness: Gathering intelligence. In M. Fine, L. Weis, L. P. Pruitt, & A. Burns, *Off white: Readings on power, privilege, and resistance* (pp. 245-256). New York: Routledge.

Galabuzi, G-E (2006). *Canada's economic apartheid: The social exclusion of racialized groups in the new century*. Toronto: Canadian Scholar's Press Inc.

Hagey, R. & McKay, R. W. (2000). Qualitative research to identify racialist discourse: towards equity in nursing curricula. *International Journal of Nursing Studies, 37*(1), 45-56.

Hall, J. A., Irish, J. T., Roter, D. L., Ehrlich, C. M., & Miller L. H. (1994). Satisfaction, gender, and communication in medical visits. *Medical Care, 32*, 1216-1231.

Health Canada (2005). *Canada's health care system*. Ottawa: Author.

Henry, F., Tator, C., Mattis, W & Rees. T. (2000). *The color of democracy: Racism in Canadian society*. Toronto: Harcourt Canada.

King, D. K. (1988). Multiple jeopardy, multiple consciousness: The context of a Black feminist ideology. *Signs: Journal of Culture, Women, and Society, 14*, 42-72.

Kirby, S., & McKenna, K. (1989). *Experience, research,nd social change: Methods from the margins*. Toronto, ON: Garamond Press.

Labonte, R., Schrecker, T., & Gupta, A. S. (2005). *Health for some: Death, disease and disparity in a globalizing era*. Toronto: Center for Social Justice.

Lock, M. (1993). The concept of race: An ideological construct. *Transcultural Psychiatry, 30*(9), 203–227.

Lorber, J. (1994). *Paradoxes of Gender*. Hartford, CT: Yale University Press.

MacIntosh, P. (1990). White privilege: Unpacking the invisible knapsack. *Independent School*, Winter, 1990, 31-36.

McGibbon, E. (2008). *Health and health care: A human rights perspective*. In Dennis Raphael (Ed.). The social determinants of health: A Canadian perspective. Toronto: Canadian Scholar's Press International.

McGibbon, E., Etowa, J. &, McPherson, C. (2008). Health Care Access as a social determinant of health. *Canadian Nurse*, 104(7), 22-27.

McGibbon, E. Calliste, A., Arbuthnot, E, Bassett, R. Cameron, C., Graham, H., & MacDonald, D. (2006) *Barriers in Access to health Services for Rural Aboriginal and African Canadians: A Scoping workshop Report*. St. Francis Xavier University, Antigonish, Nova Scotia, June, 2005.

Ministerial Advisory Council on Rural Health (2002). *Rural health in rural hands: Strategic directions for rural, remote, northern and Aboriginal communities*. Ottawa: Health Canada.

Navarro, V. (2004). *The political and social contexts of health*. New York: Baywood Publishing Company.

Pate, K. & Neve, L. (2005). Challenging the criminalization of women who resist. In Julia Sudbury (Ed.).*Global Lockdown: Gender, Race and the Rise of the Prison Industrial Complex Around the World* (pp. 19-34). New York: Routledge

Rawls, J. (1971). *A theory of justice*. Cambridge, Mass.: Belknap Press of Harvard University Press.

Rozenbaum, H. (2004). Critique of the evidence from large trials of hormone replacement therapy. *International Congress Series*, 1266, 139-150. (Advances in Fertility and Reproductive Medicine. Proceedings of the 18th World Congress on Fertility and Sterility).

Tassy, E. (2006). *Unpacking the Visible Duffel Bag: Unearned White Privilege in the Context of Unearned Black Disadvantage*. Social Justice and Multiculturalism: The Moral Imperative of Our Time. Annual Conference of the National Association of Multicultural Education, Atlanta, Georgia, USA, March 24-25, 2006.

Toumishey, H., (1995). Multicultural health care: An introductory course. In: Masi, R., Mensa, L. and Mcleod, K.A., (Eds.). *Health and Cultures. Exploring the relationships*. Rockville, MD: Wildside Press.

Wells, K., Klay, R., Koike, A., & Sherbourne, C. (2001). Ethnic disparities in unment need for alcoholism, drug abuse, and mental health care. *The American Journal of Psychiatry*, 158(12), 2027-2032.

Westra, Laura. (1999). "Environmental Racism and the First Nations of Canada: Terrorism at Oka." *Journal of Social Philosophy*, 30, 103-124.

Chapter 6

Arnold, R., Burke, B., James, C., Martin, D. A., & Thomas, B. (1991). Educating for a change. Toronto: Between the Lines Press.

Bishop, A. (2002). *Becoming and ally: Breaking the cycle of oppression in people*. Halifax: Fernwood Publishing.

Bishop, A. (2006). *Beyond token change: Breaking the cycle of oppression in institutions*. Halifax: Fernwood Publishing.

Burgess, A. (1998). *Advanced practice psychiatric nursing*. Stamford, CT: Appleton and Lange. Canadian Mental Health Association (2007). *Discussion paper: Power, paternalism and partnerships*. Retriwved October 4, 2007 from: http://www.cmha.ca/data/1/rec_docs/1336_Power%20Paternalism%20and%20Partnerships.pdf

Dei, G. S. (1996). *Anti-racism education: Theory and Practice*. Halifax: Fernwood Publishing.

Denzin, N. & Lincoln, Y. (2007). *Collecting and interpreting qualitative materials*. Thousand Oaks, CA: Sage Publications.

Green, C. (2000). *Critical thinking in nursing: Case studies across the curriculum*. New Jersey: Prentice Hall Health.

Hagey, R. & McKay, R. W. (2000). Qualitative research to identify racialist discourse: towards equity in nursing curricula. *International Journal of Nursing Studies*, 37(1), 45-56.

hooks, b. (1990). *Yearning: Race, gender, and cultural politics*. Toronto: Between the Lines.

hooks, b. (1994). *Teaching to transgress*. New York: Routledge.

Kinsman, G. (1995). The textual practices of sexual rule: Sexual policing and gay men. In M. Campbell and A Manicom (Eds.), *Knowledge, experience, and ruling relations: Studies in the social organization of knowledge* (pp. 80-95). Toronto: University of Toronto Press.

Krieger N., Chen J. T., Waterman P. D., Rehkopf, D. H., Subramanian, S. V. (2005). Painting a truer picture of US socioeconomic and racial/ethnic health inequalities: the Public Health Disparities Geocoding Project. *Am J Public Health* 2005; 95:312-323.

MacIntosh, P. (1990). White privilege: Unpacking the invisible knapsack. *Independent School*, Winter, 1990, 31-36.

McGibbon, E. (2000). The situated knowledge of helpers. In C. James (Ed.) *Experiencing difference*. Halifax: Fernwood Publishing. (p 185-200).

McGibbon, E. & McPherson C. (2007). Interpretative pedagogy in action: The St. Francis Xavier University violence and health workshop. *Journal of Nursing Education, 45*(2), 81-85.

Niemöller, M. (1946). *"First they came..."* Speech to the representatives of the Confessing Church in Frankfurt, January 6, 1946, Frankfurt, Germany.

Razack, S. (1998). *Looking white people in the eye: Gender, race, and culture in courtrooms and classrooms*. Toronto: University of Toronto Press.

Senate Canada (2004). *Mental health, mental illness and addiction: Overview of policies and programs in Canada*. Ottawa, ON: Author. Available on-line at http://www.parl.gc.ca/38/1/parlbus/commbus/senate/com-e/soci-e/rep-e/report1/repintnov04vol1table-e.htm#PDF%20FORMAT

Smith, D. (1987). *The everyday world as problematic: A feminist sociology*. Toronto: University of Toronto Press.

Smith, D. (1990a). *The conceptual practices of power*. Boston: Northeastern University Press.

Smith, D. (1990b). *Texts, facts, and femininity: Exploring the relations of ruling*. London: Routledge.

Smith, D. (1999). *Writing the social: Critique, theory and investigations*. Toronto: University of Toronto Press.

Wijeyesinghe, C., Griffin, P., & Love, B. (1997). *Racism curriculum design*. In M. Adams, L. A. Bell & Griffin, P. (Eds.). Teaching for diversity and social change (pp. 82-109). New York: Routledge.

Chapter 7

Baker, T.A. (2005) Chronic pain in older Black Americans: The influence of health and psychosocial factors. *Ethnicity & Disease, 15*(2): 179-186.

Ball, J., & Elixhauser, A. (1996). Treatment differences between Blacks and Whites with colorectal cancer. *Medical care, 34*, 970-984.

Barnwell, G. (2006). *Women and public pensions: Working toward equitable policy change*. Ottawa: Status of Women Canada.

Bensimon, E. M. & Marshall, C. (2003). Like it or not: Feminist critical policy analysis matters. *Journal of Higher Education, 74*(3), 337-349.

Breen, N., Wesley, M., Merril, R., & Johnson, K. (1999). The relationship of socioeconomic status and access to minimum expected therapy among female breast cancer patients in the Black-White Cancer Survival Study. *Ethnicity and Disease, 9*, 111-125.

Canadian Council on Social Development (2000). *Urban poverty in Canada*. Ottawa: Author.

Canadian Nurses Association (2006). *Social Justice: A means to an end and an end in itself*. Ottawa: Author.

Canadian Research Institute on the Advancement of Women (2005). *Women and Poverty Fact Sheet*, 2005. Ottawa: Author.

Cooper, G., Yuan, Z., & Rimm, A. (2000). Patterns of endoscopic follow-up after surgery for non-metastatic colorectal cancer. *Gastrointestinal Endoscopy, 52*, 33-38.

Etowa, J. & McGibbon, E. (2008). *Racism as a social determinant of health: Towards a human rights health report card for Canada.* Invited Keynote Presentation. Canadian Race Relations Foundation Fifth Annual Symposium, April 30-May 2, 2008, Calgary, AB.

Galabuzi, G. E. (2008). The economic exclusion of racialized communities—A statistical profile. In Barrington Walker (Ed.). *The history of immigration and racism in Canada: Essential readings.* Toronto: Canadian Scholar's Press.

Galabuzi, G. E. (2006). *Canada's economic apartheid: The social exclusion of racialized groups in the new century.* Toronto: Canadian Scholar's Press Inc.

Gilbert, N. (2003). *Laidlaw's perspective on social inclusion.* Canadian Council on Social Development (CCSD). Paper presented at the CCSD Conference, March 2003.

Government of Canada (1982). *Canadian Charter of Rights and Freedoms.* Ottawa: Department of Justice.

Gruskin, S., Mills, E. J., & Tarantala, D. (2007). Health and human rights I: History, principles, and practice of health and human rights. *Lancet, 370,* 449-55.

Harper, L. (2007). *Policy is poverty created.* Antigonish, NS: The Antigonish Women's Resource Center. Retrieved on December 5, 2007 from: http://www.fafia-afai.org/en/poverty_is_policy_created.

Henry, F., Tator, C., Mattis, W & Rees. T. (2000). *The color of democracy: Racism in Canadian society.* Toronto: Harcourt Canada.

Illich, I. (1976). *Limits to medicine, medical nemesis: The expropriation of health.* Middlesex, England: Penguin Books.

Laidlaw Foundation (2003). *Building inclusive communities: Social infrastructure strategy for municipalities. Final report on cross-Canada community soundings.* Ottawa: The Laidlaw Foundation.

Ministerial Advisory Council on Rural Health (2002). *Rural health in rural hands: Strategic directions for rural, remote, northern and Aboriginal communities.* Ottawa: Health Canada.

McGibbon, E. (2008). Health and health care: A human rights perspective. In Dennis Raphael (Ed.). *The social determinants of health: Canadian perspectives.* Second Edition (pp. 318-335). Toronto: Canadian Scholar's Press.

McPherson, C. (2008). *Child health networks: A case study of network development, evolution, and sustainability.* Unpublished doctoral dissertation. McMaster University, Hamilton, ON.

Mettlin, C., Murphy, G., Cunningham, M., & Menck, H. (1997). The National Cancer Database Report on race, age, and region variations in prostate cancer treatment. *Cancer, 80,* 1261-1266.

Navarro, V. (2004). Introduction: Objectives and purposes of the study. In V. Navarro (Ed.).*The political and social contexts of health.* (pp. 1-10). New York: Baywood Publishing Company Inc.

National Anti-poverty Organization (2005). *Election Sheet on Poverty in Canada,* December 2005.

Niemöller, M. (1946). *"First they came..."* Speech to the representatives of the Confessing Church in Frankfurt, January 6, 1946, Frankfurt, Germany.

Queensland Government (2008). Policy Handbook. Queensland: Department of the Premier and Cabinet, Author. Retrieved on July 20, 2008 from: http://www.premiers.qld.gov.au/About_the_department/publications/policies/Governing_Queensland/Policy_Handbook/approval/issues/

Ray, P. (2002). The political compass. Retrieved on April 7, 2006 from: http://www.politicalcompass.org/

Roy, J. (2008). Legalized racism. Toronto: Canadian Race Relations Foundation. Retrieved on April 20, 2008 from: http://www.crr.ca/content/view/224/377/lang,english/

Raphael, D. (2007).*Poverty and policy in Canada: Implications of health and quality of life.* Toronto: Canadian Scholar's Press.

Raphael, D. (2006). *Staying alive: Critical perspectives on health and health care in Canada.* Toronto: Canadian Scholar's Press.

Raphael, D. (2004). Strengthening the social determinants of health: The Toronto Charter for a healthy Canada. In Dennis Raphael (Ed.). *The social determinants of health: Canadian perspectives* (361-365).
Saloojee, A. (2002). *Social inclusion, citizenship, and diversity*. Toronto: The Laidlaw Foundation.
Schrag, D., Cramer, L., Bach, P. & Begg, C. (2001). Age and adjuvant chemotherapy use after surgery for Stage III colon cancer. *Journal of the National Cancer Institute*, 93, 850-857.
Smith, D. B. (2005a). Racial and ethnic health disparities and the unfinished civil rights agenda. *Health Affairs*, 24(2), 317-325.
Smith, D. B. (2005b). Eliminating disparities in treatment and the struggle to end segregation. New York: The Commonwealth Fund. Retrieved on July 6, 2005 from http://www.commonwealthfund.org/
Smith (1996). Addressing racial inequalities in health care: Civil rights monitoring and report cards. *Journal of Health Politics, Policy and Law*, 23(1):75-105
Shamian, J. (2001). *The policy cycle, external influence and the role of the chief nursing officer*. Global Nursing Partnerships Conference Proceedings. October 18-19, Atlanta, Georgia.
Statistics Canada (2001) Census Analysis Series. The changing profile of Canada's labor force, February 11, 2000.
Sullivan, K., Johnson, L., Cloyer, C., Beale, J., Willis, J., Harrison, J., & Welsh, K. (2003). *National indigenous palliative care needs study*. Canberra: Commonwealth of Australia. Retrieved December 12, 2003 from: http://72.14.205.104/search?q=cache:OX4GWil8b24J:www.aodgp.gov.au/internet/wcms/publishing.nsf/Content/5619BFE763995E17CA256F410011C5C3/%24File/needcov.pdf+National+indigenous+palliative+care+needs+study.+Canberra:+Commonwealth+of+Australia.&hl=en&ct=clnk&cd=1&gl=ca
United Nations International Children's Emergency Fund (UNICEF, 2005). *Child poverty in rich countries*. Florence: UNICEF Innocenti Research Center.
Wharf, B. & McKenzie, B. (2004). *Connecting policy to practice in the human services*. Don Mills, ON: Oxford University Press.
White, P. (1998). Ideologies, social exclusion and spatial segregation in Paris. In S. Musterd & W. Ostendorf. *Urban segregation and the welfare state: Inequality and exclusion in Western cities* (pp. 148-167). London:Routledge.
Wilkinson, & Pickett (2005). Income inequality and population health: A review and explanation of the evidence. *Social Science and Medicine*, 16, 1768-84.
World Health Organization (2003). *The social determinants of health: The solid facts*. Geneva, Switzerland: Author. Retrieved June 4, 2006 from: http://www.who.dk/document/e59555.pdf
Zola, I. (1972). Medicine as an institution of social control. *Sociological Review*, 4, 487-504.
Yalnazyin, N. (2005). *Canada's commitment to equality: A gender based analysis of the last ten federal budgets (1995-2004)*. Ottawa: Canadian Feminist Alliance for International Action. Available at: http://www.fafia-afai.org/images/pdf/CanadaCommitmentsEquality.pdf.

Copyright Acknowledgements

Cover photo ©iStockphoto.com/file_closeup.php?id=6398312-nurse
Chapter 1 opening photo ©iStockphoto.com/file_closeup.php?id=630209-doctor-visit-3
Chapter 2 opening photo © Dalhousie University School of Nursing
Chapter 3 opening photo © *Health Canada website and Media Photo Gallery*, Health Canada, http://www.hc-sc.gc.ca. Reproduced with the permission of the Minister of Public Works and Government Services Canada, 2008.
Chapter 4 opening photo ©iStockphoto.com/file_closeup.php?id=3586971_home_health_care
Chapter 5 opening photo ©iStockphoto.com/file_closeup.php?id=830639 -nurse-listening-to-boy-with-stethoscope
Chapter 6 opening photo ©sxc.hu/browse.phtml?f=view&id=472011
Chapter 7 opening photo ©iStockphoto.com/file_closeup.php?id=5968400 father-holding-baby-for-pediatrician-to-examine
Box 1.1: McGibbon, E. (1998). The many sides of poverty: Health issues (The Nurse is in) Racism and Health: rome Reflections. *Street Feat* — "The Voice of the Poor" June/July 1998.
Box 1.2: Spence, C. M. (2000). *The skin I'm in: Racism, sports, and education*. Halifax: Fernwood Publishing (pp. 7–8).
Box 1.4: Enang, J. (1999). *Childbirth Experiences of African Nova Scotian Women*. MN thesis, Dalhousie University, Halifax, NS.
Box 2.1: Assembly of First Nations (2008). *History of Indian residential schools*. Indian Residential Schools Unit, Assembly of First Nations. Retrieved on January 20, 2008 from: http://www.afn.ca/residentialschools/history.html.
Box 2.3: "Toward a healthy future: Second report on the health of Canadians", Health Canada, (1999). Reproduced with the permission of the Minister of Public Works and Government Services Canada, 2008.
Box 2.6: McGibbon, E. Calliste, Arbuthnot, E. Bassett, R., Cameron, C. Graham, H., & MacDonald, D. *Barriers in Access to health Services for Rural Aboriginal and African Canadians: A scoping workshop*. St. Francis Xavier University, Antigonish, Nova Scotia, June, 2005 (p. 149–150).
Figure 2.1: Adapted from Statistics Canada (2008). Ethnic origin, visible minorities, place of work and mode of transportation. *The Daily*, Wednesday, April 2, 2008.
Figure 2.2: Adapted from Statistics Canada (2008). Ethnic origin, visible minorities, place of work, and mode of transportation. *The Daily*, Wednesday, April 2, 2008.
Figure 2.3: Adapted from Statistics Canada (2001). *The changing profile of Canada's labor force*, February, 2000.
Figure 2.5: Assembly of First Nations (2007). *First Nations Regional Longitudinal Health Survey*. Ottawa author.
Table 2.1: Adapted from Statistics Canada (2008). Ethnocultural Portrait of Canada Highlight Tables, 2006 Census. Retrieved on August 20, 2008 from: http://www12.statcan.ca/english/census06/data/highlights/ethnic/SelectGeo.cfm?Lang=E&Geo=PR&Table=2

Table 2.3: Etowa, J., Bernard, W. T., Clow, B. & Oyinsan, B. (2007) Participatory Action Research (PAR): Improving Black women's health in rural and remote communities. *International Journal of Transcultural Nursing*, 18: 349–359.

Box 3.1: Nova Scotia Department of Health

Figure 3.1: Etowa, J. & Adongo, L. (2007) Cultural competence: Beyond culturally sensitive care for childbearing Black women. *Journal of the Association for Research on Mothering, 9* (2), 73–85. Originally printed/appears in *Journal of the Association for Research on Mothering*.

Box 4.2: Collins, Patricia Hill. (1990). *Black feminist thought: Knowledge, consciousness, and the politics of empowerment* (p. 221). New York: Routledge.

Box 5.1: Jim Meek (2008). The *Chronicle Herald*, Halifax, NS, Sunday, March 9, 2008. Republished with permission from The Halifax Herald Ltd.

Box 5.3: Elaine Tassy. "Unpacking the visible duffel bag: Teaching about White privilege to Philadelphia-Area community college students" March 2008, Comparative and International Education Society Teachers College, Columbia University, New York.

Figure 5.2: McGibbon, E., Etowa, J., & McPherson, C. (2008). Health Care Access as a social determinant of health. *Canadian Nurse, 104*(7), 22–27. Reprinted with permission from the Canadian Nurses Association.

Figure 5.3: Reprinted with the permission of the Canadian Association of Elizabeth Fry Societies.

Table 5.1: From HENRY. *The colour of Democracy: Racism in Canadian society*. Copyright 2006 Nelson Education Ltd. Reproduced by permission, www.cengage.com/permissions.

Box 6.6: Adele Vukic, MN, Dalhousie University School of Nursing, Halifax, Nova Scotia; Etowa, J., Foster, S, Vukic, A., & Youden, S. (2005). Recruitment and retention of minority students: Diversity in nursing education. *International Journal of Nursing Education Scholarship* 2(1).

Extended Extract, pp. 172–174: Barnwell, G. (2006). Women and public pensions: Working toward equitable policy change. Ottawa: Funded by Status of Women Canada — Western Area Women's Centres — Nova Scotia (Tri County Women's Centre — Yarmouth, Second Story Women's Centre — Bridgewater, and The Women's Place — Bridgetown).

Box 7.4: From HENRY. *The colour of Democracy: Racism in Canadian society*. Copyright 2006 Nelson Education Ltd. Reproduced by permission, www.cengage.com/permissions.

Box 7.6: McPherson, C. (2008). *Child health networks: A case study of network development, evolution, and sustainability*. Unpublished doctoral dissertation. McMaster University, Hamilton, ON.

Figure 7.2: United Nations International Children's Emergency Fund (UNICEF, 2005). Child poverty in rich countries. Florence: UNICEF Innocenti Research Center.

Index

Aboriginal peoples. *See* Indigenous peoples
accountability, 60–61, 101, 105, 190
    and social justice, 133, 135, 137–38, 189
action continuum, for social change, 13, 28, 157, 159–61, 160*f*, 162–63
African Americans
    civil rights struggle of, 100, 178
    and environmental racism, 118, 120
    health problems of, 52–55, 57–58
and slavery, 34, 52, 90
African Canadians, 35–36
    see also Black children; Black women
    and barriers to health care, 60–61
    and Black disadvantage, 127–28, 129–30
    distribution of, 40*t*, 41*f*–42*f*
    and environmental racism, 35, 121
    health knowledge/practices of, 14–15, 108, 120, 122
    as immigrants, 78–79, 103
    and racist clinical procedures, 11, 52, 89, 114, 126
    in rural/remote areas, 47, 48*t*, 49, 132–33
    and screening for diseases, 5, 54, 55, 122, 161, 186*t*
    and slavery, 78, 103
    stereotypes of, 113, 114*t*
    subordination of, 124–27
Africville (Nova Scotia), 35–36
anti-colonialism, 96, 97*t*, 213
anti-racism, 93–95, 96, 97*t*, 188*t*, 213
anti-racist framework, to guide practice, 12–13, 28, 111–38
    see also intersectionality of oppression; racism, types of
    and action for social change, 13, 28, 157, 159–61, 160*f*, 162–63
    and Black disadvantage, 127–28, 129–30
    diagram of, 13*f*, 113*f*
    and intersectionality of oppression, 128, 131–33, 134*f*
    and paths from oppression to policy, 12–13
    and paths from stereotype to oppression, 12, 112, 115
    and professional codes of ethics, 133, 135–38, 189

theoretical foundations for. *See* critical perspectives on health care
    and White privilege, 123–27, 129–30
anti-racist health care practice, 27–29, 140–63
    and action for social change, 13, 28, 157, 159–61, 160*f*, 162–63
    and biomedical dominance, 94, 105–8, 110
    and Canada Health Act, 38–39, 117, 123
    and centrality of power, 140–41
    and critical thinking, 152–53
    harsh language of, 156–57, 159*t*
    key terms in, 17–20
    and multiculturalism, 27, 64–65, 76, 180
    and myth of neutrality, 149–52, 153
    and oppression, 141–43, 144
    and policy cycle, 12–13, 28–29, 166–71
    resistance to, 6–7, 10–11, 28, 145, 153–57, 158–59*t*
    and situated practice, 147–49, 150
    White people's role in, 143–47
apartheid, 7, 24, 120, 215
    economic, 93–94, 174–75, 186*t*, 215
Apgar scale, for newborns, 52, 89, 126
Asian Canadians, 36–38, 114*t*
assimilation/acculturation, 33–35, 64, 95–96

barriers to health care, 59–61
    see also rural/remote areas
    for African Canadians, 47, 48*t*, 49, 60–61
    cost, 46–49
    and critical perspectives approach, 105, 106
    and cultural competence model, 75
    for Indigenous peoples, 49, 59, 60–61
    and lack of accountability, 60–61
    privatization, 179–80
    racism, 56–61, 76–78
    and safety issues, 60–61
Battiste, Marie, 85, 90, 95–96, 188*t*
Becker, Howard, 86–87
best practices guidelines, critical approach to, 102–5
    and nested layers of intervention, 103*f*, 103–5
bias, 12, 18, 115*f*, 209
biomedicine, culture/dominance of, 72, 82, 100–10
    and anti-racism, 94, 105–8, 110

239

and critical best practices, 102–5
and critical thinking, 152–53
and ethnocentrism, 120, 122
and medicalization, 106, 107–8, 131–32
and social determinants of health, 101–2
and social science perspective, 109–10
Black Canadians. *See* African Canadians; *see also* entries below
Black children, 19
and Apgar health scale, 52, 89, 126
and racism in sports, 7–9
and sickle cell anemia screening, 5, 55, 161, 186*t*
Black disadvantage, 127–28, 129–30
Black women
see also women
and breast cancer, 52, 54
and feminism, 90–91
in health care professions, 22–24, 117
health problems of, 52, 54–56
and intersectionality of oppression, 47–50, 48*t*, 61, 125
in maternity care, 5, 14–15, 20, 21–22, 66, 67
poverty of, 47, 48*t*, 52
in rural/remote areas, 47, 48*t*, 49, 132–33
breast cancer, 52, 54, 131

Calliste, Agnes, 10, 90, 93, 95, 188*t*
Canada Health Act (CHA), 38–39, 99, 104, 117, 123, 180
five criteria of, 210–11
Canadian Association of Elizabeth Fry Societies, 118, 119*f*
Canadian Association of Social Workers, 133, 135, 136–37
Canadian Charter of Rights and Freedoms, 65, 100, 177–78, 179, 180, 181
Canadian Human Rights Act, 177, 181
Canadian Medical Association (CMA), 133, 135, 179
Canadian Nurses Association (CNA), 133, 135–36, 137, 190
Canadian Psychological Association (CPA), 136
cardiovascular disease, 49, 52–53, 53*f*, 54, 55, 131
case study of care for, 103–5, 106
cervical cancer, 54
child poverty, 4, 43, 46–47, 49, 89, 98, 171, 172*f*, 180, 191, 206–7
Chinese Canadians, 37
civil rights, 100, 178
classism, 13, 25, 28
Collins, Patricia Hill, 24, 85, 90–91, 93, 95, 188*t*
colonialism/colonization, 9, 32, 34–35, 211
see also White privilege
and assimilation/acculturation, 34–35, 95–96
and concept of "Other," 70–71, 73
and need for education on, 95, 96
and slave trade, 34
trauma of, 57, 96, 108, 110
conflict theory, 87–88, 96, 97*t*, 213

Convention on the Elimination of All Forms of Discrimination Against Women, 100, 179
Convention on the Elimination of All Forms of Racial Discrimination, 179
Convention on the Rights of the Child, 100, 179
criminal justice system
law enforcement, 26, 129
prisons, 87, 117–18, 119*f*
critical perspectives on health care, 82–83, 88–100
see also health care, perspectives on
and anti-colonialism, 96, 97*t*, 213
anti-racist, 93–95, 96, 97*t*, 188*t*, 213
and critical theory, 82, 88–89, 96, 97*t*, 213
and critical thinking, 152–53, 154
feminist, 90–93, 96, 97*t*, 213
and human rights, 98–100, 189–91
and political economy, 98
and post-colonialism, 95–96
critical perspectives on health care, and clinical practice, 100–10
and barriers to care, 105, 106
best practices approach to, 102–5
and biomedical dominance, 72, 82, 100–10
and biomedical perspective, 109–10
case study of, 103–5, 106
and social determinants of health, 101
critical perspectives on public policy, 183–85, 190
critical theory, 82, 96, 97*t*, 213
and health care practice, 88–89, 102–5, 106
critical thinking, 152–53, 154
cultural competence, 27, 64–80
see also immigrants; racialized groups; visible minorities
definitions of, 65–66
and Eurocentrism, 15, 64, 66, 72–73
ineffectiveness of, 73–75
going beyond, 76–79
and maternity care, 66, 67, 74
measurement of, 68–69, 70–72
models/tools, 67*f*, 67–68, 73–75
and multiculturalism, 27, 64–65, 76, 180
Nova Scotia guidelines for, 77
overview of, 65–69
problems of, 69–76
as process, 67*f*, 67–68
and racism, 66–67, 69, 76–79
cultural competence, problems of, 69–76
and concept of culture, 71–72, 74*t*
and concept of "Other," 70–71, 72–73, 74*t*, 78
and health outcomes/inequities, 74–75
and ineffectiveness of models, 73–75
with measurement, 70–72
and power imbalance, 72–73, 76–77
and promotion of stereotypes, 75–76
and racism, 66–67, 69, 76–79
cultural racism, 120, 122, 214
cultural sensitivity, 60, 67*f*, 68
cultural/health literacy, 60
culture, 14–15, 17
of biomedicine, 72, 82, 100–10

and ethnicity/race, 15, 71–72, 74*t*
and stereotypes, 52, 75–76

Dalhousie University, 7, 121, 162
Dei, George Sefa, 10, 90, 93, 94, 95, 141, 188*t*
dementia, 57–58, 131
democracy, 87–88, 190
depression, 56, 57, 96, 97*t*
diabetes, 52, 53*f*, 55, 149, 169–70
Diagnostic and Statistical Manual of Mental Disorders (DSM), 107–8
disabilities, people with, 47, 49, 58
discrimination, 12, 17, 18, 209
    and cultural stereotypes, 52, 75–76
    and cycle of oppression, 114, 115*f*
    against Jews, 16
    racism as, 20, 22–23, 32–33, 78–79
Douglas, Tommy, 179, 188*t*

early childhood development, 43*t*
economic apartheid, 93–94, 174–75, 186*t*, 215
education
    about colonialism/colonization, 95, 96
    financial supports for, 172, 173–74
    of health care professionals, 66–67, 76–79, 155–56, 157, 158–59*t*
    and health promotion materials, 142–43
    and racism/segregation, 174
    as social determinant of health, 43*t*
employment, 43*t*
    of disabled, 47, 49
    of immigrants/racialized groups, 44*f*, 47, 174–75, 175*f*, 176*f*
employment insurance (EI), 172, 173
environmental racism, 35, 50, 118, 120, 121, 123, 186*t*, 214
epidemiology, 83–84, 106
ethnicity, 15–16, 17
ethnocentrism, 120, 122, 214
Eurocentrism, 15, 64, 66, 91, 125–26, 184
    and power imbalance, 72–73

family, cultural attitudes towards, 66, 67, 116, 122
    and hospital visits, 21, 66, 120, 122
    and nuclear family as norm, 79, 120, 122
    and social exclusion based on, 43, 93
feminism, 90–93, 188*t*
    and Black women's struggle, 90–91
    and health care, 92–93, 96, 97*t*, 213
    on inequality and oppression, 91–92
    intersectionality frameworks of, 45
    pioneers of, 90, 91–92
    and sexual orientation, 92, 93
First Nations, 19, 33, 35, 40*t*, 61, 120
    see also Indigenous peoples
    health conditions of, 54, 55, 57
    Regional Longitudinal Health Survey of, 42, 53, 53*f*, 59
food security, 43*t*

Galabuzi, Grace-Edward, 10, 44–45
    on economic apartheid, 93–94, 174
    on social exclusion, 184–85
geography, and intersectionality of oppression, 44–50, 46*f*, 51, 132*f*, 134*f*
    see also rural/remote areas
    for Black women, 47–50, 48*t*
    and costs of health care, 46–47
    and environmental factors, 35, 50, 118, 120, 121, 123, 186*t*, 214
    and identity, 46, 47, 48*t*, 49–50, 132–33
    for rural women, 43, 47, 48*t*, 49, 132–33
ghettoization, 50, 51
Goffman, Erving, 85, 86, 87, 107

Habermas, Jurgen, 88
health
    and access to care. *See* barriers to health care; rural/remote areas
    as human right. *See* human rights
    mental. *See* mental health
    and racism. *See* racism, in health care; racism, as social determinant of health
health care, perspectives on, 82–100
    see also critical perspectives on health care, *and entry following*
    and anti-colonialism, 96, 97*t*, 213
    anti-racist, 93–95, 96, 97*t*, 213
    and conflict theory, 87–88, 96, 97*t*, 213
    and critical theory, 82, 88–89, 96, 97*t*, 213
    epidemiological, 83–84
    feminist, 90–93, 96, 97*t*, 213
    and human rights, 98–100, 190
    and political economy, 98
    and post-colonialism, 95–96
    sociological, 84–85
    and structural functionalism/systems theory, 85–86, 96, 97*t*, 213
    and symbolic interactionism/interpretive sociology, 86–87, 97*t*, 213
health care professions, 27
    Black women's experience in, 22–24, 117
    codes of ethics for, 133, 135–38, 189
    and education/awareness about racism, 66–67, 76–79, 155–56, 157, 158–59*t*
    racial underrepresentation in, 20, 23
health education/promotion materials, 142–43
health inequity, 50, 100–1, 105, 141, 166, 212
    and distributive justice, 99, 137
    and political economy, 185
health services, as social determinant of health, 27, 43*t*
heart disease. *See* cardiovascular disease
Hispanics, 55, 57, 58, 74, 117
historical context, of racism, 32–38
    and African Canadians, 35–36
    and Asian Canadians, 36–38
    and European colonization, 32
    and immigration policy, 16, 27, 36–38

and Indigenous peoples, 33–35, 95–96,
    147–48, 183, 186t
Holocaust, 15–16
hooks, bell, 9–10, 90, 93, 141
hormone replacement therapy (HRT), 131
housing, 43t
human rights, 98–100, 177–82
    and Canadian legislation, 177–80
    and democratic racism, 180, 182
    in health care system, 189–91
    UN initiatives on, 99, 100, 177, 178, 179, 180
human rights codes and commissions, 180–82
human rights health report card, 190–91
hypertension, 52, 52–53, 53f, 55

identity, 44t, 147
identity, and intersectionality of oppression,
    44–50, 46f, 51, 132f
    for Black women, 47–50, 48t
    for disabled women, 47, 49
    and geography, 46, 47, 48t, 49–50, 132–33
    for rural women, 47, 48t, 49, 132–33
Illich, Ivan, 87, 106, 108
immigrants, 39
    see also cultural competence; racialized
        groups; visible minorities
    in health care setting, 75, 77–78, 99
    health issues of, 65, 126
    income/earnings of, 42, 47, 175, 175f
    and multiculturalism, 64–65
    and situated practice, 149
    unemployment among, 44f, 47, 174–75, 176f
immigration policy, and racism, 16, 27, 36–38
    and discrimination against Blacks, 78–79
    and point system/regulations, 79
    and multiculturalism, 64–65
income
    of immigrants/racialized groups, 42, 44–45,
        47, 48t, 49, 174–75, 175f
    as social determinant of health, 43t
income assistance, 172, 173
Indian Act, 20, 34, 71, 89
Indigenous peoples, 211
    assimilation/acculturation of, 33–35, 95–96
    and barriers to health care, 49, 59, 60–61
    Charter recognition of, 178
    and criminal justice system, 26, 117–18, 119f
    and cultural competence approach, 69
    distribution of, 39, 40t, 41f–42f
    and environmental racism, 118, 120
    health knowledge/practices of, 108, 120
    health problems of, 53, 53f, 54–58
    and historical context, 33–35, 95–96, 147–48,
        183, 186t
    and internalized racism, 116, 122
    knowledge of, 94, 96, 108, 120
    legislation governing, 20, 34, 71, 89
    and mental health, 56, 57–58, 61
    as "Others," 71
    and post-colonialism, 95–96, 147–48

racial categorization of, 19–20
racial segregation of, 35, 50, 58, 174
as refused enlistment, 37
and residential schools, 7, 20, 24, 33–34, 57,
    116, 122
in rural/remote areas, 49, 59, 61
stereotypes of, 113–14, 114t, 147–48, 149
suicide among, 89
trauma of, 57, 96, 108, 110, 183, 186t
unmet health care needs of, 38
individual racism, 7, 115–16, 122, 214
institutional racism, 19, 79, 117
internalized racism, 116, 122, 214
International Classification of Diseases, 107
International Covenant on Civil and Political
    Rights, 177
International Covenant on Economic, Cultural,
    and Social Rights, 100, 179
interpretive sociology/symbolic interactionism,
    86–87, 97t, 213
intersectionality of oppression, 13, 28, 44–50, 46f,
    51, 125, 132f
    see also oppression; women
    for Black women, 47–50, 48t, 61, 125
    and costs of health care, 46–47
    for disabled women, 47, 49
    feminist frameworks of, 45
    and geography/identity, 46, 47, 48t, 49–50,
        132–33
    and health inequity, 50
    for Indigenous peoples, 49, 50
    and poor health outcomes, 49, 52, 128,
        131–33, 134f
    and professional codes of ethics, 133, 135–38
    for rural women, 47, 48t, 49, 132–33
    White understanding of, 144
Inuit, 33, 34, 40t. See also Indigenous peoples
Irish, discrimination against, 24–25
Islam, and post 9/11 attacks on, 16
-isms, 18, 144

James, Carl, 10, 90, 94–95
Japanese Canadians, 37
Jews, 15–16, 73–74

legalized racism, 211
Lincolnville, N.S., 121
low income cut-off (LICO), 172–73, 215

MacIntosh, Peggy: *White Privilege: Unpacking the
    Invisible Knapsack*, 11–12, 123, 126, 158t
Marx, Karl, 85, 98
Marxism, 87–88, 90, 92
materialist epidemiology, 84
maternity care
    see also women
    and cultural competence approach, 66, 67, 74
    power imbalance in, 148–49
    racism/insensitivity in, 5, 14–15, 20, 21–22,
        66, 67

Index

media perpetuation, of racism/White privilege, 124, 127, 129–30, 152, 154–55
    in health education materials, 142–43
medicalization, 87, 106, 107–8, 131–32
medicare, 179
menopause, 106, 131–32
mental health, 56, 57–58, 61, 65
    biomedical approach to, 87, 107–8
    feminist perspective on, 92–93
    and Indigenous trauma, 57, 96, 108, 110
    sociological approach to, 96, 97*t*
Métis, 26, 33, 40*t*. *See also* Indigenous peoples
Mills, C. Wright, 87–88
minimum wage, 172, 173
multiculturalism, 27, 64–65, 76, 180. *See also* cultural competence

nationality, 15, 17
Navarro, Vincente, 84, 94, 166, 185
neo-conservatism, 185, 188*t*
neo-liberalism, 98, 185, 188*t*
9/11, terrorist attacks of, 16
North End Community Health Centre (Halifax), 105
Nova Scotia
    health care initiatives in, 77, 105
    homelessness in, 167–68
    poverty in, 172–73, 174, 180
Nova Scotia, Black experience in, 6–7, 121, 180
    and Africville, 35–36
    and environmental racism, 35, 121
    in health care professions, 23, 162
    and maternity care, 20, 21–22
    for rural women, 47, 48*t*

Oka crisis, 120
Ontario Human Rights Code, 181
oppression, 12–13, 18
    see also intersectionality of oppression
    cycle of, 114, 115*f*
    stories of, 141–42
    supporting vs. confronting, 157, 159–61, 160*f*, 162–63
    understanding and addressing, 141–43, 144
"Other," concept of
    and Black women, 91
    and colonization, 70–71, 73
    and cultural competence, 70–71, 72–73, 74*t*, 78
    and stories told by, 152

pain, chronic and acute, 55
palliative care, 55
Parsons, Talcott, 85–86, 87
pay equity, 172, 174
pensions, 172, 174
policy cycle, 12–13, 28–29, 166–71, 215
    see also public policy
    application of, to everyday practice, 167–68, 169
    evaluation, 168–70, 170*t*
    formulation and adoption, 167, 170*t*
    identification of issues, 167, 170*t*
    implementation, 167–68, 170*t*
    overview of, 166–67
    stages of, 167–71, 168*f*, 170*t*
"political compass," 187, 189
political economy, 98, 185
political ideology, 187, 188*t*, 189
post-colonialism, 95–96, 147–48
post-traumatic stress disorder (PTSD), 57. *See also* trauma
poverty, 4, 6–7, 46–47, 49, 59, 98, 127
    of Black women, 47, 48*t*, 52
    and "case-of-one" argument, 155, 158*t*
    and ghettoization, 50, 51
    and public policy, 171–75, 186*t*
    as social determinant of health, 41–42, 43, 101
    and social/materialist epidemiology, 83–84
poverty, child, 4, 43, 46–47, 49, 89, 98, 171, 172*f*, 180, 191, 206–7
power imbalance, and racism, 20, 61–62, 78
    critical thinking about, 153, 154
    and cultural competence model, 72–73, 76–77
    in therapeutic work, 147–49, 148*f*, 150
    understanding and addressing, 140–41
prejudice, 12, 18, 113, 115*f*, 210
prisons, 87, 117–18, 119*f*
privatization, 179–80
professional codes of ethics, 133, 135–38, 189
prosthetics, 11, 114, 120
prostrate cancer, 54
psychiatry, 92–93, 96, 97*t*. *See also* mental health
public policy, 166–92
    anti-racist, 189–91
    critical social science view of, 183–85, 186–87*t*
    cycle of, 12–13, 28–29, 166–71, 215
    and democratic racism, 180, 182
    dominant view of, 186–87*t*
    and gender inequity, 175–77
    and health as human right, 177–82
    and political ideology, 187, 188*t*, 189
    and poverty, 171–75, 186*t*
    and social determinants of health, 185, 187

race, 17, 18–20
    and health, 52–58
    as loaded term, 19, 71
    and mental health, 56, 57–58
    and sexual orientation, 151–52
    and socioeconomic status, 51–52
    understanding, 141
racial categorization, 17, 19–20
racialized groups
    see also cultural competence; immigrants; visible minorities
    health of, 49, 52–56

and health care access, 56–61
    income/earnings of, 42, 44–45, 47, 48*t*, 49, 174–75, 175*f*
    segregation of, 35, 50, 51, 58
    socioeconomic status of, 51–52
    unemployment among, 44*f*, 47, 174–75, 176*f*
racial profiling, 58, 60
racial segregation
    of Indigenous peoples, 35, 50, 58, 174
    in urban settings, 50, 51
racism, 32–33, 112
    see also White privilege
    as barrier to health care, 56–61, 76–78
    and "case-of-one" argument, 155, 158*t*
    and criminal justice system, 26, 117–18, 119*f*, 129
    as discrimination, 20, 22–23, 32–33, 78–79
    education/awareness of, 66–67, 76–79, 155–56, 157, 158–59*t*
    harsh reality of, 156–57, 159*t*
    and health care, 52–58
    historical context of, 32–38
    and human rights, 177–82
    and immigration policy, 16, 27, 36–38, 64–65, 78–79
    and intersectionality of oppression, 44–50
    key concepts of, 14–20
    media perpetuation of, 124, 127, 129–30, 142–43, 152, 154–55
    and power imbalance. *See* power imbalance, and racism
    as "quiet"/hidden, 23, 78
    and socioeconomic status, 51–52
racism, in health care, 52–58
    and anti-racist framework, 13–14
    and cultural stereotypes, 52
    and dementia care, 57–58
    education/awareness of, 66–67, 76–79, 155–56, 157, 158–59*t*
    and health care professions, 20, 23
    and health education/promotion materials, 142–43
    and mental health, 56, 57–58
    and newborns' health test, 52, 89, 126
    and prosthetics/bandages, 7, 11, 114, 120
    and refusal to acknowledge, 6–7, 10–11, 154–57, 158–59*t*
    as systemic, 5, 27
    and White privilege, 123–27
racism, as social determinant of health, 27, 32, 41–62, 80, 180
    see also social determinants of health
    and cultural stereotypes, 52
    and health care access, 56–61
    and health outcomes, 50–56
    and intersectionality of oppression, 44–50
    and power, 61–62
    and social determinants overview, 41–44
    and socio-economic status, 51–52

racism, types of
    see also systemic racism
    cultural, 120, 122, 214
    environmental, 35, 50, 118, 120, 121, 123, 186*t*, 214
    individual, 7, 115–16, 122, 214
    institutional, 19, 79, 117
    internalized, 116, 122, 214
Razack, Sherene, 95, 155
religion, 15–16, 17
residential schools, 7, 20, 24, 57
    history of, 33–34
    and internalized racism, 116, 122
rural/remote areas, 39, 43, 46, 47–50, 56
    see also barriers to health care
    African Canadians in, 47, 48*t*, 49, 132–33
    and costs of access, 46–49
    Indigenous peoples in, 49, 59, 61
    and intersectionality of oppression, 45–50, 132–33
    women in, 43, 47, 48*t*, 49, 132–33

segregation, racial
    of Indigenous peoples, 35, 50, 58, 174
    in urban settings, 50, 51
sexism, 13
    and anti-racist health care practice, 142, 144, 145
    and treatment of menopause, 131–32
sexual orientation, 43, 99, 127
    and feminism, 92, 93
    and race, 151–52
sickle cell anemia, 5, 55, 61, 161, 186*t*
situated practice, 147–49, 150
slave trade/slavery, 34, 52, 78, 90, 103
Smith, Dorothy, 85, 92–93, 142, 188*t*
Snow, John, 83
social change, action continuum for, 13, 28, 157, 159–61, 160*f*, 162–63
social democracy, as ideology, 188*t*
social determinants of health, 41–44, 98, 141
    see also racism, as social determinant of health
    acknowledgement of, 101
    and biomedical approach, 101–2
    and definitions used, 27, 32, 41–42
    health care access as, 56–61
    intersectionality of, 44–50, 46*f*, 51
    list of, 43*t*–44*t*
    and poverty, 41–42, 43, 101
    and public policy, 185, 187
social epidemiology, 83–84
social exclusion, 43*t*–44*t*, 93, 183–85, 186*t*
social justice, 98–100
    and codes of ethics, 133, 135–38, 189
social location, of authors, 22–26
social safety nets, 43
social science approach to health care. *See* critical perspectives on health care, *and entry following*; *see also* health care, perspectives on

socioeconomic status (SES), 47, 48t, 49, 51–52
sociological perspective, on health care, 84–85
South Asian immigrants, 37
sports, racism in, 7–9
stereotypes, 19, 37, 58, 112–13
    of African Canadians, 113, 114t
        cultural, 52, 75–76
        and cycle of oppression, 114, 115f
        definition of, 18, 210
        gender, 124
        in health care system, 58, 60
        of Indigenous peoples, 113–14, 114t, 147–48, 149
        and paths to oppression, 12, 112, 115
        racial, 113, 114t
stories of racism/oppression, 6, 8–9, 21–22
    and need to hear, 141–42, 151–52
storytelling/narrative therapy, 108, 152
structural functionalism/systems theory, 85–86, 96, 97t, 213
suffrage movement, 90
suicide, 89, 99
symbolic interactionism/interpretive sociology, 86–87, 97t, 213
systemic racism, 5, 7, 9, 12–13, 27, 64, 117–18, 186t
    definition of, 117, 123, 214
    and immigration policy, 78–79
    and Indigenous peoples, 117–18, 119f
    and power imbalances, 61–62, 147–49
systems theory/structural functionalism, 85–86, 96, 97t, 213

therapeutic work, power imbalance in, 147–49, 148f, 150
Toronto Charter, 27, 32, 42
transgression, teaching as, 9–10, 141
trauma, 57, 96, 108, 110
Truth, Sojourner, 90

unemployment, of immigrants/racialized groups, 44f, 47, 174–75, 176f
United Nations, 99, 100, 177, 178, 179, 180
United Nations Charter of Rights and Freedoms, 100, 178
United States, civil rights in, 100, 178. *See also* African Americans
Universal Declaration of Human Rights, 100, 179

visible minorities, 39, 40t, 41f–42f
    see also cultural competence; immigrants; racialized groups
    distribution by origin, 41f
    distribution by province, 40f, 40t

White people, and role in anti-racist struggle, 143–47
    as allies, 145–47
    consciousness-raising and healing, 144–45
    maintaining hope, 147
    and self-liberation, 145
    understanding of intersectionality, 144
    understanding of oppression, 144
White privilege, 6–9, 13f, 20, 52, 64, 90, 91, 123–27
    see also colonialism/colonization; racism
    and author's experience, 24–26, 145–47
    and Black disadvantage, 127–28, 129–30
    and concept of "Other," 70–71, 72–73, 74t, 78
    as core pillar of racism, 7, 9
    definition of, 17, 210
    and dominance, 64, 77, 124–27, 141, 151–52, 184, 186–87t
    in health care, 11–12, 73, 123–27, 158–59t, 186t
    media perpetuation of, 124, 127, 129–30, 142–43, 152, 154–55
    and not noticing, 6–7, 71, 123, 143, 157, 158–59t, 159
women
    see also Black women; intersectionality of oppression; maternity care
    and criminal justice system, 117–18, 119f
    and feminism, 45, 90–93, 96, 97t, 188t, 213
    and gender inequity, 175–77
    and menopause, 106, 131–32
    and pay equity, 172, 174
    poverty of, 47, 48t, 52, 127, 173–74
    in rural/remote areas, 43, 47, 48t, 49, 132–33
    and sexism, 13, 131–32, 142, 144, 145
    stereotyping of, 52, 124
    UN convention on, 100, 179
World Health Organization (WHO), 27, 32, 41–42, 100, 107, 178